Electrocardiography of Clinical Arrhythmias

Charles Fisch, MD

Distinguished Professor of Medicine Emeritus
Krannert Institute of Cardiology
Indiana University School of Medicine
Indianapolis, Indiana

Suzanne B. Knoebel, MD

Herman C. and Ellnora D. Krannert Professor of Medicine
Krannert Institute of Cardiology
Indiana University School of Medicine
Indianapolis, Indiana

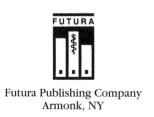

Futura Publishing Company
Armonk, NY

Library of Congress Cataloging-in-Publication Data

Fisch, Charles.
    Electrocardiography of clinical arrhythmias / by Charles Fisch and Suzanne B.
      Knoebel.
        p. ; cm.
    Includes bibliographical references and index.
    ISBN 0-87993-446-8
      1. Electrocardiography. 2. Arrhythmia—Diagnosis. I. Knoebel, Suzanne B.,
    1926- II. Title.
      [DNLM: 1. Arrhythmia—diagnosis. 2. Electrocardiography.
    WG 330 F528c 2000]
    RC683.5 E5 F52 2000
    616.1′28075—dc21

                                99-054158

Published by
Futura Publishing Company
135 Bedford Road
Armonk, New York 10504

LC#: 99-054158
ISBN#: 0-87993-446-8

Every effort has been made to ensure that the information in this book is as up to date and accurate as possible at the time of publication. However, due to the constant developments in medicine, neither the author, nor the editors, nor the publisher can accept any legal or any other responsibility for any errors or omissions that may occur.

Printed in the United States of America on acid-free paper.

Preface

The electrocardiographic diagnosis of most commonly occurring and "simple" arrhythmias requires minimal deductive reasoning; an algorithmic or rule-based approach based on standard measurements, straightforward relationships between P, P-R, and QRS, and the contour and duration of P, P-R, and QRS usually suffices. For example, a premature complex that is bizarre and not preceded by a P wave is, in most cases, a ventricular premature complex (VPC). However, differentiation of a premature ventricular complex from an aberrantly conducted premature atrial complex requires consideration of the factors that are conducive to aberrancy (preceding long R-R intervals and short coupling, among others). Thus, the degree of deductive analysis required for an accurate diagnosis serves as a practical guideline for the differentiation of "simple" and "complex" arrhythmias, gradations between the two being a continuum.

As the electrocardiogram (ECG) is essentially the only practical noninvasive technology for arrhythmia diagnosis and, as such, must be knowledgeably and competently incorporated into our clinical armamentarium, the authors' primary goal for *Electrocardiography of Clinical Arrhythmias* is to promote the deductive approach to the diagnosis of clinical arrhythmias from the surface ECG while at the same time serving as a source for quick reference to specific less complex arrhythmias. A second goal is to keep the book as practical and interesting as possible for clinicians at all levels of experience and competence. Our experience, over a combined 75 years of teaching electrocardiography, has convinced us that if required to first conquer the complexities of the electrophysiology of arrhythmias from didactic presentations before feeling confident about interpreting the surface ECG, many students at all levels are dissuaded from pursuing the subject in any depth. Furthermore, our tenet is that the essential knowledge required for the interpretation of arrhythmias is most readily acquired and retained when presented in the context of specific ECGs, repetitively presented in multiple permutations as encountered in the ECG reading room or on the wards. Thus, the book is richly illustrated.

To achieve the goals of practicality, interest, and competency the book is divided into two parts. Section I focuses primarily on the electrocardiography of the arrhythmias most frequently encountered in clinical practice and which may require differential diagnoses. Theory is kept at a minimum—only the necessary conceptual material required to develop a fundamental knowledge base is presented.

Section II provides a more in-depth discussion of ECG mechanisms of arrhythmogenesis and the deductive processes used to reach the diagnoses of complex arrhythmias. The emphasis is on the ECG manifestations of the underlying electrophysiological mechanisms as opposed to basic cellular mechanisms per se. In most cases, these are arrhythmias that display "unexpected" P, P-R, and QRS relationships, the ECG mechanisms for and diagnosis of which must be deduced. And, even here, the relevant underlying electrophysiology is presented in as nontechnical a format as possible.

It is hoped that the book's sectional presentation will permit the clinician to customize his or her information needs and interests. For some, it will provide a quick and handy reference to those arrhythmias that can be diagnosed by following a systematic or rule-based approach; for others, more in-depth discussions of electrocardiographic mechanisms and deductive and analytic approaches to complex arrhythmias are available. Finally, the authors hope that both the systematic and deductive approaches will encourage a new wave of clinical electrocardiographers and teachers to collect unusual tracings and to search for their mechanisms with the newer techniques that are certain to arise during the 21st century, techniques that will allow assessment of the electrophysiological functioning of increasingly small areas of the specialized tissues of the heart.

Acknowledgments

The authors wish to acknowledge the skillful assistance of Terri Kennedy of our staff and Joanna Levine of Futura Publishing in collecting, editing, transcribing, and encouraging the effort.

In addition, we wish to thank all of our former trainees who "collect" interesting ECGs and send them to us on a regular basis. Selected figures have been previously publisheed in Fish C. *Electrocardiography of Arrhythmias*. Philadelphia: Lea & Febiger; 1990, and reproduced with permission.

Introduction

The systematic approach to the diagnosis of cardiac rhythms and arrhythmias, whether in the research laboratory setting, in the electrophysiology laboratory, at the computer programmer's keyboard, or in the clinic, always begins with identification of the site of impulse formation coupled with rhythm rate and regularity. For example, if the P wave is of normal contour and axis, the P-R interval is constant, and the rhythm regular with a normal QRS configuration, the diagnosis is normal sinus rhythm (bradycardia or tachycardia depending on rate). If the P wave is of normal contour and axis and the rhythm irregular but there is a normal P-R interval and a fixed relationship of the P with a normal QRS complex, the diagnosis is sinus arrhythmia.

As useful as such algorithms are as a starting point, if not backed by knowledge of mechanisms of arrhythmias, normal variants, and other confounding factors, they do not foster the development of the foundation for competent ECG interpretive skills. The goal of this volume is therefore to expand the knowledge required for a clinically relevant approach to arrhythmia diagnosis. Commonly encountered variables in P wave configuration, rhythm, rate, regularity, and relationships with P-R and QRS are discussed relative to the site of origin of the initiating impulse. Is the timing between impulse initiation and ventricular activation normal or abnormal? What are the probable reasons for irregularities in rhythm, and if an impulse is blocked, where is it blocked? Illustrative ECGs with explanatory legends are presented in immediate juxtaposition to the didactic material.

When highly complex electrophysiological mechanisms are involved and the arrhythmia diagnosis is not readily apparent from a systematic approach, the reader is referred to the appropriate location in Section II for more in-depth information about such electrocardiographic mechanisms. Section II also is richly illustrated with repetitive examples of ECGs that illustrate the electrocardiographic mechanism in question.

TO

Jon, Gary, and Bruce Fisch

and

Doster Buckner, MD

Contents

Section I
Sinoatrial Node, Atrial, Junctional,
Ventricular Rhythms and
Atrioventricular Blocks

Wide QRS Tachycardias–Differential Diagnoses

Section II
Complex Arrhythmias
Diagnosis and Mechanisms Based
Primarily on Deductive Analysis

Cellular Basis
of the Electrocardiogram

The following is a simplified discussion of the cellular basis of the ECG.

Cardiac excitation originates in the sinoatrial node (SAN), activates the atria, and is registered in the ECG as the P wave. The impulse is delayed in the atrioventricular (AV) node, inscribing the P-R interval. The impulse then traverses the bundle of His, the two bundle branches, the two divisions of the left bundle, and the Purkinje system to activate the ventricular myocardium. The current generated by activation of the ventricular myocardium is responsible for the QRS complex. It is important to recognize that although an arrhythmia is often a manifestation of disordered function of the specialized conduction system, its activity is not directly reflected in the ECG waveform. Rather, the P wave and the QRS complex reflect the activation of the "working" myocardium. Consequently, an ECG diagnosis of an arrhythmia may have to be based on deductive analysis, with the abnormal behavior of the specialized conduction tissue being deduced from the electrical behavior of the atrial and ventricular myocardium. This may make the ECG diagnosis of some arrhythmias difficult.

The electrophysiological properties of the heart recorded in the ECG represent the sum of electrical behavior of the individual cardiac cells. Development of the *Ling-Gerrard* microelectrode and parallel advances in instrumentation have made it possible to study the electrical behavior of isolated cells. Consequently, considerable knowledge has accumulated regarding the basic cellular mechanism of various arrhythmias. Many of the clinical ECG concepts derived from the study of the surface ECG are being confirmed by direct observation at the cellular level.

The resting intracellular transmembrane voltage is negative, the magnitude of the negativity varying for different cells. The magnitude for the sinoatrial (SA) nodal cell and Purkinje cell, for example, are -60 mV and -90 mV, respectively. Activation of a cell is associated with a sudden and rapid reversal of the intracellular negativity, the phase 0, and the positive overshoot, phase 1. Phase 2 is fairly stable and is followed by phase 3, during which the transmembrane negativity is restored. A stable phase 4 follows. These changes define the transmembrane action potential (TAP) (Figure E-1).

Phases 0 and 1 occur when a sudden influx of sodium reverses the intracellular negativity. Any changes during phase 2 are due to slow calcium channel fluxes, which play a significant role in the generation of the TAP of the SA and AV nodal cells. Phase 3 is due to efflux of potassium, which restores the intracellular negativity. During phase 4, restitution of normal ionic concentration takes place. This is accomplished by Na^+, K^+, and Ca^{++} pumps. The process is energy consuming (Figure E-1A).

The ECG manifestations of the TAP phases are as follows: phase 0 and phase 1, the overshoot, are reflected as the QRS, phase 2 as the ST segment, phase 3 as the T wave, and phase 4 as the isoelectric baseline (Figure E-1).

Automaticity and Threshold Potential

Spontaneous loss of transmembrane resting potential (TRP) during phase 4 defines automaticity. It is largely due to the slow, inward movement of Na^+ with a gradual reversal of the intracellular negativity (Figure E-2).

In order to invoke an action potential, the TRP must be reduced to a level known as the threshold potential (TP). TRP reduced to a level less than that of the TP will, with removal of the stimulus, return to the resting state without evoking a propagated impulse. The strength of the stimulus necessary to reduce the TRP to TP defines the excitability of the cell. The stronger the stimulus required to reduce the TRP to TP, the less excitable the cell. Thus, the greater the potential difference between the TRP and TP, the less excitable the cell.

Only a stimulus of sufficient strength to reduce the TRP to TP results in a "full" propagated impulse (Figure E-3).

There are two avenues by which the TRP can be reduced to TP. One is external stimulation, and the second is a process of gradual, spontaneous loss of the TRP during phase 4. This spontaneous loss of diastolic potential defines automaticity.

The nonautomatic cell demonstrates a steady TRP until it is stimulated, while the automatic cell exhibits a gradual loss of phase 4 potential (Figure E-4).

Of the specialized conduction tissue, the SAN exhibits automaticity normally. The AV node, the His-Purkinje system, and perhaps specialized atrial tissues exhibit latent automaticity. The myocardial cells, on the other hand, are nonautomatic and require an external stimulus for depolarization. The cell with the most rapid spontaneous loss of phase 4 potential, normally an SA nodal cell, acts as the primary pacemaker and controls the heart. The heart rate depends on the slope of phase 4. The greater the slope, the more rapid the heart rate; the lower the slope, the slower the heart rate.

The effect of atropine on the slope of phase 4 and its clinical correlate are demonstrated in Figure E-5. Under the influence of atropine, the rate of phase 4 depolarization increases, the TRP reaches TP more rapidly, and the ECG demonstrates an acceleration of the sinus rate.

Latent automaticity in subsidiary sites provides a mechanism for escape when the primary pacemaker fails. AV junctional escape and its electrophysiological correlate are shown in Figure E-6. Cessation of stimulation in the top panel allows the TRP to reach the TP, and an action potential is recorded. On the ECG shown, the SA pacemaker is suppressed by an atrial premature systole. This allows for slow diastolic depolarization of a lower latent automatic pacemaker and an escape.

Under the influence of a variety of pharmacologic agents and pathophysiological aberration, cells with latent pacemaking properties may develop rapid phase 4 depolarization and become the dominant pacemaker. Such an example is demonstrated in Figure E-7. The top panel displays a Purkinje fiber which, when exposed to acetylstrophanthidin, develops spontaneous phase 4 depolarization. A clinical correlate is shown in the bottom panel. A patient with atrial fibrillation recorded in the top row demonstrates the emergence of nonparoxysmal junctional tachycardia (NPJT) and ventricular tachycardia (VT) in the middle and bottom rows, respectively.

Conduction

Several cellular variables that may differ quantitatively from tissue to tissue affect conduction differently. In general, however, the prime determinant of conduction velocity is the rate of upstroke of phase 0, which in turn depends on the magnitude of the TRP at the time of stimulation (the so-called take-off potential). The rate of upstroke of phase 0 declines as the take-off potential is decreased. The reduced velocity of phase 0 results in decreased amplitude of the action potential. The lower amplitude action potential becomes a less efficient stimulus to the surrounding tissue, and speed of conduction is reduced. There is finally a point at which the take-off potential is reduced to a critical level, the cell is unexcitable, and the stimulus fails to elicit a propagated response (Figure E-8).

Stimulation of the cell before recovery of the TRP results in slow upstroke of phase 0, a low amplitude action potential that propagates poorly or may be blocked completely. The difference in response of the two cells in Figure E-9 is due to the different level of the take-off potential at the time of stimulation. An atrial premature systole which excites the bundles prior to full recovery results in aberrant intraventricular conduction (Figure E-9).

The mechanism of potassium-induced atrioventricular nodal (A-V) block is shown in Figure E-10. Panel A shows two action potentials with expanded phase 0, recorded approximately 1 mm apart. After infusion of KCl the TRP (phase 4) is reduced from -90 mV to -70 mV, and the rate of rise of phase 0 and the amplitude of the TRP are also reduced. This results in depression of conduction clearly demonstrated as an increase in the distance between the two TAPs. The surface tracing demonstrates A-V block due to potassium (Figure E-10).

The disturbance in conduction described above is largely voltage-dependent; the delay in conduction is due to premature stimulation prior to electrical recovery and, consequently, at a reduced take-off potential. However, in the AV node, for example, as the impulse propagates there is a progressive decrease in the rate of rise of phase 0 and in the amplitude of the TAP until a point is reached at which the TAP fails to stimulate the adjoining tissues and propagation ceases. This form of gradual depression of conduction due to generation of a progressively weaker impulse has been defined as decremental conduction.

Refractory Period

The variables responsible for refractoriness are not yet fully understood. With this reservation, the following section attempts to briefly define this period.

Refractoriness is that interval during which a stimulus does not elicit a normal response. The cell may be absolutely refractory and fail to respond to any stimulation, or it may respond with a local, nonpropagated action potential. The interval that includes the absolute refractory period and the time during which a nonpropagated response may be elicited is the effective refractory period. The interval during which the cell responds to 1) a stronger than normal stimulus or 2) a normal stimulus with delayed conduction defines the relative refractory period. In the normal cell, refractoriness is a function of the recovery of the TAP—that is, the cell must recover to a certain transmembrane potential before it can be reexcited. Refractoriness that is determined by the recovery of TAP is said to be voltage-dependent.

Reentry

An ectopic impulse may be due to enhanced automaticity of a latent automatic fiber. It may also result from unequal depression of conduction, with the most common mechanism being localized unidirectional block (Figure E-11).

This can be illustrated by assuming that an impulse proceeds normally along one limb of a Y-shaped Purkinje fiber, but is blocked in the other limb. The normally conducted impulse participates in the activation of the heart. It also reenters the blocked fiber in a retrograde direction and exits through the normally conducting branch. The second activation of the heart is registered as an ectopic impulse. The impulse is able to reenter the blocked branch of the fiber because the block is unidirectional, namely, in the antegrade direction only. Perpetuation of the reentrant conduction results in a reentrant tachycardia.

In contrast to an automatic rhythm, which is an independent rhythm, reentry of an impulse depends on a previous dominant impulse for its genesis, and is thus coupled to the dominant impulse.

Triggered Activity

The normal rhythm of the heart is initiated and maintained by the spontaneous, automatic generation of electrical activity in cells of the SAN. Slow diastolic (phase 4) depolarization of the cells, if of sufficient strength and duration, brings the TRP of the tissue surrounding the SAN to the threshold for excitation, and a cardiac impulse results. Then the automatic diastolic depolarization process begins again, the transmembrane potential once more reaches threshold, and the cycle repeats itself. Suppression of the sinus node by vagal stimulation, an atrial premature complex (APC), or an artificial stimulus is followed by resumption of the sinus rhythm after a pause equal to or longer than the basic sinus node cycle because of membrane effects that alter this phase 4 depolarization process. Occasionally, the pause that follows sinus node suppression is relatively long and is terminated by an escape complex from another focus.

At times, usually in a well defined milieu, such as following the administration of digitalis, the pause following interruption of a dominant automatic pacemaker is paradoxically short. The impulses responsible for the unexpectedly short cycles are thought to arise from another form of impulse-generating activity commonly referred to as afterdepolarization. Abnormal afterdepolarizations may appear either early, during phase 2 or 3, or they may be delayed and occur during phase 4 of the parent action potentials. The impulses resulting from these depolarizations are said to be "triggered," and arrhythmias so initiated are referred to as "triggered" arrhythmias (Figure E-12).

His bundle electrocardiography is discussed briefly in Chapter 5.

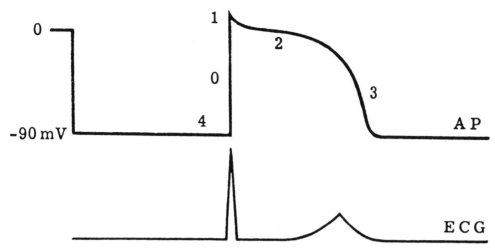

Figure E-1. Action potential (AP) and the surface ECG. The AP resting potential (phase 4) is followed by a rapid upstroke depolarization (phase 0) followed by repolarization, which includes an early, relatively rapid phase 1, a slow phase 2 (plateau), and a second, rapid phase 3. On the surface ECG, phase 4 represents the diastolic isoelectric period, phase 0 represents the R wave, phase 2 represents the ST segment, and phase 3 represents the T wave.

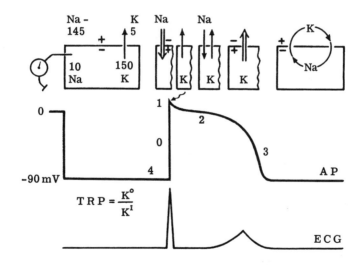

IONIC BASIS OF TRANSMEMBRANE AP

1. IONIC CONCENTRATION GRADIENT
2. ELECTRICAL CONCENTRATION GRADIENT
3. MEMBRANE PERMEABILITY

Figure E-1A. Ionic basis for the AP. The top row reflects: 1) equilibrium of ionic concentration during phase 4; 2) influx of sodium during phase 0; 3) efflux of potassium during phase 1; 4) efflux of potassium during phase 3; and 5) restitution of ionic concentration gradient. For correlation of the different phases of the action potential and the surface ECG, see Figure E-1.

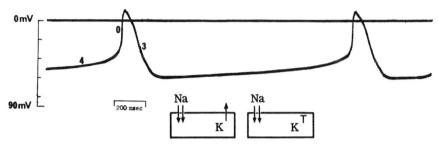

Figure E-2. Automaticity. An automatic SAN fiber showing gradual spontaneous loss of phase 4 transmembrane voltage. When the declining transmembrane voltage reaches the threshold level, a propagated action potential is generated.

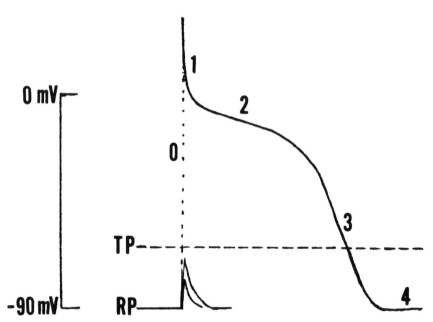

Figure E-3. TAP and the TP. The subthreshold stimuli are simulated and superimposed. When the resting transmembrane potential (RP) of −90 mV is reduced to a TP potential of approximately −60 mV, a propagated action potential is generated. When the stimulus is subthreshold (does not reach the TP), the transmembrane potential returns to baseline.

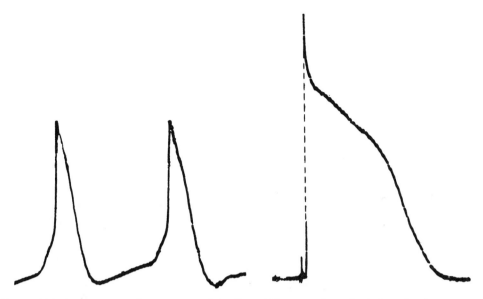

Figure E-4. Automatic and nonautomatic cells are illustrated on the left and right, respectively. The automatic cell exhibits a gradual loss of phase 4 potential. The nonautomatic cell requires a stimulus to generate a propagated potential.

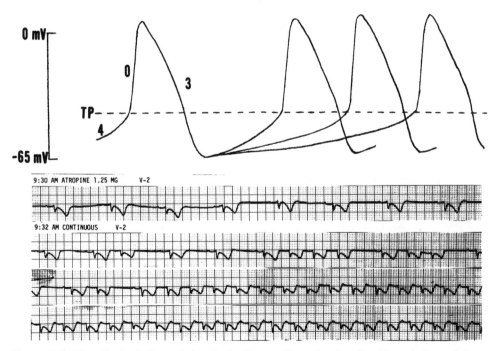

Figure E-5. The effect of phase 4 depolarization on the rate. Acceleration of phase 4 depolarization increases the heart rate. The increase in the steepness of reduction of phase 4 is due to atropine. The tachycardia due to atropine is illustrated in the bottom panel.

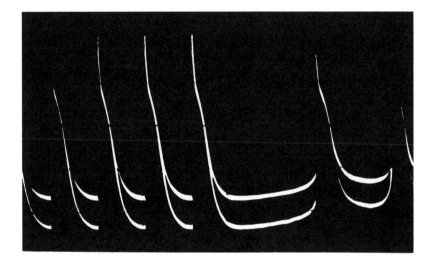

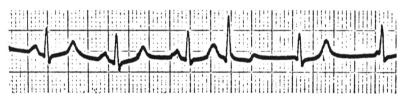

Figure E-6. Electrophysiology of escape and its clinical correlate. Slowing of the rate by cessation of stimulation in the top panel and suppression of SA nodal rhythm by atrial premature stimulation allows the phase 4 potential of the subsidiary pacemaker to reach the TP, resulting in an escape complex.

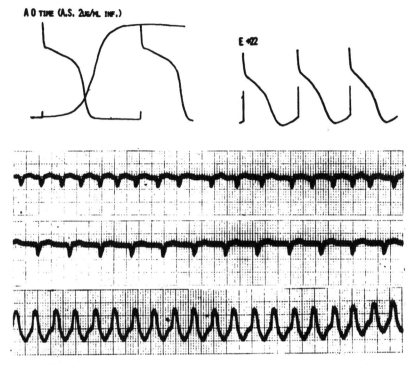

Figure E-7. Latent automaticity. Under the influence of acetylstrophanthidin, the Purkinje fiber exhibits enhanced automaticity of phase 4 and assumes the role of a dominant pacemaker. The clinical correlate demonstrates atrial fibrillation, which, under the influence of toxic doses of digitalis, develops NPJT (middle row) and ventricular tachycardia (bottom row).

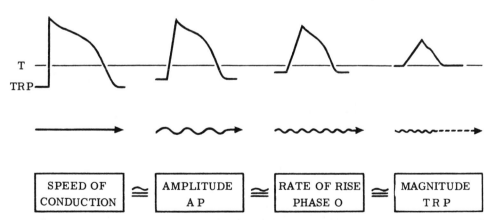

Figure E-8. Conduction. Schematic presentation of the relation of the speed of conduction to the magnitude of the take-off potential of phase 4. As the take-off potential is reduced, the amplitude of the action potential and the speed of rise of phase 0 are also reduced. These changes, in turn, result in slowing or failure of conduction.

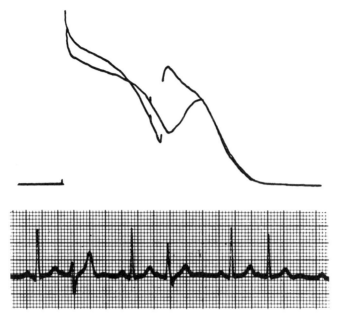

Figure E-9. Resting potential and conduction. Premature activation results in a depressed phase 0 and poor action potential amplitude. Such an action potential may propagate at a decreased rate or be blocked completely. The clinical correlate demonstrates APCs with varying degrees of depression of conduction and/or block in the right bundle.

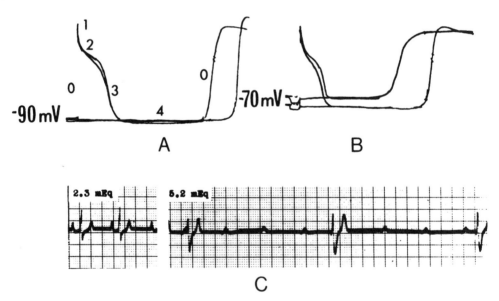

Figure E-10. Effect of potassium on conduction. The ECG (**C**) demonstrates A-V block due to K$^+$ in a digitalis-intoxicated dog and the electrophysiological mechanism responsible for the block (**A** and **B**). The two control action potentials recorded at the left in **A** are approximately 1 mm apart. Phase 0 is shown enlarged on the right. After infusion of KCl (**B**), the phase 4 potential is reduced from −90 to −70 mV; the rate of change of voltage (dV/dt) of phase 0 is reduced: the amplitude of the action potential is reduced and the conduction between the two microelectrodes is greatly delayed, as indicated by an increase in the distance between the two action potentials (**B**, right). From Fisch C. Relation of electrolyte disturbances to cardiac arrhythmias. *Circulation* 1973;47:408–419.

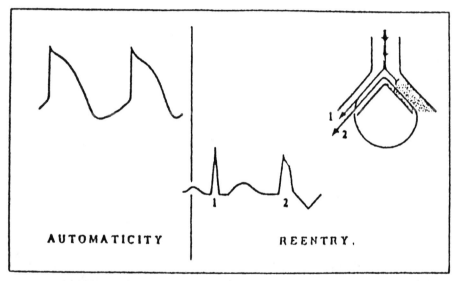

Figure E-11. Mechanisms responsible for most ectopic arrhythmias. Automaticity is manifested by a gradual loss of resting membrane potential (phase 4), which on reaching the TP generates a propagated action potential. In reentry, an impulse arrives at an area of unidirectional block. It is conducted normally along one pathway and takes part in ventricular activation, which gives rise to the normal QRS. Following cardiac excitation, the impulse enters the blocked area in a retrograde direction and reenters the tissue via the normally conducting pathway, giving rise to the second, or reentrant, or ectopic, QRS complex. From Fisch C. Electrophysiological basis of clinical arrhythmias. *Heart Lung* 1974;3:51–56.

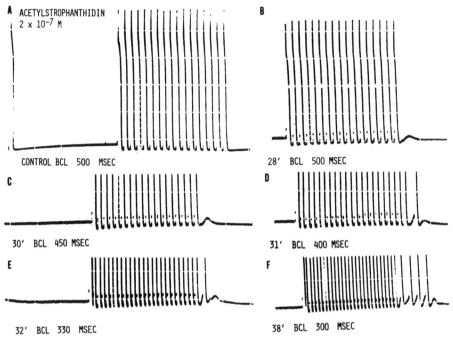

Figure E-12. Triggered automaticity. A cell superfused with acetylstrophanthidin is paced at increasing rates with foreshortening of the basic cycle from 500 to 300 ms. In **B** and **C,** cessation of stimulation is followed by an afterdepolarization; in **D** and **E** by a triggered action potential and an afterdepolarization; in **F** by four consecutive triggered action potentials and an afterdepolarization. From Fisch C, Knoebel SB. Triggered activity and AV junctional arrhythmias. In Rosen MR, Janse MJ, Wit AL (eds): *Cardiac Electrophysiology.* Mount Kisco, NY: Futura Publishing Co., Inc.; 1990:333–340. Courtesy of Dr. John C. Bailey.

Section I

Sinoatrial Node, Atrial, Junctional, Ventricular Rhythms, and Atrioventricular Blocks

---

1

Sinoatrial Rhythms

Normal Sinus Rhythm
Sinus Tachycardia
Sinus Bradycardia
Sinus Arrhythmia
    Phasic (Respiratory) Sinus Arrhythmia
    Nonphasic (Nonrespiratory) Sinus Arrhythmia
    Ventriculophasic Sinus Arrhythmia
Sinoatrial Arrest
Sinoatrial Block
    Type I (Wenckebach)
    Type II (Mobitz)
Sinoatrial Node Suppression
Sinoatrial Nodal Premature Complexes
Sinoatrial Nodal Reentrant Tachycardia
Escape

Normal Sinus Rhythm

The P Wave

The normal impulse that originates in the SAN, located high in the right atrium, traverses the atria in a wavelike "front" with a velocity of approximately 1000 mm/s. The P wave is a record of that process. Depolarization of the right atrium, an anterior chamber, is directed anteriorly and inferiorly. This is followed by depolarization of the left atrium, to the left, posteriorly and inferiorly. For practical purposes, normal atrial activation or depolarization because of the dominance of the inferior and posterior forces can be expressed by a vector oriented inferiorly, to the left and posterior. When projected on the Einthoven triangle, the vector is most parallel to lead II followed by leads III and I. Consequently, the P wave amplitude is the greatest in lead II followed by leads III and I. The P wave configuration is constant as long as the site of origin of the P wave is constant. If the site of origin of the P wave is high in the sinus node, as in the case of tachycardia, the amplitude of the P wave is increased. With shift of the site of the pacemaker lower within the SAN, as with sinus bradycardia, the amplitude is diminished.

The P-R Interval and QRS

Delay of the impulse in the AV junction is manifest on the surface ECG as the P-R interval. Following the delay in the AV junction, initial ventricular depolarization is that of the septum from left to right. Septal depolarization is followed by the simultaneous depolarization of the right and left ventricular walls from endocardium to epicardium, with the basal portions being the last to be depolarized. Thus, for practical purposes, ventricular activation can be expressed by two vectors. The initial vector reflects septal activation from left to right and is oriented to the right, anteriorly and inferiorly and occasionally superiorly. This initial vector also may include early activation of the right ventricle. The second and dominant vector reflects left ventricular activation and is oriented to the left, inferiorly and posteriorly.

Sinus Tachycardia

As the slope of phase 4 of the TAP steepens, the rate of SAN discharge increases (see Cellular Basis of the Electrocardiogram). When the rate reaches and exceeds 100 per minute, sinus tachycardia is said to be present. During maximal exercise the sinus rate may approach and occasionally exceed 200 per minute. At that rate it may be difficult to differentiate sinus tachycardia from rapid supraventricular ectopic tachycardias (Figure 1-1).

Sinus Bradycardia

As the slope of phase 4 of the TAP decreases, it takes longer for the phase 4 potential to reach TP, and the rate of SA discharge slows. Sinus bradycardia is said to be present when the rate is 60 per minute or less. The range is, as a rule, 40 to 60 per minute. On rare occasions, the rate may be as low as 30 per minute (Figure 1-2).

Sinus Arrhythmia

In sinus arrhythmias, the sinus rhythm is irregular, the P wave and P-R interval are normal, and the P-P interval varies by more than approximately 0.16 seconds. Three types of sinus arrhythmias are recognized. These include phasic or respiratory, nonphasic or nonrespiratory, and ventriculophasic.

Phasic (Respiratory) Sinus Arrhythmia

With phasic sinus arrhythmia, the rate is dependent on the respiratory cycle, increasing during inspiration and decreasing during expiration. The pacemaker site within the SAN shifts with respiration. As the pacemaker site moves higher in the SAN, the heart rate and P wave amplitude in leads II, III, and AVF increase. As the pacemaker shifts lower in the SAN, the P wave amplitude and the heart rate decrease. The heart rate changes rhythmically and gradually, thus differentiating this from nonphasic arrhythmia. In healthy individuals, pauses up to 20 seconds may occur normally (Figures 1-3 and 1-4).

Nonphasic (Nonrespiratory) Sinus Arrhythmia

In nonphasic (nonrespiratory) sinus arrhythmia, the P wave and P-R interval are normal but the P-P intervals vary at random and independently of any physiological function (Figure 1-5).

Ventriculophasic Sinus Arrhythmia

Ventriculophasic sinus arrhythmia is noted in the presence of A-V block. The P waves and the P-R interval are normal. The P-P intervals encompassing a QRS complex are shorter than the P-P intervals without an intervening QRS complex. Two mechanisms have been proposed to explain the effect of the intervening QRS complex on the P-P interval. One is that the mechanical pressure of the ejected blood on the sinus node accelerates the sinus node discharge. Another is that the prolongation of the P-P interval may be due to a vagal effect initiated by the carotid sinus reflex in response to systolic ejection (Figure 1-6).

Sinus Arrest

Failure of the SAN to generate an action potential because of depression of automaticity is manifest in the ECG by a transient absence of P waves that may last longer than 2.0 seconds. The pause is referred to as a sinus pause or arrest. The P-P intervals are not a multiple of the basic sinus cycle but are random in duration (Figures 1-7, 1-8, and 1-9).

Sinoatrial Block

SA block differs from sinus arrest in that the SAN generates an action potential but its exit is blocked (exit block) in the sinus node or the perinodal tissue, thus failing to inscribe a P wave. When the rhythm is regular and the pause a multiple of the basic sinus cycle, the exit block is Mobitz Type II (Figures 1-10, 1-11, 1-12, and 1-13). If the P-P intervals are irregular and exhibit repetitive group beating with a progressively shorter P-P interval and a long pause that is shorter than two preceding P-P intervals, the exit block is Type I or Wenckebach block (Figure 1-14). The Wenckebach sequence is diagramed in Figure 1-15.

Sinoatrial Node Suppression

The effect of an ectopic premature complex on the SAN is to discharge and reset or suppress its intrinsic pacemaker activity. The compensatory pause may equal or be longer than the basic sinus cycle.

Suppression of the SAN may be due to vagal influence, APCs (Figure 1-16) or VPCs with retrograde conduction (Figure 1-17), ectopic tachycardias, or pacing. Suppression of the SAN by an APC was recognized before the advent of the ECG (Figures 1-16 and 1-17) and has been substantiated experimentally and clinically. The compensatory pause is longer with more rapid overdrive impulses. It has been suggested that an APC may induce Stokes-Adams attacks due to SA nodal suppression.

Bradycardia-Tachycardia Syndrome

Paroxysms of supraventricular tachycardia (SVT) alternating with periods of bradycardia or arrest are referred to as bradycardia-tachycardia syndrome. The prolonged pause is most probably due to overdrive suppression of the sinus node (Figures 1-18, 1-19, and 1-20). The duration of the post-tachycardia suppression is presumed to be related to concomitant SA nodal disease.

Sinoatrial Nodal Premature Complexes

Premature SA nodal complexes are characterized by premature P waves that are identical in configuration to the sinus rhythm P waves or are only minimally altered. The P-R interval in premature SA nodal complexes is normal. It may be difficult if not impossible to differentiate SA nodal premature complexes from sinus rhythm with a 3:2 Wenckebach exit block from the sinus node (Figures 1-21 and 1-22).

Sinoatrial Reentrant Tachycardia

SA reentrant tachycardia satisfies the criteria for reentry (see Chapter 10), using the SAN as part of the atrial reentrant loop. The P waves may be identical to the sinus P waves or may differ slightly, but are upright in leads II, III, and AVF and, as such, differ from most other forms of supraventricular reentrant tachycardias. The rate may vary from 80 to 140 per minute with an average rate of approximately 100 to 110 per minute. The episodes of tachycardia are brief, and termination is usually abrupt, although occasionally there may be a gradual slowing before the tachycardia ceases (Figures 1-23, 1-24, and 1-25).

Escape

Normally, the SAN is the dominant cardiac pacemaker, with a rate varying from 60 to 100 per minute. With slowing of the heart rate because of sinus bradycardia, sinus arrest, or exit block, other areas of the heart with intrinsic automaticity at slower rates than the SAN may assume the role of the dominant pacemaker. The most usual site is the junction. It may manifest as a single escape (Figure 1-26) or as a sustained escape rhythm (Figure 1-27). With failure of the AV junction to assume the role of pacemaker, the site of the pacemaker shifts to the Purkinje (ventricular) fibers (Figure 1-28). The rate of Purkinje (ventricular) pacemaker is approximately 30 to 40 per minute. The shift of pacemaker site reflects a passive, physiological response of standby pacemaker.

When the QRS complex is normal, the escape is junctional. When the QRS complex is aberrant and the escape rate is between 30 and 40 beats per minute, the escape is most likely ventricular in origin. The escape intervals are constant. At times, however, as in atrial fibrillation, the escape intervals may not be equal. This is due to displacement of the escape impulse by concealed fibrillatory atrial impulses (see Concealed Conduction, Chapter 6).

Escape and escape rhythms are discussed more fully in Chapter 3 with junctional rhythms.

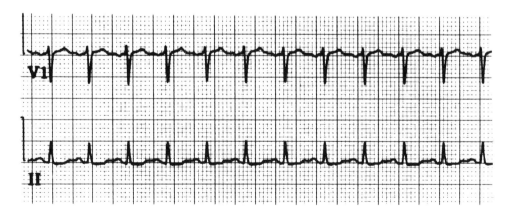

Figure 1-1. Sinus tachycardia. The P waves, P-R interval, and QRS complex are normal. The rate is 158 per minute.

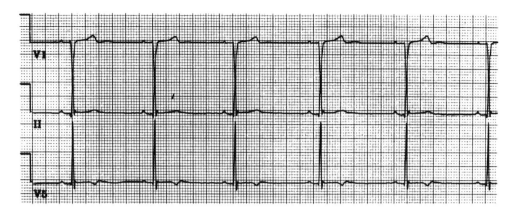

Figure 1-2. Sinus bradycardia. The rate is 50 per minute. The site of origin of the P wave is in the sinus node with a normal sequence of atrial activation; thus, a normal configuration of the P wave.

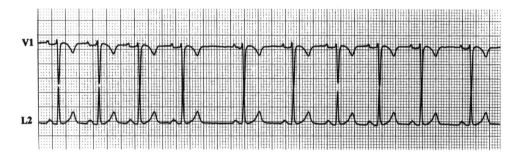

Figure 1-3. Sinus arrhythmia. The P waves, P-R interval, and QRS complex are normal. The rate varies from 65 to 100 per minute in synchrony with respiration, increasing with inspiration, and decreasing with expiration.

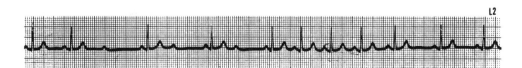

Figure 1-4. Sinus arrhythmia. The P waves, P-R interval, and QRS complex are normal. The rate varies from 103 to 65 per minute in synchrony with respiration. The block of the third, fifth, and seventh P waves is probably vagal in origin.

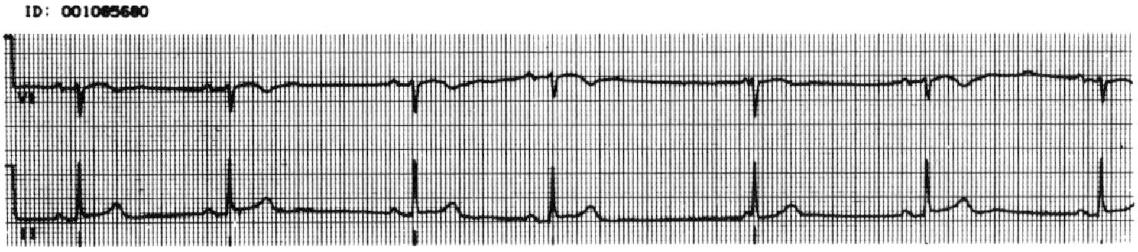

ID: 001085680

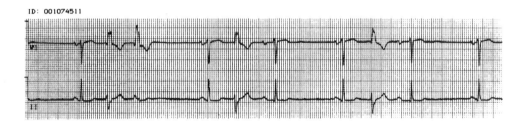

Figure 1-5. Nonphasic sinus arrhythmia. The P waves, P-R interval, and QRS complex are normal. The rate changes at random rather than being phasic as in Figures 1-3 and 1-4. There is a junctional escape following the fourth sinus P wave.

ID: 001074511

Figure 1-6. Ventriculophasic sinus arrhythmia. Sinus rhythm at a rate of approximately 50 to 60 per minute is interrupted by VPCs. The P-P intervals encompassing a VPC are shorter than the P-P interval without an intervening VPC. This relationship is characteristic of ventriculophasic sinus arrhythmia.

V1

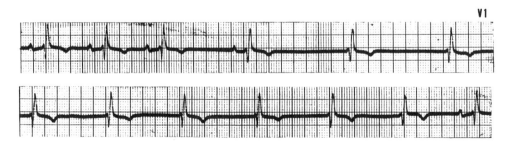

Figure 1-7. Sinus arrest. The P waves are normal with a P-R interval of 240 ms and right bundle branch block. Atrial standstill with a junctional escape rhythm follows the fourth P wave. The initial slower escape rhythm is probably due to a vagal effect. The two strips are continuous.

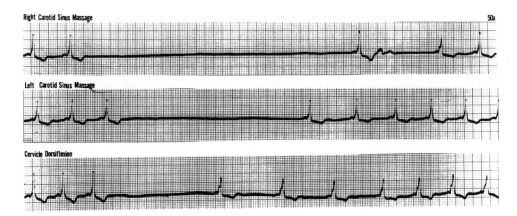

Figure 1-8. Sinus arrest and Wolff-Parkinson-White syndrome. The arrest is due to a sensitive carotid sinus and is initiated by right carotid sinus massage (top strip), left carotid sinus massage (middle strip), and cervical dorsiflexion (bottom strip).

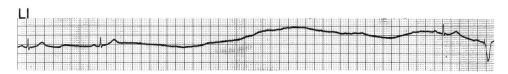

Figure 1-9. Sinus arrest. The first two sinus P waves at a rate of 37 per minute are followed by sinus arrest manifest by the absence of P waves. The sinus rhythm resumes at the end of the strip and is followed by electronic pacemaker stimulation.

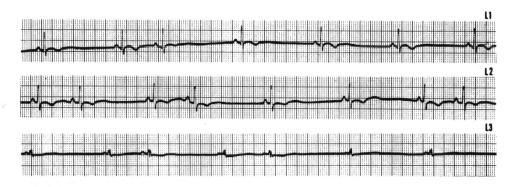

Figure 1-10. SA Mobitz II block. The basic sinus rate is 80 per minute. The longer cycles are a multiple of the basic cycle, indicating that even though a sinus potential was generated, it failed to exit from the sinus node; thus, the longer cycles are an exact multiple of the basic P-P. This is an example of Mobitz Type II SA block.

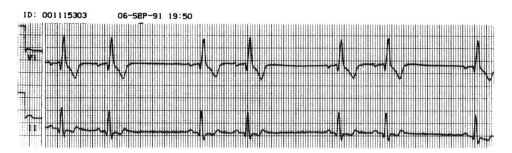

ID: 001115303　　06-SEP-91 19:50

Figure 1-11. SA block. The basic sinus rate is 80 per minute with right bundle branch block. The long pauses are a multiple of the sinus cycle indicating Mobitz Type II SA block (see Figure 1-10).

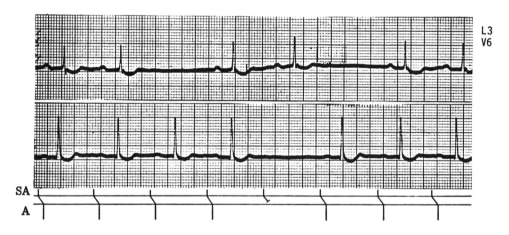

Figure 1-12. SA block. The basic sinus rate is 61 per minute with a P-R interval of 280 ms. The QRS complex is normal with ST segment depression. The long pauses are an exact multiple of the basic sinus cycles, indicating a 2:1 Type II A-V block. The Lewis diagram illustrates failure of a sinus impulse to exit and to excite the atrium (A) and, thus, absence of the P wave.

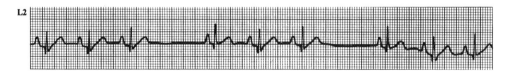

Figure 1-13. SA block. The basic rate is 85 per minute. The longer pauses are an exact multiple of the sinus cycle, indicating Type II exit block (see Figures 1-10, 1-11, and 1-12).

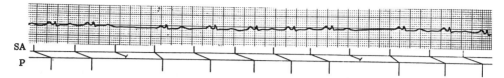

Figure 1-14. SA block. As illustrated in the Lewis diagram, the conduction time from the sinus node (SA) to the atrium (P) is gradually longer until a sinus impulse fails to activate the atrium. The long pause that follows is shorter than the sum of the two preceding cycles, a feature characteristic of the Wenckebach Type I structure (see Figure 1-15).

WENCKEBACH PERIODICITY

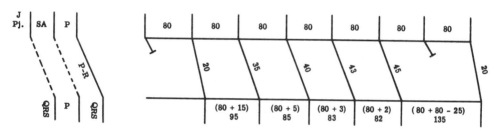

Figure 1-15. Wenckebach periodicity. The diagram shows a gradual prolongation of the P-R interval from 200 to 450 ms with block of the sixth P wave. The maximum prolongation occurs after the second P wave. The long cycle is shorter than the sum of the two preceding cycles. This is a Wenckebach structure and is applicable to all pacemakers and to A-V conduction.

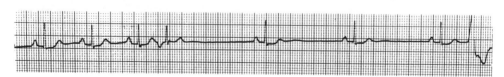

Figure 1-16. Sinus node suppression. The first three sinus P waves are followed by an APC which depresses the sinus node automaticity resulting in a prolonged P-P interval. The two long P-P intervals that follow are twice the length of the basic sinus P-P, and indicate a 2:1 SA exit block. The differential between a junctional and an APC is based on the duration of the P-R interval. A P-R interval shorter than 0.12 seconds indicates a junctional premature complex. A P-R interval longer than 0.12 seconds indicates an APC.

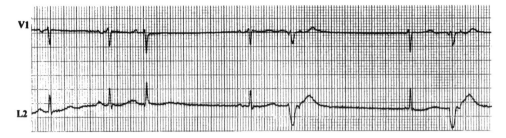

Figure 1-17. Sinus node suppression. The first two sinus P waves are followed by an APC with suppression of the sinus node and a compensatory pause longer than the sinus cycle. The premature ventricular complexes conduct retrogradely, inscribing the negative P wave. The retrograde atrial impulse suppresses the sinus node, and the long cycle that follows is terminated by a junctional escape.

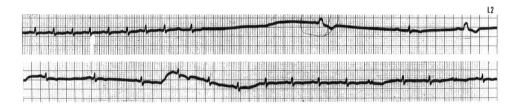

Figure 1-18. Sinus node suppression. Cessation of an SVT is followed by a long period of atrial quiescence with a gradual resumption and acceleration of the sinus rhythm.

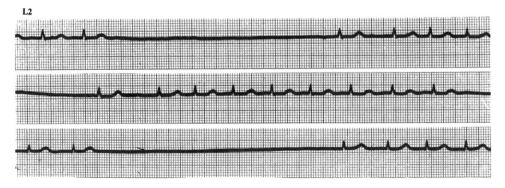

Figure 1-19. Bradycardia-tachycardia syndrome. Episodes of SVT are interrupted by periods of atrial standstill and junctional escapes.

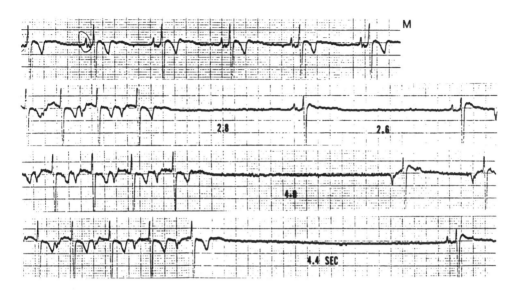

Figure 1-20. Bradycardia-tachycardia syndrome. In the top strip, the P-R interval is 180 ms. In the second, third, and bottom strips, the P-R interval is prolonged at 260 ms. In parallel with the duration of the atrial tachycardia, the pause that follows increases gradually from 2.8 to 4.0 and to 4.4 seconds.

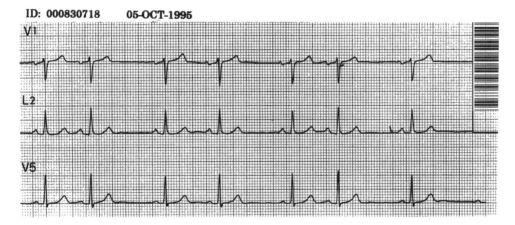

Figure 1-21. Sinus node bigeminy. The bigeminal rhythm is characterized by premature P waves similar in appearance to the sinus P wave with a normal P-R interval. The cycle that differentiates a 3:2 Wenckebach exit block from atrial bigeminy is the last P-P of 1000 ms. This is a full sinus cycle and equals the compensatory pauses following the premature P waves. Were this a 3:2 exit block, this 1000-ms cycle would be shorter than the compensatory pause following the sinus premature.

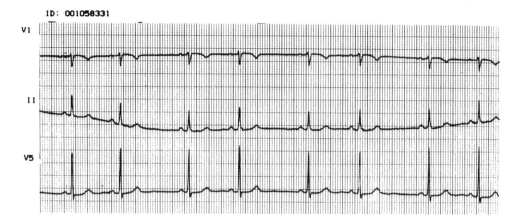

Figure 1-22. Sinus node bigeminy. The P waves are the same as the sinus P waves in appearance with a normal P-R interval. In this instance, differentiation between sinus bigeminy and Wenckebach with a 3:2 exit block is not possible because a full sinus cycle without a "premature" is not recorded (see Figure 1-21).

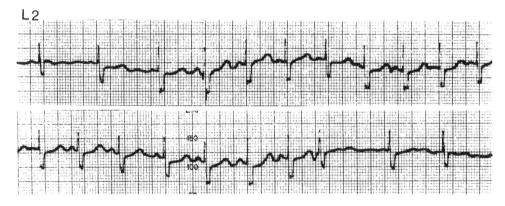

Figure 1-23. SA nodal reentrant tachycardia. The sinus rhythm at a rate of 67 per minute is followed by an abrupt onset of a more rapid rhythm at a rate of 100 per minute. The order of depolarization of the ectopic and sinus P waves is the same. Thus, both are similar in configuration. The tachycardia is terminated by a junctional premature complex. The termination is abrupt, in keeping with reentry.

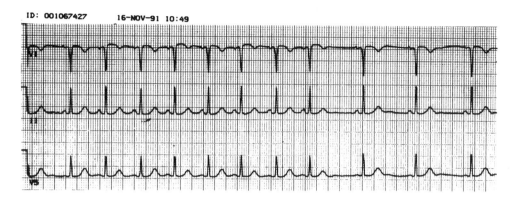

Figure 1-24. SA nodal reentrant tachycardia. The tachycardia at a rate of 100 per minute is followed by sinus rhythm at a rate of 64 per minute. The characteristic feature of sinoatrial nodal reentrant tachycardia is similarity of the P waves and, frequently, an abrupt onset and termination of the tachycardia.

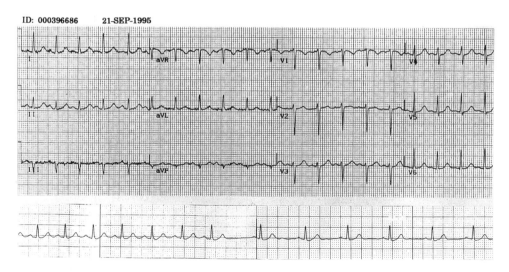

Figure 1-25. SA reentrant tachycardia. The 12-lead tracing illustrates a sinus tachycardia at a rate of 115 per minute. Were it not for the bottom strip, in which the tachycardia terminates abruptly and is followed by sinus rhythm at a rate of 80 per minute, the diagnosis would have been sinus tachycardia.

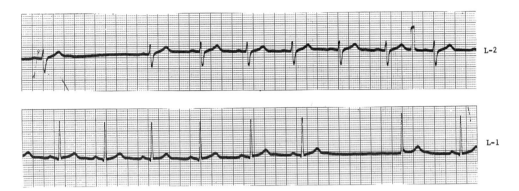

Figure 1-26. SA arrest. The sinus rhythm at a rate of 55 per minute is interrupted by prolonged cycles that are not a multiple of the basic cycle. The second long cycle is terminated by a junctional escape. The long cycles are not a multiple of the sinus rate and, thus, differentiate SA arrest from SA block.

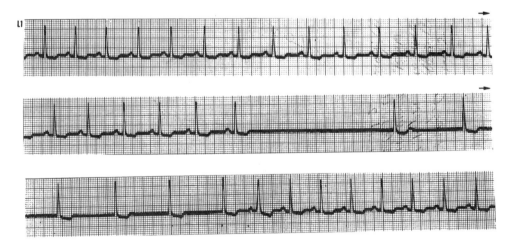

Figure 1-27. Sinus arrest. Sinus rhythm at a rate 83 per minute is interrupted by atrial standstill and a junctional escape rhythm with gradual acceleration of the junctional escape rate. Resumption of sinus rhythm is recorded in the bottom strip.

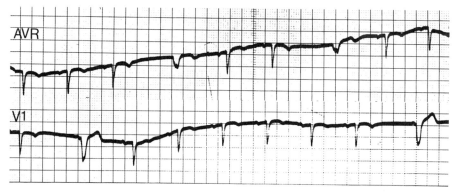

Figure 1-28. Escape. The sinus rhythm at a rate of 86 per minute is interrupted by sinus pauses of 1.0 second in duration terminated by ventricular escapes.

2

Atrial Arrhythmias

Atrial Premature Complexes
    Conducted
    P-R, R-P Relationship
    Nonconducted
    Interpolated
    Compensatory Pause (Return Cycle)
    Postextrasystolic Aberration
    Shift of Pacemaker Site
    With Aberration
    Multifocal Atrial Premature Complexes
Multifocal Atrial Tachycardia
Ectopic Rhythm
Ectopic Tachycardia
    With Block (Paroxysmal Atrial Tachycardia)
Atrial Flutter
    Typical, Atypical
    Type I, Type II
    Atrioventricular Conduction: 1:1, 2:1
      Variable: Type I, Type II
      Complete Atrioventricular Block
Atrial Fibrillation
Interatrial Dissociation; Dissimilar Atrial Rhythms
Atrial Parasystole

Atrial Premature Complexes

The site of origin of APCs is outside the SAN, and is thus ectopic. The diagnostic feature of an APC is prematurity and alteration of P wave configuration. Most often the pause that follows is noncompensatory (see below). The closer the origin of the atrial premature P wave to the SAN, the more the APC resembles the sinus P wave. APCs may differ in amplitude, duration, direction, and configuration. An APC originating low in the atrium may have a low amplitude or negative P in leads II, III, and AVF and a low amplitude or isoelectric P in lead I (Figure 2-1). Differentiation from junctional P waves is based on the P-R interval, a P-R interval for junctional premature complexes (JPCs) being 120 ms or less.

Depending on the degree of prematurity, an APC may conduct to the ventricle with a normal or prolonged P-R interval (Figure 2-2). As a rule, the shorter the R-P (coupling), the longer the P-R. Similarly, the longer the R-P, the shorter the P-R interval (Figures 2-3 and 2-4). An APC falling within the effective (absolute) refractory period of the AV node will fail to conduct (nonconducted APC) (Figure 2-5). On very rare occasions, an atrial premature impulse is interpolated and does not disturb the normal sinus rhythm. This happens when the tissue surrounding the SAN is abnormal and prevents the atrial premature impulse from reaching and discharging the SAN (entrance block) (Figures 2-6 and 2-7) (see Chapter 13).

When an ectopic P wave discharges the SAN, resetting it, the pause that follows often but not always equals the basic sinus cycle. The sum of the coupling interval and the APC to the next P wave interval is usually less than two basic sinus cycles, and is thus noncompensatory. On occasion, however, an APC may suppress the sinus node rather than simply resetting it, and the pause that follows is longer than the basic sinus cycle. This is also true when the entrance time of the APC to the sinus node and the exit time from the node are included with the post ectopic interval. Under such circumstances, fortuitously, the pause may equal two sinus cycles and is thus compensatory. It has been estimated that approximately 50% of APCs are followed by a full compensatory pause. This makes the utility of the compensatory pause as an aid in differentiating APCs from VPCs unreliable.

An APC may be followed by postextrasystolic aberration of the P wave (Figure 2-8) or a shift of the site of origin of the ectopic P (Figure 2-9).

A pause due to failure of the dominant sinus rhythm may be terminated by an atrial escape, with the escape P wave differing in appearance from the sinus P wave (Figure 2-10). An APC reaching the bundle branch system during its effective (absolute) or relative refractory period will result in right bundle branch block (RBBB) aberration (Figures 2-11 and 2-12). Since the refractory period of the right bundle is longer than that of the left bundle, in the normal heart the aberration is nearly always that of RBBB and only rarely that of left bundle branch block (LBBB) (Figure 2-13). Occasionally, when the heart rate accelerates or the APC follows an abruptly shorter R-P interval, the refractory period of the left bundle may exceed that of the right, resulting in LBBB aberration (crossover of refractory periods) (see Chapter 7, Figure 7-14).

When APCs originate from at least three different foci as indicated by varying configurations of the P wave, the arrhythmia is multifocal (Figure 2-14).

Multifocal Atrial Tachycardia

When multifocal APCs are present in the setting of a rapid rate without identifiable, dominant P waves and with varying P-P, R-R, R-P, and P-R intervals, the arrhythmia is referred to as multifocal (chaotic) atrial tachycardia (Figure 2-15).

Ectopic Atrial Rhythm and Tachycardia

Ectopic atrial rhythms originate outside the SAN and are recognized by an altered configuration of the P wave and usually a normal or, at times, a prolonged P-R interval. The appearance of the P wave depends on the site of origin of the ectopic rhythm. The P wave may simply be of decreased amplitude, or it may be biphasic or negative in leads II, III, and AVF. The rhythm is regular, the shortest run consisting of three consecutive ectopic P waves. The heart rate of the ectopic rhythm is 100 per minute or less (Figures 2-16, 2-17, 2-18, and 2-19).

Ectopic rhythms with the above features but with heart rates of 100 per minute or greater are defined as ectopic atrial tachycardia (Figures 2-20 and 2-21).

Atrial (Ectopic) Tachycardia with Block

Because of the rapid rate, ectopic tachycardia is frequently associated with A-V block and is referred to as atrial (ectopic) tachycardia with block.

As in the case of ectopic rhythms or tachycardias, atrial tachycardias with block originate outside the SAN. The heart rate may vary from as low as 100 per minute to as high as 240 per minute. Most often, the rate is below 200 per minute. The P wave contour depends on the site of origin. The closer the site or origin to the SAN, the more normal the appearance of the P waves. With a focus lower in the atrium, the P wave may be of diminished amplitude, or it may be biphasic or inverted (Figures 2-20, 2-21, and 2-22).

A-V conduction of the atrial complexes depends on the duration of AV nodal refractoriness and on the heart rate. A 1:1 A-V ratio can be maintained up to a rate of approximately 240 per minute. At higher rates, 1:1 conduction suggests the presence of an accessory pathway (WPW) (Figure 2-23). Because of the rapid rate, attempted conduction during the AV nodal effective (absolute) refractory period will fail, resulting in A-V block. The block is nearly always at the level of the AV node. The A-V ratio is usually 2:1 (Figures 2-24 and 2-25), although higher ratios (Figures 2-26 and 2-27), frequently with Wenckebach block, are common (Figures 2-19, 2-22, 2-28, and 2-29).

Wenckebach block is manifest by a gradual prolongation of the P-R interval but at decreasing increments. As a result the R-R interval shortens. The longest increment of P-R prolongation is that of the second P-R interval of the sequence. The longest P-R interval precedes the blocked P wave, the shortest follows the pause, and the long cycle encompassing the blocked P wave is shorter than the sum of two basic sinus P-P cycles (see Figures 1-15, 2-19) (see Wenckebach Periodicity, Chapter 19).

Lown-Ganong-Levine Syndrome

Sinus rhythm with a short P-R interval, normal QRS complex, and supraventricular arrhythmias is known as the Lown-Ganong-Levine syndrome. It may be due to the presence of a bypass, such as the James fibers, thus eliminating AV nodal delay (Figures 2-30 and 2-31).

Atrial Flutter

Atrial flutter is due to a circus movement with the impulse traveling along the interatrial septum and the right ventricular free wall. The impulse may proceed counterclockwise or clockwise, most commonly at a rate of 300 per minute.

Atrial flutter can be divided into typical flutter with a negative sawtooth appearance in leads II, III, and AVF (Figure 2-32), and atypical with low amplitude positive flutter waves in leads II, III, and AVF and more prominent positive flutter waves in lead V_1 (Figure 2-33).

In typical flutter, the circus movement is counterclockwise with the impulse traveling caudocranially in the interatrial septum and cranocaudally in the free right ventricular free wall. In atypical flutter, the pathway is the same but the impulse travels clockwise.

Flutter is also divided into Type I or classical, with an atrial rate of 240 to 340 per minute (Figure 2-32), and Type II, manifesting rates of 340 to 430 per minute (Figure 2-34). Type II is rare, and information regarding this arrhythmia is meager.

Classical (Type I) atrial flutter is characterized by a constant configuration of the flutter waves with a regular rate varying, as stated above, from 240 to as high as 340 per minute. In nearly all instances, however, the flutter rate is approximately 300 per minute. Under the influence of antiarrhythmic drugs, the flutter rate may be as slow as 160 per minute (Figures 2-35 and 2-36). As a rule, the A-V ratio is 2:1 or 4:1. Odd ratios are rare and usually are recorded in patients treated with drugs such as digitalis. In such instances, the A-V ratio may be 3:1 or, rarely, 5:1. Wenckebach block with ratios 3:2, 4:3 (Figure 2-37), or higher are not infrequent (Figure 2-38). Only rarely is there a 1:1 flutter-to-QRS complex ratio (Figures 2-39 and 2-40) or complete heart block (Figure 2-38).

In the vast majority of patients, the flutter waves are best seen in leads II, III, and AVF, and have a "sawtooth" or "picket fence" appearance. Because of the rapid rate of the reentrant wave, there is rarely an isoelectric period separating the flutter waves.

With 2:1 A-V conduction, one of the flutter waves may be superimposed on the QRS complex or recorded immediately after the QRS complex, making the diagnosis difficult (Figures 2-38 and 2-41). Careful inspection of lead V_1 may disclose a small upright flutter wave at the end of the QRS complex. This combined with a regular ventricular rate of 150 per minute will point to atrial flutter. Application of carotid sinus pressure by increasing the degree of A-V block will unmask the flutter waves (Figure 2-41) and, thus, clarify the diagnosis.

Atrial Fibrillation

The site of impulse formation in atrial fibrillation is the atrial myocardium. The SAN is not involved. The electrical activity is completely disorganized, with 400 to 600 atrial wavelets per minute. The ECG records atrial wavelets ("f" waves) of varying amplitude, duration, and orientation. The f waves may be fine and, at times, hardly visible. Such fine f waves are most often seen in hypertensive or coronary heart disease. Coarse f waves are seen more often with valvular heart disease (Figure 2-42).

The characteristic feature of atrial fibrillation is a random ventricular rhythm. In untreated individuals with normal A-V conduction, the ventricular rate may be as high as 200 per minute but most often varies from 140 to 170 per minute (Figure 2-43). Fibrillation may be precipitated by an atrial premature impulse falling in the vulnerable period of the atria (Figure 2-44).

In the presence of atrial fibrillation, isolated prolonged pauses all of the same duration indicate junctional (Figure 2-45) or ventricular escape (Figure 2-45).

Normalization of the ventricular rhythm, especially in the course of administration of digitalis, indicates digitalis excess. A regular ventricular rhythm at a rate of approximately 70 to 130 per minute with normal QRS complexes indicates NPJT (Figures 2-46 and 2-47). When the QRS complex is prolonged during normalization of the rhythm in atrial fibrillation, the most likely diagnosis is VT.

Because of the vagal effect of digitalis on the AV node, a slow regular rhythm may be present, suggestive of complete A-V block due to the digitalis. However, minimal physical activity inhibits the vagal effect on A-V conduction and there is a prompt increase in heart rate.

Dissimilar Atrial Rhythms

Dissimilar atrial rhythms were produced experimentally in the dog by Scherf,[1] and have been rarely reported in humans.[2,3] The usual dissociation consists of atrial flutter in one atrium, atrial fibrillation in the other atrium, or, rarely, sinus rhythm (Figure 2-48). With the advent of cardiac transplantation, the dissociation is manifest by two atrial rhythms. One P wave originates in the vestige of the atrium of the recipient's heart and the other in the atrium of the donor's heart (Figure 2-49).

Atrial Parasystole

Classical parasystole is a protected, independent, automatic focus, and is most often regular (Figure 2-50) (see Chapter 9).

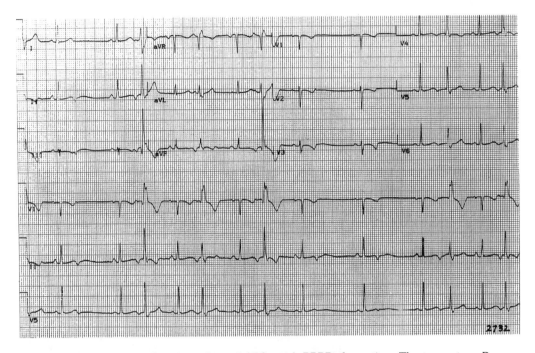

Figure 2-1. Nonconducted and conducted APCs with RBBB aberration. The premature P waves are inverted in leads II, III, AVF, V_4, V_5, and V_6. Some are conducted while some are nonconducted. The inversion of the P waves in leads V_4, V_5, and V_6 indicates a left atrial origin of the APCs. The RBBB pattern reflects aberration due to attempted conduction during the bundle's refractory period.

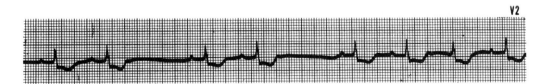

Figure 2-2. Conducted and nonconducted APCs. The basic rhythm is sinus with a P-P interval of 800 ms and P-R interval of 240 ms. The first and second APCs are nonconducted while the third conducts with the P-R interval of 360 ms.

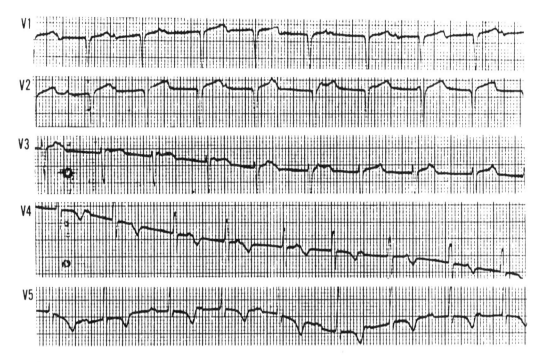

Figure 2-3. The P-R and R-P relationships. The basic rhythm is sinus with a P-R interval varying from 240 to 560 ms. APCs interrupt the sinus rhythm. The duration of the P-R intervals is inversely proportional to the preceding R-P intervals. The shorter the R-P interval, the longer the P-R interval and, conversely, the longer the R-P interval, the shorter the P-R interval (see Figure 2-4).

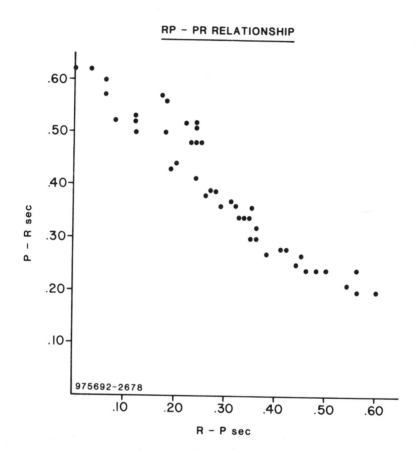

Figure 2-4. R-P-P-R relationship. The R-P interval is indicated on the abscissa and the P-R interval on the ordinate. The inverse relationship of the P-R interval with the R-P interval is nearly linear. The shorter the R-P interval, the longer the PR. This relationship is one of the basic fundamental principles of A-V conduction (see Figure 2-3).

AVF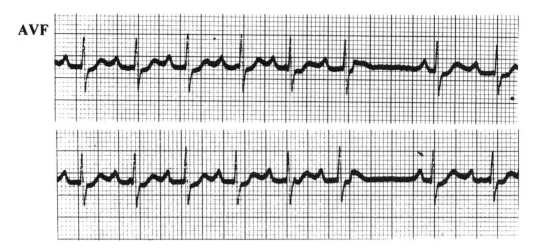

Figure 2-5. Nonconducted APCs. The sinus rhythm at a rate of 125 per minute is interrupted by closely coupled APCs that fail to conduct. The return cycle, the pause between the APC and the next sinus complex, is considerably longer than the basic P-P, indicating that the APCs not only discharged but also suppressed the sinus node.

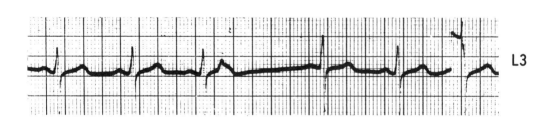

L2

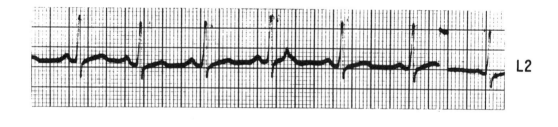

L3

Figure 2-6. APCs with entrance block to the SAN. The APC in lead L3 is nonconducted. The APC in lead L2 is similarly nonconducted. The return cycle, the pause between the APC and a subsequent sinus P wave in lead L2, is considerably shorter than the sinus P-P, indicating that the APC failed to reach and to discharge the sinus node. This is an example of entrance block where the APC fails to enter and to alter the SAN rhythmicity.

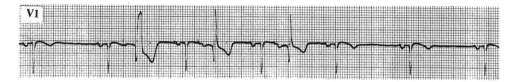

Figure 2-7. APCs with SA nodal entrance block. The APCs with right bundle branch aberration are interpolated and do not disturb the rhythmicity of the sinus node, which discharges at a rate of 50 per minute. The APCs failing to reach the sinus node do not disturb its rhythmicity, and exemplify entrance block to the SAN.

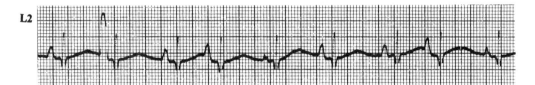

Figure 2-8. APCs with postextrasystolic aberration. The sinus rhythm at a P-P interval of 800 ms is followed by an APC. This, in turn, is followed by an altered appearance of the sinus P reflecting postextrasystolic aberration. The return cycle following the APC is 800 ms, equal to the basic sinus cycle length.

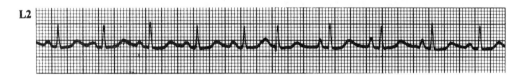

Figure 2-9. APCs with displacement of the atrial pacemaker. The sinus rhythm with a P-P of 600 per minute is interrupted by an APC, and this in turn is followed by three altered P waves reflecting either postextrasystolic aberration or a shift of the site of origin of the atrial pace-

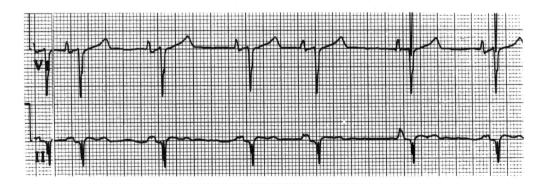

Figure 2-10. Atrial escape. The sinus rhythm is interrupted by an APC. The APC is followed by a prolonged pause terminated by a P wave of different configuration than the sinus P wave. This altered P wave reflects an atrial escape.

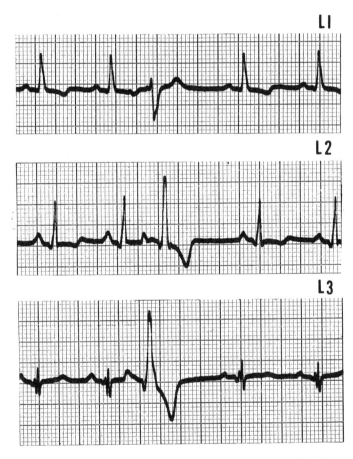

Figure 2-11. APCs with aberration. The APCs conduct with RBBB and left posterior fascicular block aberration.

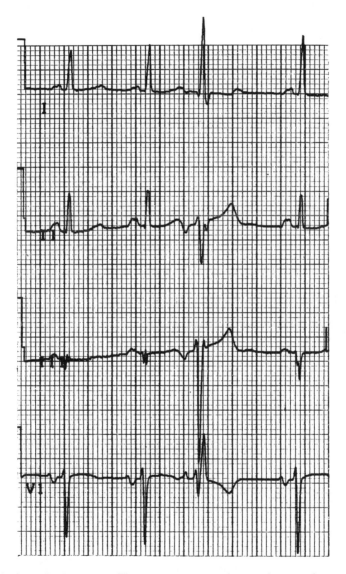

Figure 2-12. APCs with aberration. The premature impulses, either atrial or junctional, conduct with RBBB and left anterior fascicular block aberration.

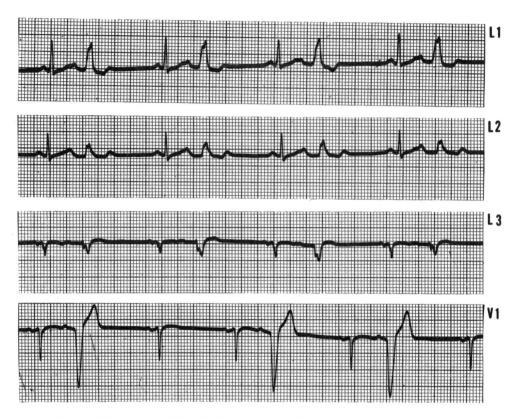

Figure 2-13. Atrial bigeminy with LBBB aberration. LBBB aberration is relatively rare and is usually indicative of an abnormal state of the Purkinje system.

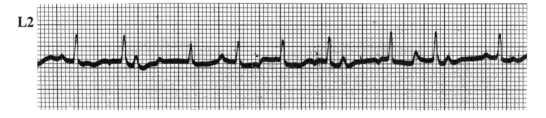

Figure 2-14. Multifocal APCs. Three or more APCs with different configuration are indicative of multifocal or multiform APCs.

ID: 001053160

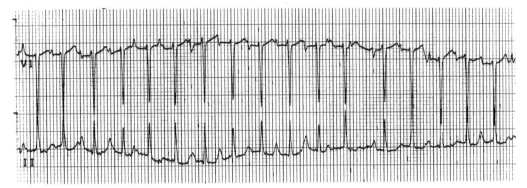

Figure 2-15. Multifocal atrial tachycardia. The presence of multiform and multifocal APCs with a heart rate of greater than 100 per minute and no discernible sinus rhythm classifies this as a multifocal atrial tachycardia.

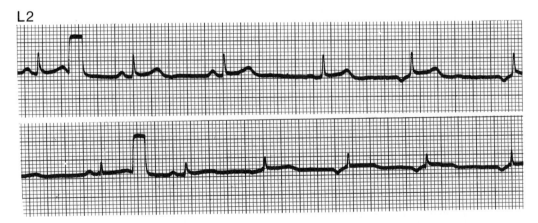

Figure 2-16. Atrial escape rhythm (lead II). The sinus rhythm at a P-P of 800 ms is followed by a pause of 1080 ms and an escape complex. The fourth P wave in the top row, the first of the escape rhythm, is a fusion between the sinus and the inverted escape P wave. In the bottom row, the third P wave is also a fusion. The assumption that the rhythm is atrial rather than a junctional escape is based on the P-R interval of 160 ms.

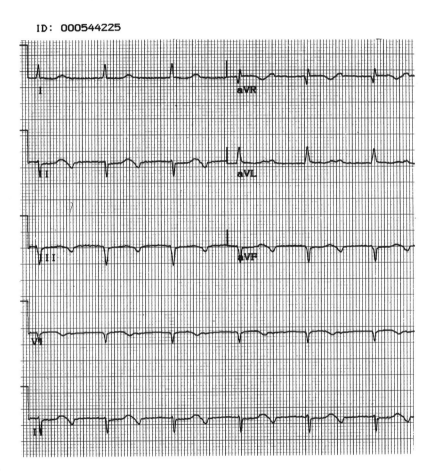

Figure 2-17. Ectopic atrial rhythm. Ectopic atrial rhythm, a P-R interval of 320 ms, and a rate of 75 per minute. The P is inverted in leads II, III, and AVF with left anterior fascicular block of the QRS complex.

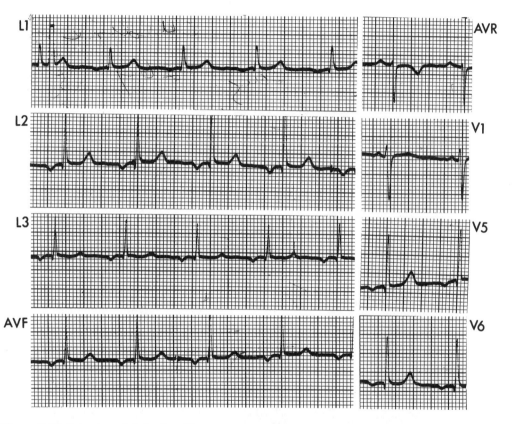

Figure 2-18. Ectopic atrial rhythm. The rate is 75 per minute. The P waves are inverted in leads II, III, AVF, V$_5$, and V$_6$, with a P-R interval of 160 ms. The inversion of the P waves in the precordial leads indicates that the rhythm originates in the left atrium.

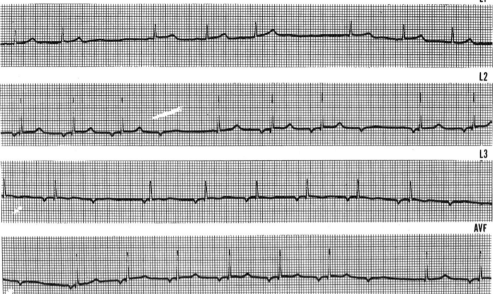

Figure 2-19. Junctional rhythm with Wenckebach block. The P wave is isoelectric in lead I and inverted in leads II, III, and AVF. The rate is 70 per minute. In lead III, the P-R interval of 100 ms gradually increases to 200 ms prior to block. The assumption of junctional rhythm rather than atrial is based on the short initial P-R interval of 100 ms.

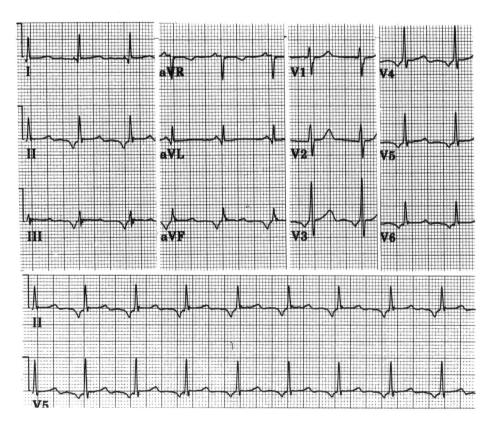

Figure 2-20. Ectopic atrial tachycardia. The rate is 94 per minute. The P wave is isoelectric in lead I and inverted in leads II, III, AVF, V_3, V_4, V_5, and V_6, indicating a left atrial origin of the tachycardia.

AVF

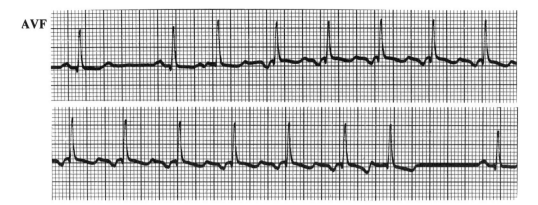

Figure 2-21. APCs with shift of the pacemaker site. Following the first two sinus P waves, an APC initiates an ectopic atrial tachycardia at a rate of 100 per minute with inverted P waves and a P-R interval of 140 ms. The tachycardia is terminated by a premature atrial impulse. The assumption that the origin is atrial rather than junctional is based on the P-R interval of 140 ms.

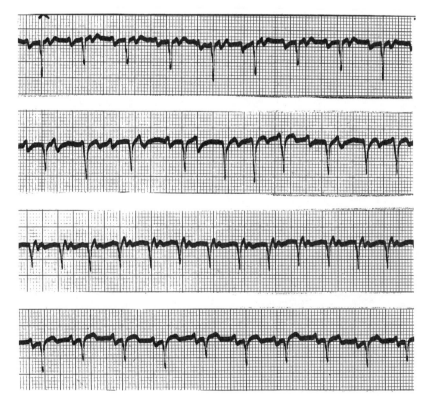

Figure 2-22. Atrial tachycardia with block. The atrial rate varies from 214 with 2:1 A-V block per minute in the top row to 150 per minute in the third row. In the second row, conduction is that of Wenckebach sequence with 3:2 and 4:3 ratios. In the third row, the conduction is 1:1 with a P-R interval of 240 ms. In the bottom row, normal sinus rhythm resumes. Characteristic features of atrial tachycardia with block are ectopic P waves resembling sinus P waves, and A-V block with varying ratios of A-V conduction with or without Wenckebach structure.

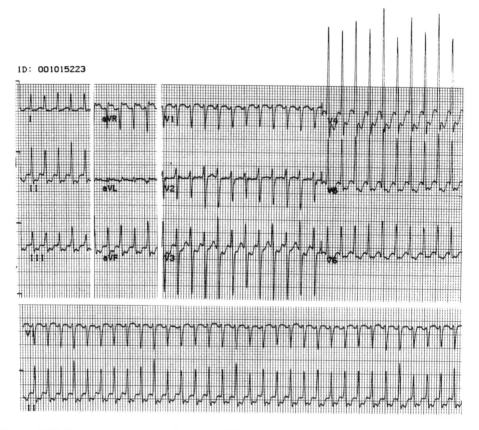

ID: 001015223

Figure 2-23. Supraventricular tachycardia. The rate is approximately 300 per minute with nonspecific ST-T changes. The QRS complex is normal. SVT at this rate suggests strongly that the mechanism may be concealed, retrograde reentry along an accessory pathway (Wolff-Parkinson-White).

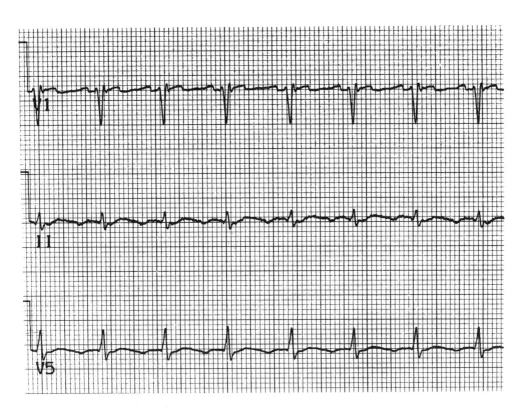

Figure 2-24. Atrial ectopic tachycardia. The P waves are upright in V_1 and inverted in L_2 and V_5, suggesting that the origin of the tachycardia is in the left atrium. The rate of the tachycardia is 214 per minute with 2:1 A-V conduction.

ID: 000753369

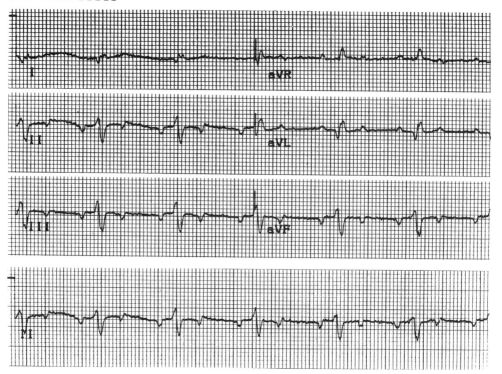

Figure 2-25. Ectopic atrial tachycardia. The rate is approximately 150 per minute with a P-R interval of 170 ms and 2:1 A-V conduction. The P waves are isoelectric in lead I and inverted in II, III, and AVF.

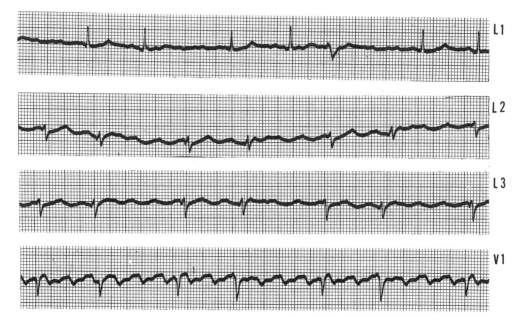

Figure 2-26. Atrial tachycardia. The rate is 188 per minute with A-V conduction ratios of 2:1 and 3:1 with Wenckebach sequence.

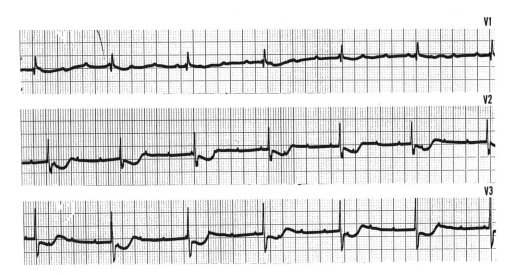

Figure 2-27. Atrial tachycardia with AV dissociation and A-V block. The atrial rate is approximately 150 per minute and regular. The ventricular rate is approximately 47 per minute, regular, and junctional in origin. There is no correlation between the P wave and the QRS complex, indicating AV dissociation due to A-V block.

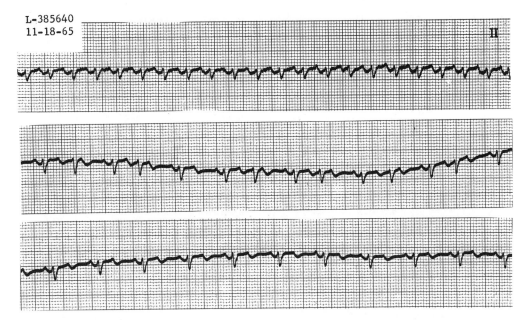

Figure 2-28. Atrial tachycardia. The rate is 188 per minute with 1:1, 2:1, and 3:2 Wenckebach conduction in the top, bottom, and middle tracings, respectively.

ID: 000996611

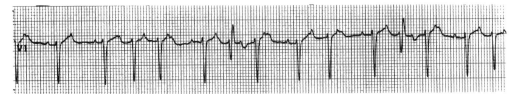

Figure 2-29. Atrial tachycardia. The atrial rate is 167 per minute with 3:2 and 4:3 Wencke-bach A-V block. The latter is exemplified by a sequence beginning with the fourth P wave with a P-R interval of approximately 120 ms prolonging gradually to 220 ms prior to block. Two P waves, each following a long pause, conduct with right bundle branch aberration (Ashman phenomenon).

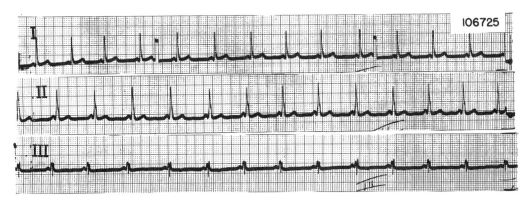

Figure 2-30. Lown-Ganong-Levine syndrome. This syndrome is characterized by short P-R interval, normal QRS complex, and frequent SVT. In this instance, the sinus rate is 65 per minute, the P-R interval is 80 ms, and the QRS complex is normal.

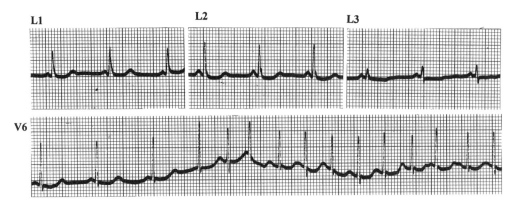

Figure 2-31. Lown-Ganong-Levine syndrome. The basic rhythm is sinus with a P-R interval of 80 ms, normal QRS complex, and an SVT in lead V_6.

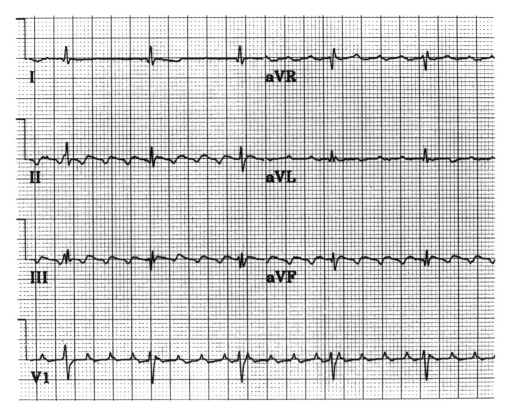

Figure 2-32. Atrial flutter. Atrial flutter at a rate of 240 per minute, with a typical "saw-tooth" pattern, is illustrated in leads II, III, and AVF. The ratio of the flutter to the QRS complex is 4:1.

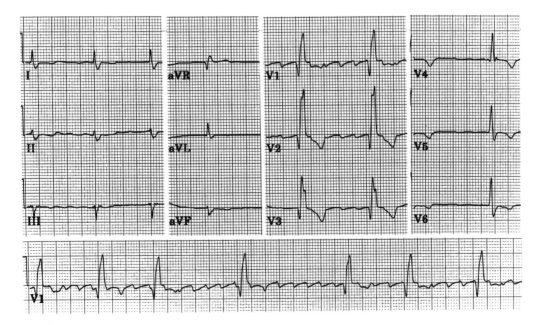

Figure 2-33. Atypical atrial flutter. The pattern of the QRS complex is that of left anterior fascicular block, RBBB, and septal myocardial infarction. The atypical form of atrial flutter is characterized by the absence of discrete flutter waves in leads II, III, and AVF and prominent flutter waves in leads V_1 and V_2.

L2

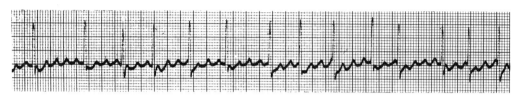

Figure 2-34. Atrial flutter Type II. Atrial flutter with a rate of approximately 400 per minute indicates Type II flutter.

FLUTTER
RATE

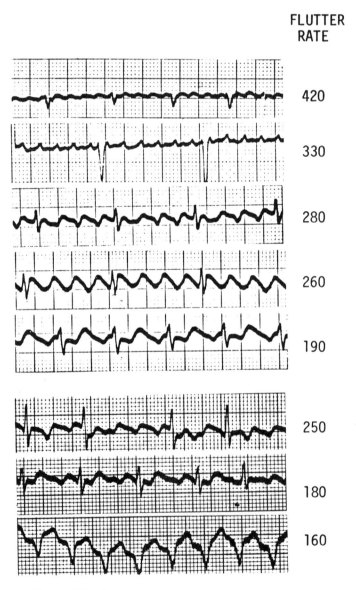

Figure 2-35. Atrial flutter. The flutter rates vary. Although the usual atrial flutter rate is 300 per minute, it may, under the influence of drugs or other interventions, slow to as low as 160 per minute. This collage of atrial flutter illustrates rates varying from 420 per minute in the top tracing to as low as 160 per minute in the bottom tracing.

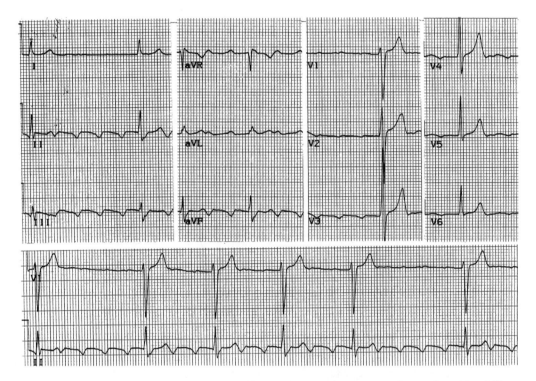

Figure 2-36. Atrial flutter. The flutter rate slowed after administration of quinidine. The A-V ratio varies from 3:1 to as high as 5:1. The flutter is typical, with a sawtooth appearance in leads II, III, and AVF.

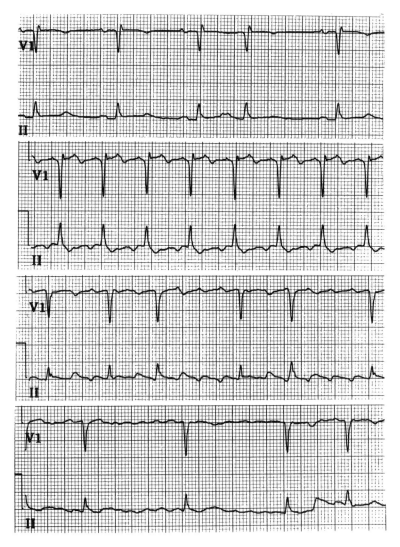

Figure 2-37. Atrial arrhythmias. This spectrum of atrial arrhythmias was recorded in one patient. APCs are noted in the top panel, 2:1 atrial tachycardia in the second panel, flutter in the third panel, and fibrillation in the bottom panel.

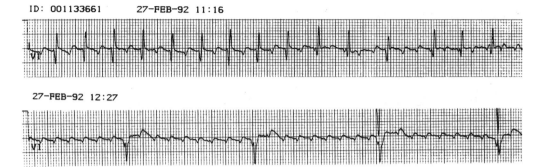

ID: 001133661   27-FEB-92 11:16

27-FEB-92 12:27

Figure 2-38. Atrial flutter. Atrial flutter with 2:1 A-V conduction is recorded in the top tracing and complete A-V block with a regular ventricular rate of 33 per minute is recorded in the bottom tracing.

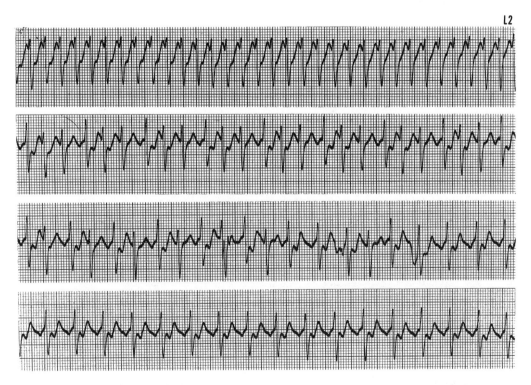

L2

Figure 2-39. Atrial flutter. The A-V conduction ratio is 1:1, 4:3, 3:2, and 2:1 in the top, second, third, and bottom tracings, respectively. The ventricular rate during 1:1 flutter is 300 per minute.

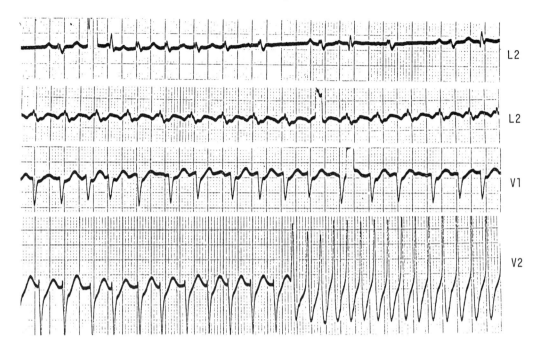

Figure 2-40. APCs, flutter, and fibrillation. Sinus rhythm, APCs, and a short run of atrial tachycardia are recorded in the top row, atrial flutter with 2:1 conduction in the second row, and atrial fibrillation in the third row. In the bottom tracing, atrial fibrillation changes to atrial flutter with 1:1 A-V conduction with a ventricular rate of 300 per minute. All strips were recorded from the same patient.

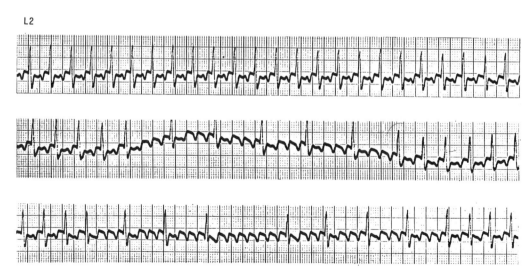

Figure 2-41. Atrial flutter. Atrial flutter with 2:1 A-V conduction was recorded in the top tracing, 2:1 and 4:1 in the middle tracing, and 2:1, 4:1, and 8:1 in the bottom tracing. The increase in A-V block was induced by vagal stimulation.

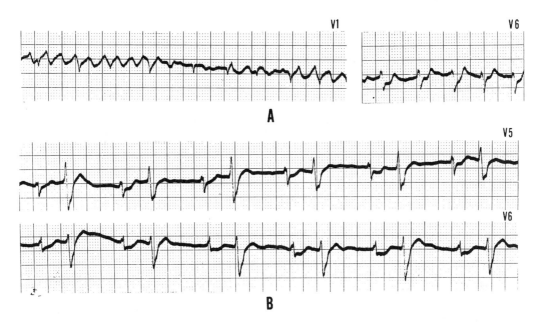

Figure 2-42. A. Coarse atrial fibrillation. B. Junctional rhythm with ventricular bigeminy. The coupling of the VPCs in this panel is fixed while the configuration varies, suggesting unifocal VPCs with a varying direction of exit.

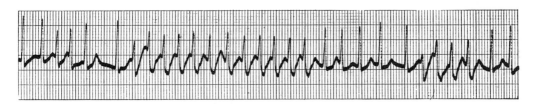

Figure 2-43. Atrial fibrillation with right bundle branch aberration. The onset of aberrant complexes is preceded by a relatively longer R-R interval in keeping with the Ashman phenomenon. The rate of the aberrant complexes is approximately 300 per minute. There is no compensatory pause such as would be expected with ventricular arrhythmias.

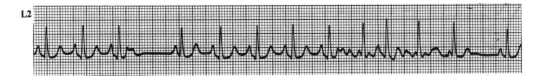

Figure 2-44. Atrial fibrillation. Following the first three sinus P waves, there is a nonconducted APC followed by a junctional escape. The P-R interval is too short to conduct. Half way down the strip, there is an early APC that falls within the vulnerable period of the atrium, initiating atrial fibrillation. The atrial fibrillation is short in duration and a sinus impulse is noted at the end of the strip.

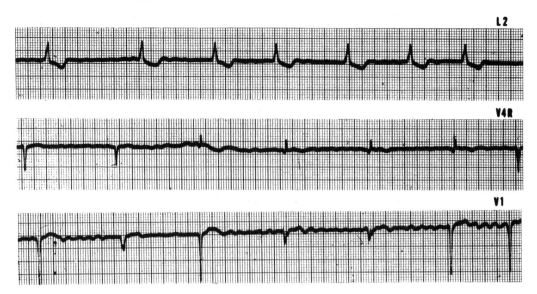

Figure 2-45. Atrial fibrillation with ventricular escape rhythm. Following the second supraventricular QRS complex in lead V_4R, the QRS configuration changes, indicating a ventricular escape rhythm. Since the escape QRS complex is narrow, the escape focus is probably high in the septum or in one of the fascicles. Similar escape complexes are noted in lead V_1.

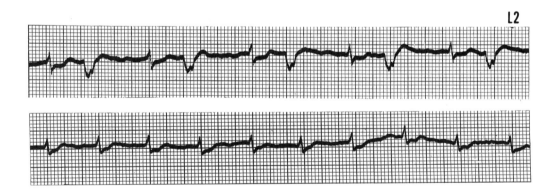

Figure 2-46. Atrial fibrillation with junctional tachycardia. Ventricular bigeminy with a regular junctional R-R of 1200 ms and atrial fibrillation is recorded in the top tracing. In the bottom tracing, the R-R of 600 ms is also regular, indicating a junctional tachycardia (NPJT). In the top tracing, the R-R of the junctional rhythm is exactly twice the length of the R-R in the bottom tracing, indicating a single site of origin of both. The PVCs in the top tracing interfere with the expression of every other junctional impulse, but do not disturb the rhythmicity of the junctional pacemaker.

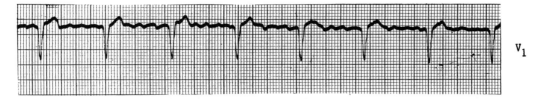

V_1

Figure 2-47. Atrial fibrillation with junctional rhythm. The ventricular rhythm is regular, at a rate of 67 per minute, indicating a junctional tachycardia (NPJT). From Fisch C, McHenry PL, Knoebel SB. Cardiac Arrhythmias. In *Tice's Practice of Medicine*. Philadelphia: Harper and Row; 1970:1–29.

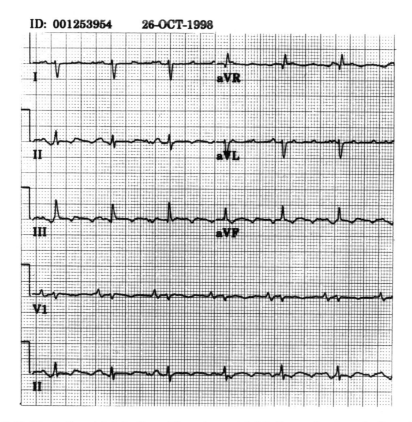

Figure 2-48. Dissimilar atrial rhythms. There is an atrial flutter and a sinus rhythm with a P-P of 800 ms. The flutter and the sinus rhythm are dissociated, with the flutter being that of the recipient atrium and the sinus that of the donor atrium.

ID: 001060408

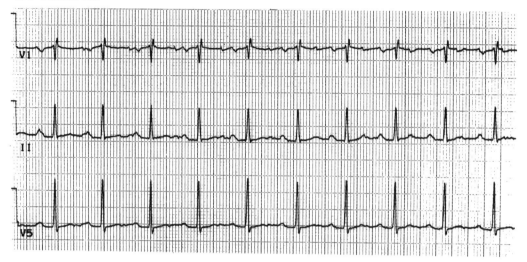

Figure 2-49. Dissimilar atrial rhythms. The findings are similar to those illustrated in Figure 2-48. The sinus P-P measures 600 ms, and the P-P arising from the recipient's atrium measures slightly less than 600 ms. The two different P waves and the interatrial dissociation are best seen in lead V_1.

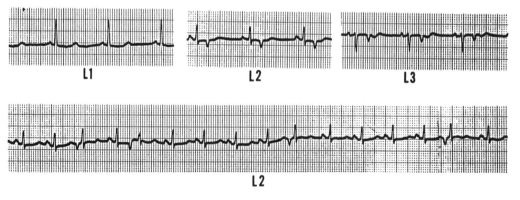

Figure 2-50. Atrial parasystole. Atrial bigeminy is recorded in the top row with deeply inverted P waves in leads II and III, and of low amplitude in lead I. In the bottom row, lead II, the coupling of the ectopic P waves to the preceding sinus wave varies. Failure of the parasystolic P wave to manifest when expected is due to local refractoriness. The fixed interectopic interval, derived from the first two parasystolic waves in the bottom row, is 960 ms.

References

1. Scherf D, Siedeck H. Uber block zwischen beiden vorhofen. *Z Klin Med* 1934;127:77.
2. Cohen J, Scherf D. Complete interatrial and intraatrial (atrial dissociation). *Am Heart J* 1965;70:23.
3. Zipes DP, DeJoseph RL. Dissimilar atrial rhythms in man and dog. *Am J Cardiol* 1973;32:618.

Atrioventricular Junctional Rhythms

It is often difficult or impossible to differentiate between complexes originating in the AV node proper from those originating low in the atrium, in the bundle of His, or in the coronary sinus. Similarly, it is impossible to estimate the effect of differing anterograde and retrograde conduction on the P-QRS complex relationships. For these reasons, it seems appropriate, from the ECG standpoint, to refer to impulses originating at any of these sites as junctional rhythms.

Mechanisms of Junctional Rhythms

Junctional rhythms are due to either enhanced automaticity or reentry. The specialized cells within the junction are capable, under certain conditions, of becoming automatic. The characteristic feature of automaticity is a gradual loss of the diastolic resting potential. When the resting potential is reduced to the level of the TP, a propagated impulse is generated. The rate of the junction, like that of the SAN, is governed by the slope of diastolic depolarization. The steeper the slope, the faster the rate (see Automaticity).

Requirements for reentry include: 1) functional longitudinal dissociation of conduction in the junction; 2) dissociation limited to the upper region; 3) dissociation that extends to the atrial margin of the AV node (some believe that reentry cannot occur without activation of an atrial bridge); and 4) a refractory period of the "final common pathway" that governs the return "trip." The dissociation may be due to: 1) pathological lesions strategically located in the junctional tissue; 2) anatomically separate pathways; or 3) variation in the duration of refractoriness of the different pathways.

Electrocardiography of Junctional Rhythms

Classically, a junctional impulse exciting both the atria and ventricles is recognized by: 1) a normal QRS complex originating above the bifurcation of the bundle of His, in the absence of bundle branch block (BBB) or aberration; 2) a negative P wave in leads II, III, AVF, low or isoelectric in lead I, and upright in AVR. The general direction of atrial activation is cephalad, forward and to the left, resulting in a mean P wave axis varying from -30 to -70. The P wave may precede, appear simultaneously with, or follow the QRS complex. If the atria and ventricles are activated simultaneously, the P wave is not recognizable, being superimposed on the QRS complex. In the absence of A-V conduction disturbances, the P-R and R-P intervals average approximately 0.12 and 0.19 seconds, respectively (Figures 3-1 and 3-2). The junctional impulse may fail to conduct to the ventricle, inscribing an isolated negative P wave (Figure 3-3).

Classification of Junctional Rhythms

Junctional rhythms are usually classified as: 1) passive, reflecting physiological function of the junctional tissues; and 2) active or accelerated rhythms most often reflecting an abnormal state of the junctional tissue.

The inherent pacemaker activity of the junction is normally held in abeyance by a more rapidly discharging "higher" focus. Failure of such an impulse, whether due to sinus bradycardia, SA suppression, or block, allows the inherent automaticity of the junction to become manifest. A junctional focus may escape for a single beat (junctional escape) or for a number of cycles (junctional escape rhythm) (Figures 3-4 and 3-5). The escape rhythm is regular, rarely irregular, the latter simulating sinus arrhythmia (Figure 3-6).

The inherent, physiological rate of a junctional pacemaker varies from 40 to 50 per minute and may be as low as 30 per minute; however, it is rarely higher than 60 per minute (Figures 3-4, 3-5, and 3-7). Allowing for a "gray zone" between 60 and 70, any rate above 70 per minute should be considered, based on electrophysiological properties of the junction, as an accelerated junctional rhythm or junctional tachycardia (Figure 3-8).

Passive Rhythms

Junctional Escape

As noted above, failure of the dominant pacemaker is followed by a pause terminated by an escape of a subsidiary pacemaker, most often junctional. In the absence of an intraventricular conduction defect, the escape QRS complex is normal.

There are two types of junctional escapes: passive and accelerated. The former is a physiological response to failure of a dominant pacemaker. Its rate is 40 to 60 per minute with a cycle longer than 1.0 second (Figures 3-4, 3-5, and 3-7). An accelerated escape is a pathological phenomenon, and the rate of the escape is greater than 60 per minute with a cycle length shorter than 1 second (Figure 3-9).

The escape may be manifest by a single complex followed by resumption of control by the dominant pacemaker, or the escape may be followed by a series of regularly spaced junctional complexes referred to as junctional escape rhythm (Figures 3-10 and 3-11). The escape QRS complex is usually normal or slightly aberrant. The junctional focus may control the atria and a negative P wave in leads II, III, and AVF may precede, be superimposed on, or follow the QRS complex (Figure 3-1). Should the atria remain under the control of a pacemaker other than the junctional, AV dissociation is present (Figure 3-12).

An interesting form of junctional escape, known as escape-capture bigeminy, is present when the sinus rhythm is slower than the escape interval. The junctional focus may escape because of sinus bradycardia, SA block, or A-V block above the site of the junctional escape. The ECG feature of escape-capture bigeminy is one of repetitive junctional escape followed by an atrial capture (Figures 3-13 and 3-14).

Active Rhythms

Junctional Premature Systoles

A junctional premature systole is recognized by early appearance and a negative P wave in leads II, III, and AVF either preceding or following a normal or aberrant QRS complex. Most often a junctional P wave precedes the QRS complex. At times, the P wave is superimposed on the QRS complex and, thus, is not recognizable (Figure 3-1). On occasion, the premature impulse may be blocked during its retrograde conduction, and a QRS complex without a P wave is recorded. Similarly, the ectopic impulse may fail in its transmission to the ventricles, and a retrograde P without a QRS complex is recorded (Figures 3-3 and 3-15). In rare instances, the impulse may be blocked in both directions, and the junctional discharge is recognized only because of its effect on the subsequent impulse (see Concealed Conduction, Chapter 6). It may be difficult, if not impossible, to differentiate a junctional premature impulse from a low atrial P wave. Similarly, when the P wave follows the QRS complex, it may be difficult, if not impossible, to differentiate it from a septal VPC with normal or nearly normal QRS complex and retrograde conduction to the atria. Admittedly, this combination is extremely rare.

Junctional Parasystole

Junctional parasystole is identified by varying coupling of junctional complexes to the dominant impulse, a common interectopic interval, and fusion complexes. The rate nearly always exceeds 40 per minute, with an average rate of 60 per minute. In the rare case of junctional parasystole with negative P waves preceding the QRS complex, the junctional parasystole cannot be differentiated with certainty from an atrial parasystole. Similarly, ventricular parasystole originating in the septum and, thus, inscribing a narrow QRS complex cannot be differentiated from junctional parasystole (Figure 3-16) (see Chapter 11).

Atrioventricular Nodal Reentrant Tachycardia

AV nodal reentrant tachycardia (AVNRT) is the most common mechanism of paroxysmal SVT (PSVT) and accounts for approximately 60% of PSVTs without a recognizable mechanism.

In AVNRT, the resting ECG is normal in the absence of BBB or aberration. Rarely, two different P-R intervals are recorded, indicating dual A-V conduction or functional longitudinal dissociation within the junctional tissue (see Chapter 17). The onset of AVNRT is usually abrupt following an APC with a prolonged P-R interval. The onset is predicated on longitudinal dissociation within the junction, with the "anterograde slow" pathway refractory period being shorter than the refractory period of the "retrograde fast" pathway. The rate is usually 150 to 240 per minute and rarely is as high as 250 per minute. Termination of the AVNRT also is abrupt. Often the atria and the ventricles are activated simultaneously and a distinct P wave is not present. If present, the P wave is negative in leads II, III, and AVF (Figures 3-17 and 3-18). As a rule, the P wave appears close to the QRS complex, within an R-P interval of 60 ms or less, often inscribing a pseudo S wave in the limb leads and a pseudo r' in lead V_1 (Figures 3-19 and 3-20). These changes are characteristic of the typical form of AVNRT, that is, one with fast retrograde and slow anterograde conduction.

In the presence of retrograde P waves, an R-P interval shorter than the P-R interval is consistent with AVNRT or AV reentrant tachycardia (AVRT) with Wolff-Parkinson-White (WPW) (Figure 3-21), or a junctional or low atrial tachycardia with a prolonged P-R interval (Figure 3-22). In AVNRT, the retrograde P may be superimposed on the QRS complex, be recorded as the terminal part of the QRS complex, or it may appear shortly after the QRS complex (Figures 3-23 and 3-24). The mean ventricular to high right atrium (V-HRA) interval is 59 ± 42.12 ms for AVNRT as compared with the V-HRA interval of 172 ± 36 ms in WPW and 157 ± 37.7 ms in the presence of a concealed accessory pathway. A V-HRA interval shorter than 90 ms excludes WPW or concealed accessory pathway.

An R-P interval longer than the P-R interval is consistent with: 1) an unusual form of AVNRT with a rapidly conducting anterograde limb and slowly conducting retrograde limb; 2) a rare form of incessant reciprocating tachycardia; 3) a junctional or low atrial tachycardia; 4) AVRT utilizing an accessory pathway (Figure 3-21); and 5) sinus node reentry.

In approximately 10% of AVNRT cases, the findings are atypical in that the retrograde conduction is slow and anterograde conduction fast, resulting in a prolonged R-P interval that reflects the slow retrograde conduction (Figure 3-25). The differential diagnosis from other arrhythmias with a long R-P interval may be difficult. These include, among others, ectopic (paroxysmal) atrial tachycardia, sinus node reentry, permanent junctional reciprocating tachycardia, automatic junctional tachycardia, and NPJT.

Atrioventricular Reentrant Tachycardia

AVRT is a reentrant arrhythmia in which the circus movement involves the AV junction and an accessory pathway. In the vast majority of AVRT cases, the antegrade conduction is along the AV junction and retrograde conduction via the accessory pathway. In a very small number of cases, the anterograde conduction is along the accessory pathway and retrograde along the junction.

With anterograde conduction via the AV junction and retrograde along the accessory pathway, the QRS complex, in the absence of aberration or preexisting BBB, is normal. The P wave is separated from the QRS complex by an average R-P interval of 80 to 120 ms; it is, however, never shorter than 70 ms. The R-P to P-R ratio is less than 1.0 (Figure 3-26).

In the presence of preexisting BBB or aberration, the QRS complex is usually that of RBBB (Figure 3-27).

In the presence of anterograde conduction along the accessory pathway and retrograde via the AV junction, the QRS complex is bizarre and there are no discernible P waves (Figures 3-28 and 3-29).

In the 20% of AVRT cases in which the accessory pathway conducts retrogradely only, the QRS complex is normal and an accessory pathway (WPW) pattern is not recorded. The presence of a concealed accessory pathway is suspected because of the rapid heart rate, with rates often reaching or exceeding 250 per minute (See Figure 2-23).

In some instances, in the course of AVNRT, the P wave is not recorded. This suggests that the atrium is not always a necessary component of the reentrant loop (Figure 3-30).

Automatic Junctional Tachycardia

Automatic junctional tachycardia is very rare (Figures 3-31 and 3-32). Its rate varies from 120 to 200 per minute and it is difficult if not impossible to differentiate from other forms of junctional rhythms with retrograde P waves. The automatic nature of the tachycardia becomes clear in the presence of AV dissociation.

Atrioventricular Junctional Tachycardia (Nonparoxysmal Junctional Tachycardia)

NPJT is characterized by a moderate acceleration of the heart rate, the ventricular rate varying from 70 to 130 per minute. Occasionally, the atria are under the control of the junctional pacemaker, with retrograde P waves recorded in II, III, and AVF. More often, however, the atria exhibit an independent rhythm such as SA rhythm or atrial tachycardia, flutter, or fibrillation (Figure 3-33). If the atria are controlled by the SAN and the ventricles by the junction both with an almost similar rate, with variation of the sinus rate due to sinus arrhythmia there may be a gradual shift of the control of the ventricle from the SAN to the junction. In fact, this gradual emergence and disappearance is one of the characteristic features of NPJT. In NPJT with retrograde activation of the atria, the gradual shift of control from junction to the SAN or SAN to the junction may result in various degrees of atrial fusion. Such a gradual emergence of the NPJT without an accurate coupling to the sinus P wave suggests enhanced automaticity rather than reentry as the mechanism.

In the presence of ectopic atrial tachycardia or flutter, NPJT is diagnosed by a normal QRS complex with a regular rhythm and a lack of temporal relationship to the atrial waves. Similarly, in the presence of atrial fibrillation, a regular ventricular rhythm with a rate within the range of NPJT suggests this diagnosis (Figures 3-34, 3-35, and 3-36).

NPJT with a 1:1 exit from the ectopic focus with a regular and rapid ventricular rate and a normal QRS complex poses few diagnostic problems (Figures 3-35 and 3-36). However, in the presence of an exit block with varying R-R intervals, the diagnosis may be difficult (Figure 3-37) (see Chapter 15).

An NPJT with aberrant intraventricular conduction may be difficult to differentiate from VT.

Reentry (Reciprocation) (Figure 3-38)

Assuming that there is no preexisting BBB or aberration, an impulse originating in the AV node conducts to the ventricles, inscribing a normal QRS complex. It then conducts retrogradely (reenters) to the atria, inscribing a negative P wave in leads II, III, and AVF and, in turn, reenters the ventricle, inscribing a second, normal QRS complex. The reentry time does not vary more than 60 ms in any given tracing. Junctional reentry was once described as an inverted P wave "sandwiched" between two normal QRS complexes (Figures 3-39, 3-40, and 3-41).

Reentry may also originate in the atrium or the ventricle. In the case of the former, the ECG inscribes a normal upright P wave followed by a QRS complex, a reentrant negative P wave, and, in turn, ventricular reentry (Figure 3-42).

Reentry originating in the ventricle is manifest by an abnormal QRS complex followed by a negative P wave and a reentrant normal QRS complex (Figures 3-43 and 3-44).

Supraventricular Tachycardia, Not Otherwise Identified

This diagnosis is appropriate for narrow QRS tachycardia when the mechanism of the tachycardia is unclear. It has been suggested that approximately 20% of narrow QRS tachycardias may be incorrectly classified on the basis of the ECG alone (Figure 3-45).

See Table 3-1 for a guide to the diagnosis of SVTs.

Table 3-1

Supraventricular Tachycardias

With a Normal QRS
Sinus Tachycardia
SANRT (SA nodal reentrant tachycardia)
Atrial Flutter 2:1, 1:1 A-V Conduction
Atrial Flutter With Varying A-V Block
Atrial Fibrillation
Multifocal Atrial Tachycardia
Nonparoxysmal Junctional Tachycardia (NPJT)
Retrograde P Wave With an RP < PR
AVNRT (AV nodal reentrant tachycardia)—typical
AVRT (atrioventricular reentrant tachycardia, WPW)
Ectopic Atrial Tachycardia With 1° Block
With an RP > PR
AVNRT (AV nodal reentrant tachycardia)—atypical
Ectopic Atrial Tachycardia
Permanent AVNRT
Junctional Tachycardia (automatic?)

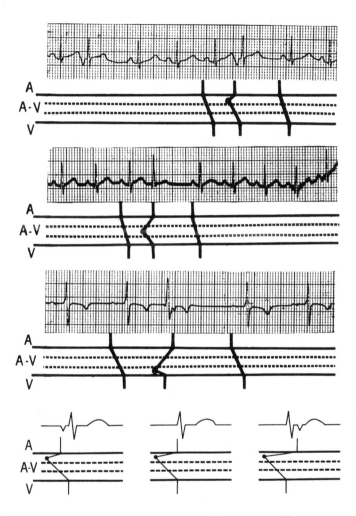

Figure 3-1. JPCs with site of origin in the AV node. The top row illustrates an upper nodal pacemaker with the P wave preceding the QRS complex. The middle row shows a middle nodal pacemaker with the P wave superimposed in the QRS complex. The third row illustrates a lower nodal pacemaker with the P wave falling after the QRS complex. The concept of upper, middle, lower site of origin is no longer tenable since it does not consider the conduction time within the AV node. As shown in the bottom diagram, an upper nodal pacemaker may inscribe the P wave preceding, superimposed on, or following the QRS complex, respectively, depending on conduction time. From Zipes DP, Fisch C. Premature A-V junctional contractions. *Arch Intern Med* 1971;128:633–635.

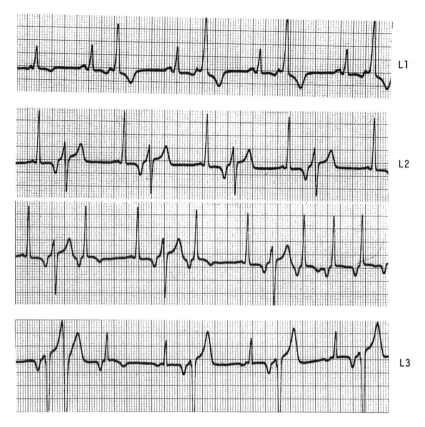

Figure 3-2. Junctional premature complexes. The P waves are negative in L2 and L3 and are of low amplitude in lead I. The JPCs conduct with left anterior fascicular block. A short run of junctional tachycardia is recorded in the third row. Left anterior fascicular block follows only the longer preceding cycles in keeping with the Ashman phenomenon (see Chapter 7).

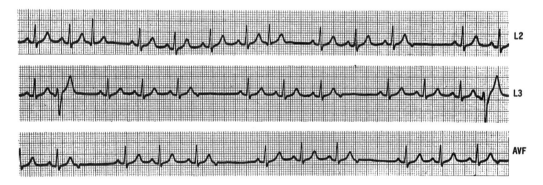

Figure 3-3. Conducted and blocked JPCs. The P waves are inverted in L2, L3, and AVF. The P waves conduct with a P-R interval of less than 100 ms and with left anterior fascicular block. A number of the JPCs are nonconducted. Fortuitously, the sum of the coupling and compensatory pause equals two sinus cycles and, thus, is fully compensatory, a feature usually associated with VPCs.

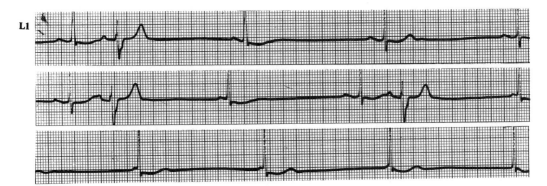

Figure 3-4. APCs with junctional escape and junctional escape rhythm. In the top row, the first APC is followed by a P-R interval that is too short to conduct; thus, the QRS complex is a junctional escape. The next two impulses are sinus in origin. In the second row, the first APC is followed by a junctional escape, sinus impulse, an APC, and again by a junctional escape. The bottom row illustrates a junctional escape rhythm at a rate of 30 per minute. The P waves maintain a close relationship with the QRS complex, indicating AV dissociation with synchronization. The APCs conduct with RBBB.

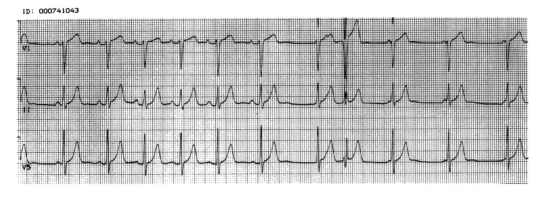

Figure 3-5. Junctional escape rhythm. The sinus rhythm at a rate of 88 per minute is followed by a junctional escape rhythm at a rate of approximately 62 per minute. A sinus capture (complex number 7) follows the first junctional escape. The P wave and the QRS complex maintain a close relationship indicative of synchronization.

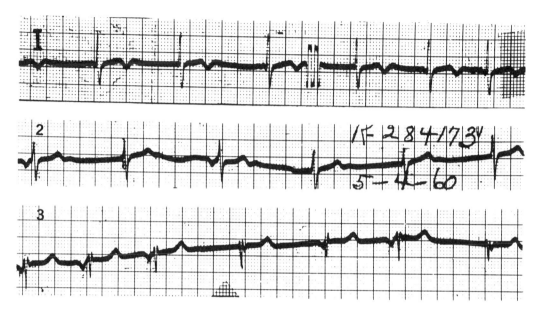

Figure 3-6. Junctional rhythm with "respiratory variation." The P wave is isoelectric in lead I, inverted in II, III, and AVF with a P-R interval of approximately 120 ms. The rate varies from 100 to as low as 80 per minute. This unusual record resembles sinus arrhythmia. As a rule, however, junctional rhythms are regular.

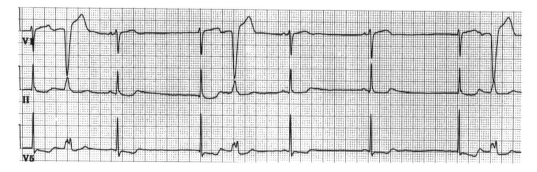

Figure 3-7. APCs with LBBB, entrance block, and junctional escape. The compensatory pause following the APC is considerably shorter than the basic P to P interval, indicating failure of the premature complex to disrupt the sinus rhythmicity, an example of entrance block. The junctional escape cycle is approximately 1600 ms.

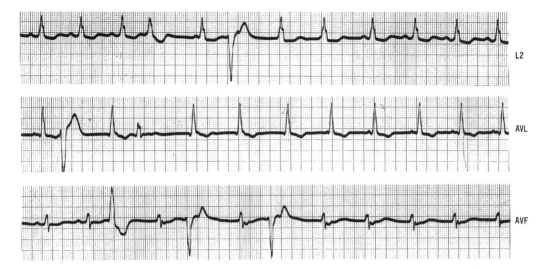

Figure 3-8. Junctional escape rhythm. In L2 the three sinus impulses are followed by a VPC with the compensatory pause terminated by a junctional escape. The second VPC, with retrograde conduction suppressing the sinus node, is followed by three consecutive accelerated junctional escapes at an R-R interval of 800 ms. Sinus rhythm resumes at the end of the record. In AVL the first VPC is followed by a junctional escape. The next VPC is followed by a junctional escape tachycardia, probably NPJT, at an R-R interval of 800 ms. In AVF the compensatory pause following the VPC is 900 ms. The VPCs with retrograde P waves suppress the sinus node, allowing for an accelerated junctional escape tachycardia.

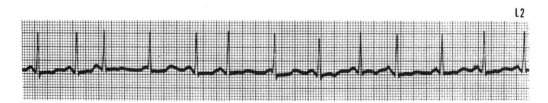

Figure 3-9. Accelerated junctional escape. The APCs suppress the sinus node with a return cycle longer than the sinus P to P interval. This longer return cycle allows for an accelerated junctional escape (QRS 4, 7, 11).

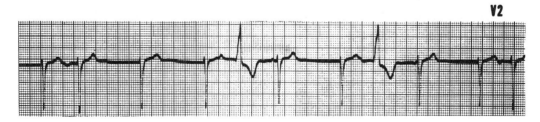

Figure 3-10. Junctional rhythm with sinus captures. The regular junctional rhythm at an R-R of 1140 ms is interrupted by supraventricular impulses conducting with either a normal QRS complex or RBBB aberration.

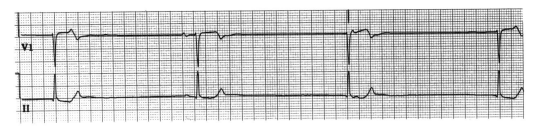

Figure 3-11. Junctional rhythm. The junctional rhythm is regular, with an R-R interval of 2560 ms. There are four irregularly spaced P waves, none of which conduct to the ventricle. It is unlikely that the second P wave conducts since it does not alter the R-R interval.

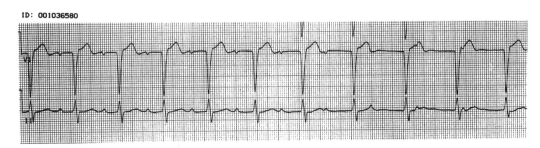

Figure 3-12. Wenckebach Type I A-V conduction followed by junctional rhythm. The basic rhythm is sinus with a P-P of 880 ms. The P-R interval prolongs gradually from 240 to 320 ms, at which point a junctional rhythm at an R-R of 1000 ms assumes control of the heart. The atrial and ventricular rhythms are dissociated with the P waves falling within the absolute refractory period of the AV node. The result is AV dissociation with synchronization, i.e., the QRS complex and P waves maintain a close 1:1 relationship.

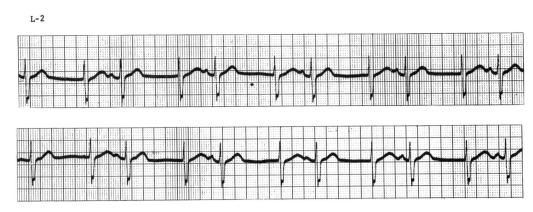

Figure 3-13. Escape-capture bigeminy. The sinus bradycardia at an R-R of 1560 ms allows for junctional escape at an interval of 1000 ms. The repetitive escape-capture results in a bigeminal rhythm. From Fisch C, Knoebel SB. Junctional rhythms. *Prog Cardiovasc Dis* 1970;13:141–158.

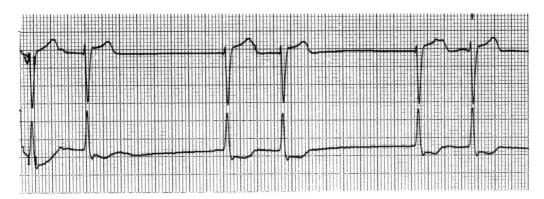

Figure 3-14. Escape-capture bigeminy. The sinus bradycardia with a P-P of 1880 ms and the shorter junctional cycle of 1640 ms results in a repetitive junctional escape. The repetitive escape-capture results in a bigeminal rhythm.

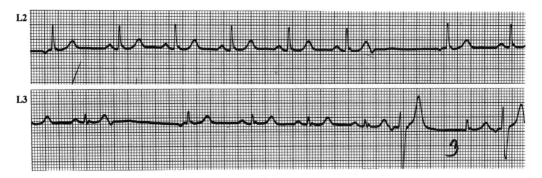

Figure 3-15. JPCs, sinus node suppression, and junctional escapes. JPCs with inverted P waves in leads L2 and L3 and a short 120-ms P-R interval suppress the sinus node as evidenced by a prolonged compensatory pause terminated by a junctional escape. The two conducted JPCs in L3 conduct with aberration, probably RBBB and left anterior fascicular block.

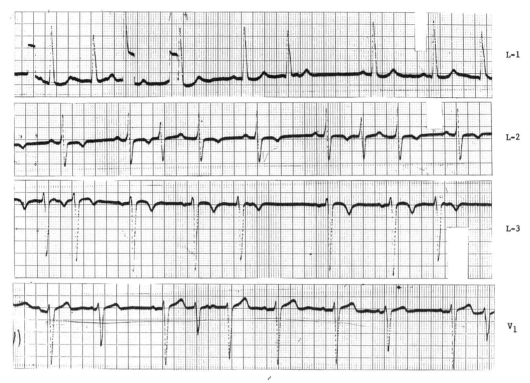

Figure 3-16. Junctional parasystole. The features of parasystole include variable coupling of the parasystolic QRS complex to the preceding sinus QRS complex, a fixed interectopic interval of 1820 ms, and fusion, as illustrated by the second and eighth complexes in lead V_1. Failure of the parasystolic impulse to manifest when expected is due to refractoriness of the tissue, and is illustrated by the expected third parasystolic complex in lead V_1. From Fisch C, Knoebel SB. Junctional rhythms. *Prog Cardiovasc Dis* 1970;13:141–158.

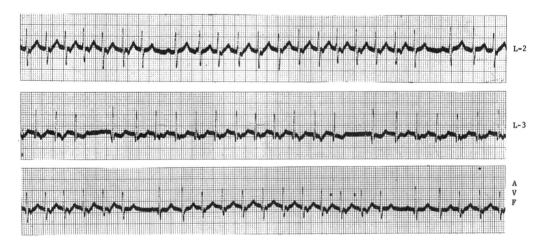

Figure 3-17. Reentrant AVNRT. AVNRT is suggested by the retrograde P waves superimposed on, or very close to, the QRS complex. As the tachycardia progresses, the R-P interval gradually lengthens, in a Wenckebach mode, with ultimate failure of retrograde conduction. Each episode of tachycardia is initiated by a premature atrial complex but without the usual feature of AVNRT of a prolonged P-R interval.

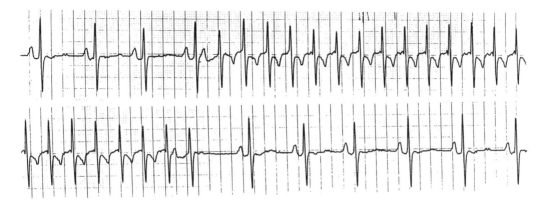

Figure 3-18. AVNRT with delayed retrograde conduction (atypical AVNRT). The sinus rhythm at a rate of 75 per minute is followed by an APC with a prolonged P-R interval and an AVNRT with a prolonged R-P interval. The latter suggests atypical AVNRT. The reentrant tachycardia is terminated by an APC.

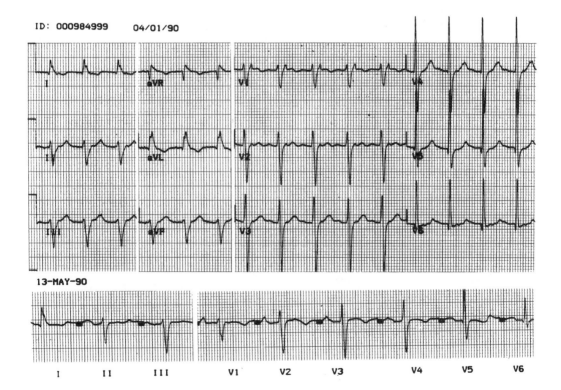

Figure 3-19. AV nodal reentrant tachycardia. The rate is 125 per minute. A retrograde P wave is recorded at the end of the QRS complex clearly visible in lead V_1 where it simulates an r'. The r' is not present during normal sinus rhythm (bottom panel). The QRS configuration is that of an intraventricular conduction defects and left anterior fascicular block.

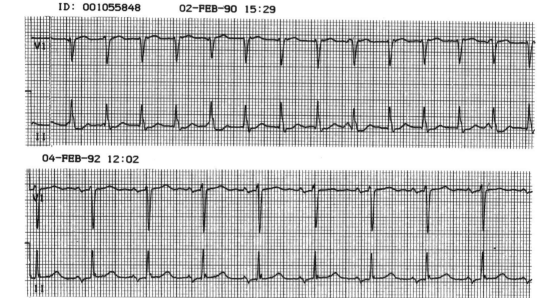

Figure 3-20. AV nodal reentrant tachycardia. The reference tracing (bottom panel) depicts sinus rhythm at a rate of 79 per minute, a P-R interval of 180 ms, and a normal QRS complex. The top panel illustrates AVNRT with a rate of 136 per minute and a sinus bradycardia at a rate of 30 per minute. The diagnosis of AVNRT is supported by retrograde P waves recorded at the end of the QRS complex in lead II and an r' in lead V_1. Their absence during sinus rhythm proves that these are retrograde P waves. The sinus P waves do not disturb the rhythmicity of the nodal rhythm, supporting an intranodal reentry. The occasional failure of retrograde conduction to engage the atrium, and without any change in the nodal rhythm, suggests that the P wave is not always a necessary link for AVNRT.

ID: 001110819

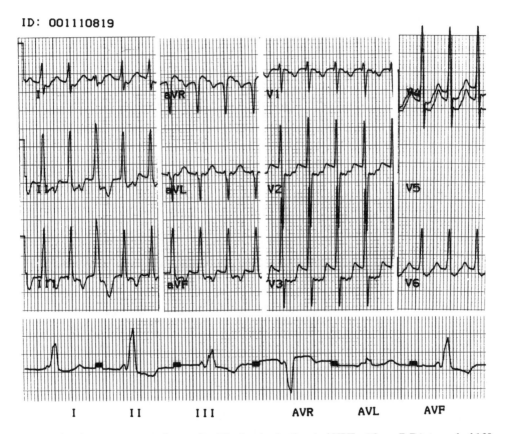

Figure 3-21. AV reentrant tachycardia. The basic rhythm is AVRT with an R-P interval of 160 ms and nonspecific ST-T changes. The bottom tracing reveals a normal sinus rhythm with a WPW pattern, supporting the diagnosis of AVRT in the top panel.

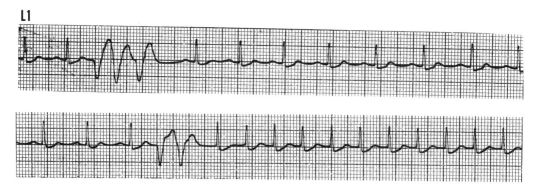

Figure 3-22. AV nodal reentrant tachycardia. In the top tracing, the basic rhythm is sinus, interrupted by three consecutive VPCs. In the bottom tracing, the ventricular couplet with V-A conduction and prolonged P-R interval initiates an AVNRT. The retrograde P wave may be superimposed on the QRS complex.

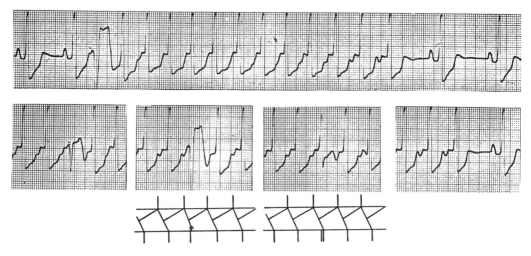

Figure 3-23. Reentrant tachycardia with retrograde, ventriculoatrial, Wenckebach conduction. The basic rhythm is sinus, with an R-R interval of 880 ms and a P-R interval of 160 ms. In the top tracing, an interpolated VPC prolongs the P-R interval to approximately 260 ms and initiates a reentrant tachycardia, with the QRS complex followed by a retrograde P wave and with a gradual prolongation of the R-P interval from 260 to 360 ms. The gradual delay of retrograde conduction, with ultimate failure of the retrograde impulse to reach the atrium or the final common pathway in the AV node, terminates the tachycardia. This is a rare form of AV nodal reentry in that the retrograde pathway conducts slowly and the anterograde conducts rapidly. The R-P interval is longer than the P-R interval. The bottom tracings illustrate ventricular fusion complexes between VPC and the supraventricular complexes. The fusions do not disturb the rhythmicity of the tachycardia, indicating that the VPCs do not reach the site of the reentrant rhythm. This arrhythmia may also be an example of an "incessant" reciprocating tachycardia, with AV nodal-like properties. From Fisch C, Knoebel SB. Junctional rhythms. *Prog Cardiovasc Dis* 1970;13:141–158.

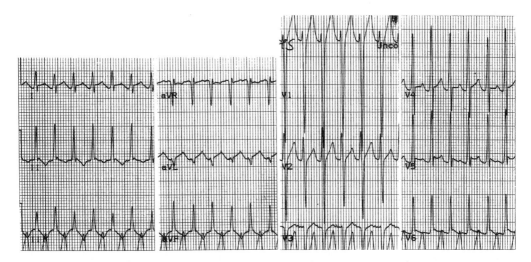

Figure 3-24. SVT, either AVNRT or AVRT. The basic rhythm is an SVT with an R-R of 280 ms. There are no visible P waves. Alternans of the QRS complex and nonspecific ST-T changes are present. It is difficult to differentiate between AVNRT and AVRT, although the alternans of the QRS complex and ST-T suggests an AVRT.

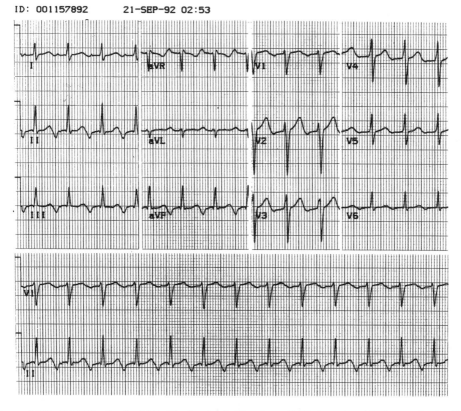

Figure 3-25. AVNRT, atypical (?). The basic rhythm is an SVT at a rate of 125 per minute. The P waves are inverted in II, III, AVF, V_4, V_5, and V_6, with a prolonged RP. Although this arrhythmia suggests an atypical AVNRT, it must be differentiated from ectopic atrial tachycardia, a permanent form of AVNRT and, on occasion, automatic junctional tachycardia.

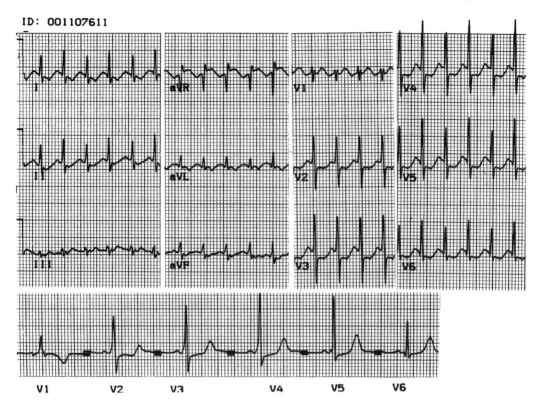

Figure 3-26. AV reentrant tachycardia. The rate of the AVRT is 214 per minute with a retrograde P wave, an R-P interval of approximately 140 ms, and alternans of the QRS complex. WPW with sinus rhythm is recorded in the bottom tracing.

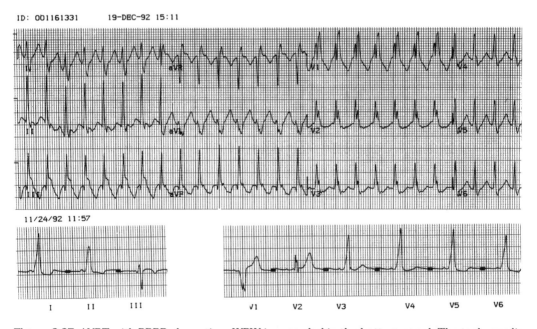

Figure 3-27. AVRT with RBBB aberration. WPW is recorded in the bottom panel. The tachycardia at a rate of 167 per minute is followed by an inverted P wave with an R-P interval of approximately 160 ms, best seen in lead II. The conduction is retrograde along the accessory pathway and anterograde via the AV node (orthodromic). The RBBB reflects acceleration-dependent aberration.

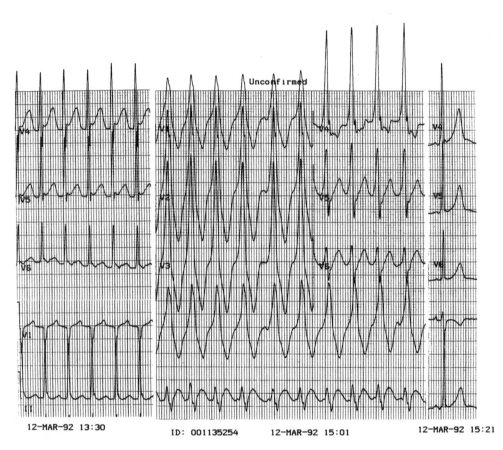

Figure 3-28. WPW with AVRT. AVRT with negative P waves is seen best in lead V_6 of the left panel. The R-P interval is approximately 140 ms. The reentry proceeds retrogradely along the bypass and anterogradely though the AV node (orthodromic). In the middle panel, the conduction is antidromic, with anterograde conduction along the accessory pathway at a rate of approximately 150 per minute. The wide QRS complexes suggest that the entire ventricle is activated via the bypass. WPW is recorded in the right panel.

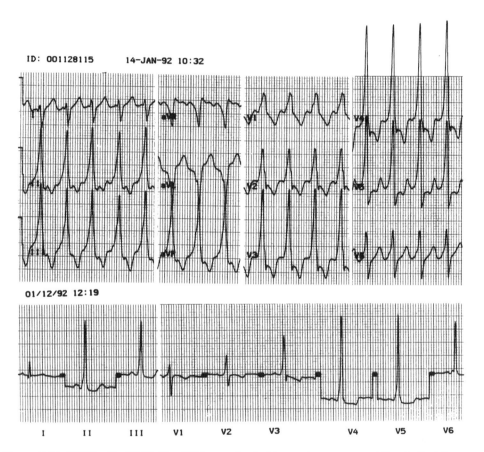

Figure 3-29. WPW with AVRT. The QRS complex is bizarre because most if not all of the ventricle is activated via the accessory pathway (antidromic). WPW is recorded in the bottom panel.

IUMC-1905

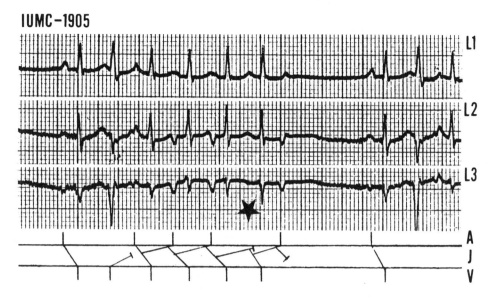

Figure 3-30. Atypical, concealed AVNRT. The three leads were recorded simultaneously. The first P wave, sinus in origin, is followed by an interpolated JPC with aberration. The next, prolonged P-R interval is followed by AVNRT. The delayed retrograde conduction suggests an atypical AVNRT. Despite the fact that the atrium is not activated (*) following the fifth QRS complex, the R-R interval remains constant. Failure to engage the atrium suggests that the atrium is not always a component of the reentrant pathway.

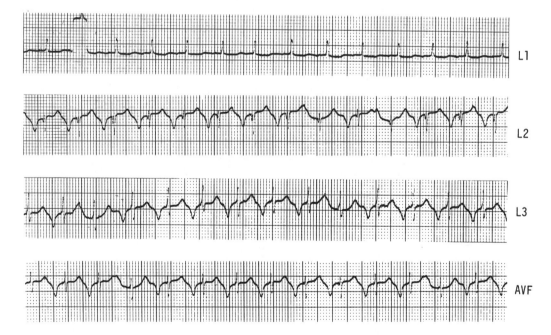

Figure 3-31. AVNRT, atypical (?). The ventricular rate is 136 per minute. The P waves are inverted in L2, L3, and AVF, and are isoelectric in L1. There is an occasional supraventricular P wave that blocks retrograde conduction but does not disturb the rhythmicity. The most likely explanation is intranodal reentry with failure to reach the atrium because of a refractoriness induced by the immediately preceding supraventricular P wave. This is an example of concealed intranodal reentry which favors an AVNRT rather than other tachycardias with prolonged R-P interval.

L2

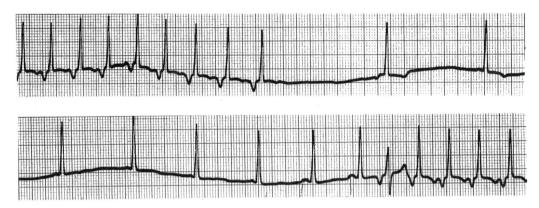

Figure 3-32. Junctional tachycardia. The tachycardia with a rate of 136 per minute, inverted P waves, and a P-R interval of 120 ms indicates a junctional tachycardia. The tachycardia is terminated with carotid pressure. The sinus rhythm accelerates gradually with recurrence of the tachycardia. The first QRS complex of the tachycardia is aberrant, consistent with the Ashman phenomenon. This tracing may be an example of an automatic AV nodal tachycardia.

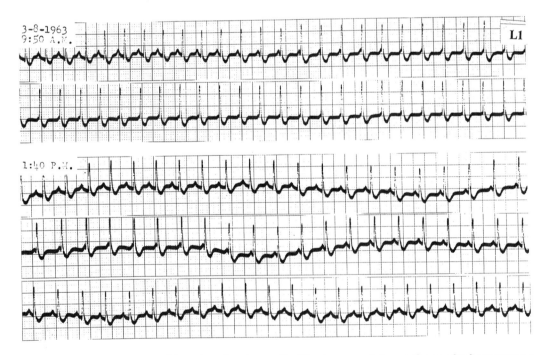

Figure 3-33. Nonparoxysmal junctional tachycardia. The top panel shows the gradual emergence of a junctional tachycardia at a rate of 165 per minute. The bottom panel illustrates a gradual emergence of the sinus rhythm and disappearance of the NPJT. The gradual interchange between the sinus and junctional tachycardia is characteristic of an automatic arrhythmia.

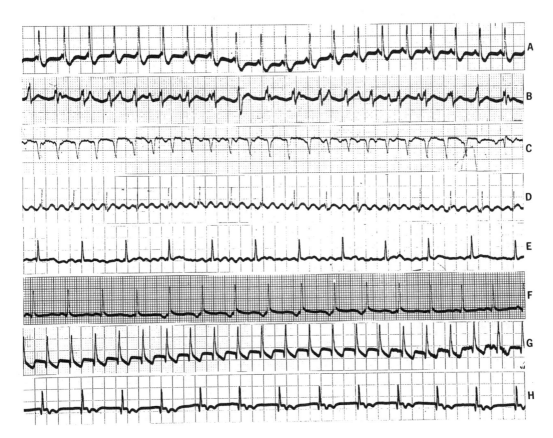

Figure 3-34. Nonparoxysmal junctional tachycardia. A. Sinus tachycardia with AV dissociation with P-QRS synchronization. B. NPJT with AV dissociation and sinus tachycardia. C. NPJT with AV dissociation and atrial tachycardia. D. NPJT and atrial flutter. E. NPJT and atrial fibrillation. F. NPJT with retrograde P waves with the third and probably the fourth, 12th, 13th, and 14th P waves being fusions. G. NPJT with no evidence of atrial activity. H. NPJT with retrograde conduction manifest by inverted P waves following the QRS complex. From Fisch C, Knoebel SB. Junctional rhythms. *Prog Cardiovasc Dis* 1970;13:141–158.

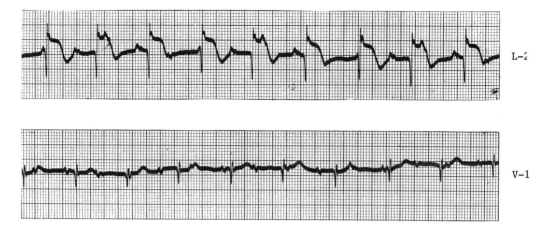

Figure 3-35. NPJT with atrial tachycardia and AV dissociation. There is an NPJT at a rate of 83 per minute with an atrial tachycardia at a rate of 125 per minute with AV dissociation. The AV dissociation is maintained by the more rapid junctional rate and probably by attempted anterograde conduction of the P wave. The combination of the two results in AV dissociation. At appropriate P-R intervals, some of the P waves should conduct to the ventricle. Failure to do so suggests that both the depressed A-V conduction and NPJT contribute to the A-V dissociation.

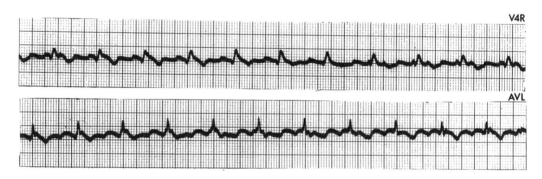

Figure 3-36. Nonparoxysmal junctional tachycardia. The flutter and the junctional rates are 250 and 85 per minute, respectively.

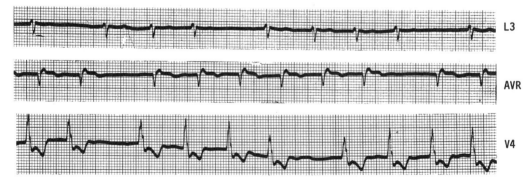

Figure 3-37. NPJT with Wenckebach Type I exit block. A group beating with the R-R shortening gradually and with the long pause less than the sum of the two preceding cycles is recorded. This is a typical Wenckebach structure. There is an intraventricular conduction defect and nonspecific ST-T changes.

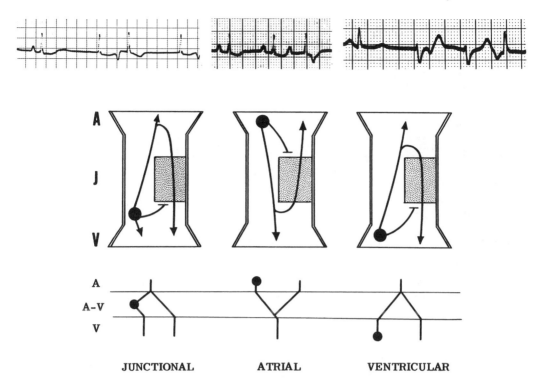

Figure 3-38. Reentry (reciprocation). The top left panel shows a junctional reentry manifest by a normal QRS complex, an inverted P wave, and a normal QRS complex. This is also illustrated in the middle and bottom panels. The middle tracing of the top panel represents atrial reentry manifest by an APC with a prolonged P-R interval, normal QRS complex, and a retrograde negative P wave. The diagrams in the middle and bottom panels illustrate the atrial reentry. The top right panel shows a ventricular reentry. The reentry is manifest by a ventricular ectopic impulse followed by a retrograde P wave with gradual prolongation of the R-P interval and a normal QRS complex. The middle and bottom panels illustrate the ventricular reentry.

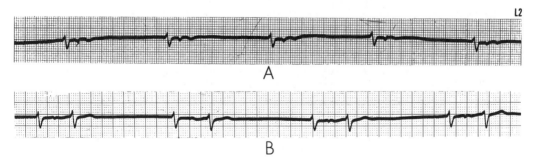

Figure 3-39. Junctional reentry. A. Junctional rhythm at a rate of 33 per minute with retrograde, negative P waves. The R-P interval is 240 ms. B. The junctional QRS complexes are followed by retrograde P waves and a normal QRS complex. This is the original description of nodal reentry, namely two normal QRS complexes with an inverted P wave "sandwiched" in between.

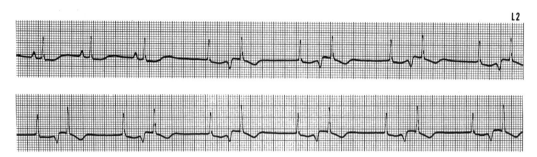

Figure 3-40. AV nodal reentry. The junctional reentry is manifest by a normal QRS complex, then an inverted P wave followed by a normal QRS complex. The R-P and RR intervals are approximately 320 ms and 1120 ms, respectively.

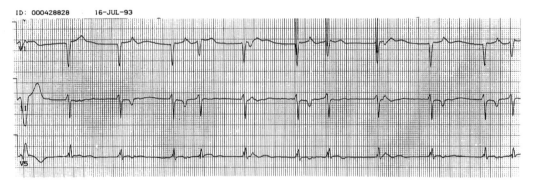

Figure 3-41. Junctional reentry. The junctional rhythm at a rate of 60 per minute is followed by retrograde P waves with an R-P interval of 320 ms. The junctional reentry is manifest by a normal QRS complex, a negative P wave, and a normal QRS complex. The reentrant R to next junctional R is shorter than the basic junctional R-R interval. This is because the reentry discharges the junctional pacemaker 140 ms before the R wave is inscribed.

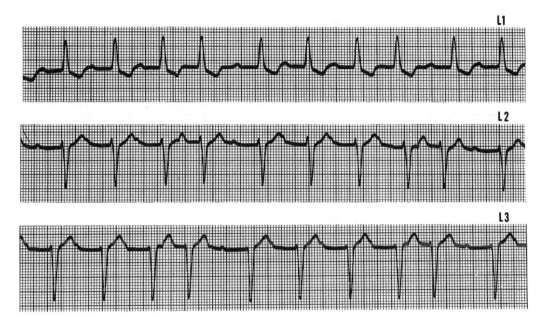

Figure 3-42. Ventricular reentry. In lead L2, beginning with the fifth P wave with a P-R interval of 360 ms, there is a slight but gradual prolongation of the P-R interval to 400 ms. The longest P-R interval is followed by an atrial and ventricular reentry. The reentry is manifest by a QRS complex with left anterior fascicular block, a retrograde P wave, and a normal QRS complex. Nonspecific ST-T changes are also noted.

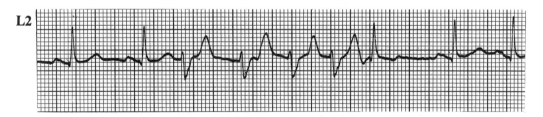

Figure 3-43. Ventricular reentry. The two sinus impulses at a rate of 107 per minute are followed by a run of VT with retrograde P waves. As the R-P interval prolongs from 140 to 340 ms, ventricular reentry follows.

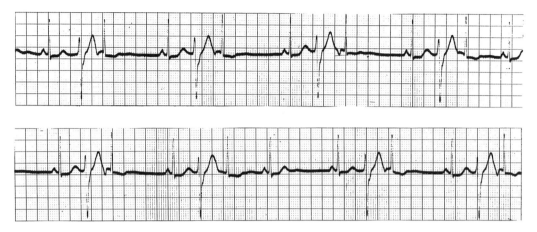

Figure 3-44. Ventricular reentry. The basic rhythm is sinus with ventricular bigeminy. Reentry is manifest by a VPC, a retrograde P wave, and a normal QRS complex. The retrograde P wave following the fourth VPC in the top row and that following the second VPC in the bottom row are nearly isoelectric and represent a fusion between the supraventricular P wave and the retrograde P wave. From Fisch C, Knoebel SB. Junctional rhythms. *Prog Cardiovasc Dis* 1970;13:141–158.

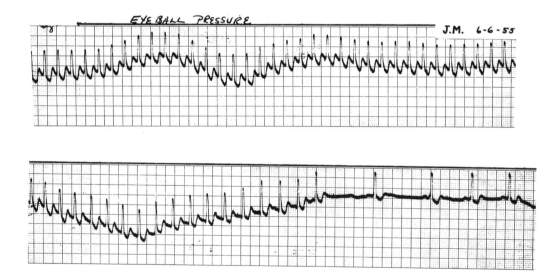

Figure 3-45. Supraventricular tachycardia. Tachycardia not otherwise identified is referred to as SVT. In this instance, the rate is approximately 210 per minute and the tachycardia is terminated by vagal pressure. The gradual slowing of the heart rate prior to cessation of the arrhythmia suggests an atrial tachycardia.

4

Ventricular Rhythms

Ventricular Premature Complexes

VPCs are premature with respect to the basic sinus interval. Since the site or origin of VPCs is ventricular, the QRS complex is abnormal in configuration and duration. Importantly, a VPC is not preceded by a P wave, or if it is, the P-R interval is too short to allow conduction to the ventricles.

In general, VPCs originating in the right ventricle resemble LBBB (Figure 4-1) and VPCs originating in the left ventricle resemble RBBB (Figure 4-2). VPCs with a superior axis originate near the left posterior fascicle (LPF), those with right axis originate near the left anterior fascicle (LAF) (Figure 4-2), those with anterior orientation originate at the base of the heart, and those with posterior orientation originate in the apical area. There is, however, considerable overlap of configuration and the site of origin of VPCs. Consequently, the configuration of a VPC does not always accurately define its site of origin.

Occasionally a VPC may be relatively narrow or, in fact, normal in duration. In such instances, the site of origin is in the septum with normal conduction along the two bundles (Figures 4–3 and 4–4). Similarly, a narrow ventricular complex may be a fusion between a VPC originating on the side of a bundle branch and the impulse being conducted along the contralateral normal bundle branch (Figure 4-5) (see Chapter 8).

The frequency and distribution of VPCs varies. The prematures may manifest as a couplet (two consecutive complexes), as bigeminy, trigeminy, or quadrigeminy (Figure 4-6). A VPC falling on the T wave, referred to as R on T, may initiate VT, ventricular flutter, or ventricular fibrillation (Figures 4–7 and 4–8).

On occasion, a long R-R interval is followed by a VPC, a compensatory pause, a supraventricular QRS complex, and, again, a VPC. The relationship of the long compensatory pause, QRS complex, and VPCs may be maintained indefinitely and is referred to as the rule of bigeminy.

The term "rule of bigeminy," coined by Langendorf, Pick, and Winternitz, refers to a VPC that appears after a prolonged cycle. The prolonged cycle may be due to atrial fibrillation (Figure 4-9), or to sinus arrhythmia, or it may be a compensatory pause following a supraventricular premature impulse. It may be caused by SAN arrest, SAN exit block, or A-V block. The appearance of a premature complex following a long cycle with a fixed coupling interval and uniform pattern supports reentry as the mechanism of the VPC.

All VPCs attempt to conduct retrogradely to the atria, but only approximately 50% reach the atria and discharge the SAN (Figure 4-3). If a VPC fails to disturb the sinus rhythm, the distance from the sinus P wave to the next sinus P wave encompassing the coupling interval (distance from the sinus QRS complex to the premature complex) and the compensatory pause equals two sinus cycles. Such a return cycle is said to be fully compensatory (Figure 4-1). When the above defined distance is shorter than two sinus cycles, the compensatory pause is said to be noncompensatory.

On occasion, a VPC does not interfere with conduction of the subsequent sinus impulse and is referred to as an interpolated VPC (Figure 4-1).

In the vast majority of cases, the coupling of VPCs is constant, rarely varying more than 60 to 80 ms. When the pattern of the premature complexes and the coupling interval are constant, they are assumed to originate from the same focus and to be unifocal (Figures 4-10 and 4-11). When the coupling interval and the ventricular premature pattern varies, it is assumed that they originate from different foci, and they are said to be multifocal (Figure 4-12). Rarely, coupling is constant but the prematures are of varying configuration. It is assumed that in this case VPCs are unifocal with varying direction of ventricular activation (Figure 4-13).

Ventricular Escape and Idioventricular Rhythm

When the dominant rate slows below that of the inherent rate of the ventricular pacemaker, the latter may escape. The slowing of the primary pacemaker may be due to marked sinus bradycardia, sinus arrest, or exit block or A-V block (Figure 4-14). The escape may be a single QRS complex or a series of ventricular complexes. As a rule, three or more escape complexes comprise idioventricular rhythm. Most often, however, escapes are junctional in origin unless junctional automaticity is impaired.

Ventricular Parasystole

VPCs with varying coupling suggest ventricular parasystole. Parasystole, with some exceptions, is a protected, independent, automatic, and regular ectopic rhythm. The protection is manifest by failure of extraneous impulses to disrupt the rhythmicity of the parasystolic focus. The mechanism of the protection is not clear. The classic electrocardiographic features of parasystole include: 1) variable coupling of the ectopic parasystolic impulse to the dominant rhythm; 2) a common interectopic interval; 3) fusion between the parasystolic and the nonparasystolic complexes; and 4) failure of the parasystolic complex to manifest because of physiological refractoriness of the surrounding myocardium (Figures 4-15 and 4-16). See Chapter 9.

Paroxysmal (Monomorphic) Ventricular Tachycardia

VT is defined as three or more consecutive ventricular complexes. It is characterized by a sudden onset and termination. If the VT lasts more than 30 seconds it is referred to as sustained VT (Figure 4-17), if the duration is less than 30 seconds it is referred to as nonsustained (Figure 4-18). The rate varies from 130 to 170 per minute but may be as low as 100 per minute and as rapid as 250 per minute. The QRS complexes are bizarre but uniform in contour (monomorphic), 140 ms or longer in duration, and often with marked left axis deviation. On rare occasions, VT may manifest narrow or normal QRS configuration. The site of origin of such a VT, as in the case of VPCs, is either high in the septum or in one of the fascicles. Fascicular VT is usually characterized by an upright QRS complex in V_1 and V_2 and left anterior fascicular block (LAFB). The diagnosis of VT is based most often on fusions and captures (Figures 4–19, 4–20, 4–21, and 4–22) (see Chapter 8).

QRS complexes that are positive in all of the precordial leads (positive concordance) are highly specific for VT. QRS complexes that are negative in all of the precordial leads (negative concordance) are less specific. Positive concordance, while most often an indicator of VT, can, however, also be present with WPW.

The site of origin of VT, when based on QRS configuration, is not always reliable. The diagnosis of VT is supported by the finding of VPCs with the same configuration as that of VT recorded either in the same tracing or in previous records. Two criteria with a high specificity but a very low sensitivity for a diagnosis of VT are fusions and captures (Figure 4-23). Similarly, a normal QRS complex at an R-R shorter than the bizarre QRS complex excludes aberration and preexisting BBB and, thus, is diagnostic of VT (Figure 4-24).

A fusion complex, either atrial or ventricular, results from simultaneous activation of the atria or ventricles by two or, rarely, several impulses originating in the same or different chambers of the heart. A capture is a supraventricular complex that opportunistically reaches and excites part or all of the ventricles in the presence of dominant junctional or ventricular rhythm (see Chapter 8).

Idiopathic Left and Right Ventricular Tachycardia

Idiopathic left VT is seen in the absence of heart disease and is manifest by RBBB with superior axis (Figure 4-25). It is generally accepted that the tachycardia is due to reentry involving the LPF.

Idiopathic right VT, also seen in the absence of significant heart disease, originates in the outflow tract of the right ventricle. The mechanism is unclear. The QRS complex is of left bundle branch (LBB) configuration with an inferiorly oriented axis (Figure 4-26). There are a few cases of idiopathic VT with RBBB and abnormal right axis deviations (Figure 4-27). The origin of this tachycardia is probably in the LAF of the left bundle.

Bidirectional Ventricular Tachycardia

Bidirectional VT was once considered to be NPJT with RBBB and alternating LAFB and left posterior fascicular block (LPFB) responsible for the changing frontal axis. Subsequent studies, however, revealed that the arrhythmia is a VT originating near the bifurcation of the LBB with alternate conduction along the LAF and LPF (Figure 4-28).

Polymorphic Ventricular Tachycardia

This arrhythmia is characterized by changing pattern, amplitude, and polarity of the QRS complex. It is initiated by a VPC. The rate is usually between 200 and 250 per minute, but it may range from 150 to as high as 300 per minute. QRS complex and T waves are difficult to separate because of the rapid rate (Figures 4-29 and 4-30).

Torsades de Pointes

Torsades de pointes is a variant of polymorphic VT associated with a prolonged QT interval. Torsades de pointes is a descriptive term indicating a 180° change in the direction of the QRS axis. In most cases, the arrhythmia is initiated by a VPC falling within the prolonged QT interval. As a rule, the differential diagnosis is that of polymorphic VT and torsades de pointes (Figures 4–31 and 4–32).

Accelerated Idioventricular Rhythm

Accelerated idioventricular rhythm resembles the slow idioventricular rhythm but with a more rapid rate, which varies from 55 to 110 per minute. The onset is generally gradual. The rhythm usually appears late in diastole when the rate of the ectopic ventricular focus exceeds that of the sinus or other dominant rhythm. The first complex is frequently a fusion complex (Figures 4–33, 4–34, and 4–35). The episodes are usually short in duration (up to 30 cycles) and most often complicate acute myocardial infarction. Termination may be due to acceleration of the dominant rhythm or to slowing or failure of the ventricular focus.

Parasystolic Ventricular Tachycardia

VT may manifest features of parasystole, including: 1) variable coupling of the parasystolic impulse to the dominant rhythm; 2) a common interectopic interval; 3) fusions; and 4) failure of the parasystolic complex to manifest because of physiological refractoriness of the surrounding tissue (Figures 4–36 and 4–37) (see Chapter 9).

Ventricular Flutter and Fibrillation

The rate of ventricular flutter is approximately 200 per minute. It differs from VT in that in ventricular flutter individual components of the QRS-ST-T complex can no longer be identified (Figures 4–38 and 4–39).

In ventricular fibrillation, the deflections are chaotic and vary in configuration and amplitude. In fibrillation, as in flutter, the individual components of the ECG cannot be identified (Figures 4-40, 4-41, and 4-42).

Wide QRS Tachycardia: A Differential Diagnosis

Wide QRS tachycardia includes SVT with aberration, SVT with preexisting BBB (Figures 4-43 and 4-44), SVT with preexcitation (Figures 4-45 and 4-46), and VT. The problems encountered in the differential diagnosis of the two were stressed by Lewis during the early days of electrocardiography. Despite numerous studies, the differential diagnosis may sometimes be difficult if not impossible.

The ECG variables that are helpful in the differential diagnosis of SVT with aberration from VT include fusions and captures, AV dissociation, the duration of the QRS complex, the QRS axis, the QRS pattern, QRS concordance, and presence or absence of WPW and preexisting BBB.

The markers with a high specificity for VT include fusions and captures, present in only 5% of patients, AV dissociation, recorded in approximately 25% or patients, and a monomorphic right bundle branch (RBB) pattern with a QRS duration longer than 140 ms. A QRS complex of 140 ms or shorter strongly favors aberration. Positive concordance, but less so negative concordance, is highly specific for VT (Figures 4-47 and 4-47A). Occasionally, positive concordance may be present with WPW syndrome. LBBB with extreme left or right axis favors VT.

Table 4-1

Diagnosis of Ventricular Tachycardia (VT)

ECG Markers of VT

QRS complex similar to VPC during sinus rhythm in the same or previous tracings
Regular or slightly irregular rhythm
Wide QRS at R-R intervals longer than R-R intervals with normal QRS
QRS prolonged to 0.14 seconds or longer
Superior axis
Abrupt onset with fixed coupling, if repetitive
Atrioventricular dissociation
Fusions
Captures
Wide QRS with right bundle branch block configuration:
  Monophasic R in V_1
  qR in V_1
  Deep S in V_6
  R taller than r^1 in V_1
Wide QRS with left bundle branch configuration:
  R wave in V_1 of $\geq$30 ms
  Slurred downstroke of S wave in V_1, V_2
  Duration $\geq$70 ms from onset of QRS to the nadir in V_1, V_2
  Any Q wave in V_6
  Positive QRS concordance

In wide QRS tachycardia, aberration is favored by a triphasic rSR in lead V_1 and a qRS in lead V_6. VT is favored by a monophasic R, a biphasic qR, QR, and RS, and a triphasic Rsr in lead V_1. In lead V_6, VT is suggested by a QRS complex with an R/S ratio of less than 1, a QS, or a qR (Figure 4-48).

In LBBB pattern, a wide QRS complex with an R wave of 30 ms or longer, a prominent notch on the downstroke in lead V_1, and a qR, QS pattern or QrS in lead V_6, favor VT (Table 4-1) (Figures 4-49 and 4-50).

Preexisting BBB does not alter the sensitivity and specificity of the different markers of VT because it does not alter the ventricular excitation induced by an ectopic ventricular pacemaker. However, a rapid supraventricular rhythm with a preexisting BBB or aberration may make a differential diagnosis of "wide QRS tachycardia" virtually impossible.

The differential diagnosis of SVT and VT based on the 12-lead ECG is possible in approximately 90% of patients.

Compensatory Pause

The pause following a premature impulse may be compensatory, in which the P-P interval encompassing the premature complex equals two sinus cycles. When the P-P interval encompassing the premature complex is either shorter or longer than two sinus cycles, the pause is noncompensatory.

The time from the premature complex to the next sinus complex (the return cycle) is included in the assessment of the compensatory pause. As discussed above, an APC discharges the SAN, which promptly begins to depolarize and, thus, the return cycle equals the sinus cycle. The sum of the return cycle and the coupling interval of an APC is less than two sinus cycles and the pause is noncompensatory. However, since the duration of the return cycle following an APC is determined not only by the duration of phase-4 depolarization of the SAN but may also be influenced by the conduction time from the site of the APC to the SAN, the duration of suppression of the SAN by the APC, and the duration of the exit time from the SAN, the return cycle is frequently longer than the basic P-P interval and is, fortuitously, compensatory.

It is evident that the mechanism of the full compensatory pause following an APC differs from that of a JPC or VPC. The prevalence of a full compensatory pause following an APC is estimated to be as high as 50%. A return cycle shorter than the basic P-P indicates an interpolated APC or sinus node reentry. In case of sinus node reentry, the configuration of the premature P wave will be the same or very similar to that of the sinus P wave (Figures 4-51 and 4-52).

Since a VPC originates in a different chamber than the sinus impulse, it does not interfere with rhythmicity of the sinus node, and it is followed by a full compensatory pause. If there is retrograde conduction of the VPC to the atrium, it may alter the rhythmicity of the SAN, and the effect may be similar to that of an APC. The return cycle may be equal to or longer than the sinus interval and, therefore, noncompensatory.

Following an interpolated VPC, the P-R interval is prolonged, the subsequent R-P interval short, and the P wave blocked. This rare phenomenon is referred to as "postponed" compensatory pause (Figures 4-53 and 4-54). Less commonly, a VPC or JPC may initiate an AV Wenckebach sequence (Figure 4-55).

LI

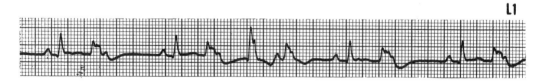

Figure 4-1. Interpolated VPCs. VPCs are manifest by a bizarre appearance of the QRS complex and absence of P wave. The second VPC is interpolated and does not interfere with conduction of the next sinus impulse. However, the P-R interval is prolonged, and measures 400 ms. The prolongation is due to concealed conduction of the VPC into the AV node which thus delays conduction of the sinus impulse.

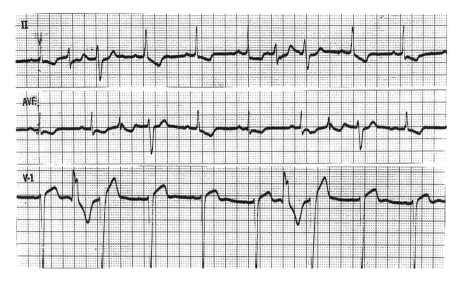

Figure 4-2. Interpolated VPCs. The P-R interval following the interpolated VPC is prolonged. The configuration of the sinus QRS complex that follows the interpolated VPC is that of LAFB.

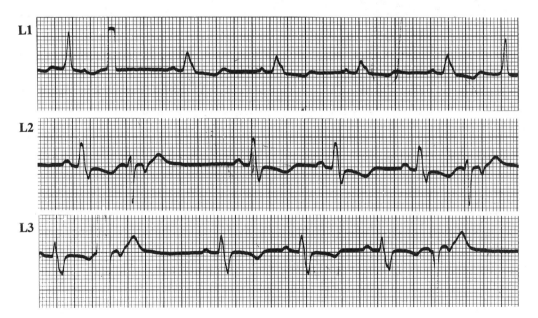

Figure 4-3. VPCs with normal QRS duration. Lead I shows sinus rhythm at a rate of 60 per minute with LBBB. The VPCs, two in each lead, are accurately coupled to the preceding sinus impulse and are followed by a retrograde P wave. The normal configuration of the VPC is due to the fact that the site of origin is high in the septum or in the LPF.

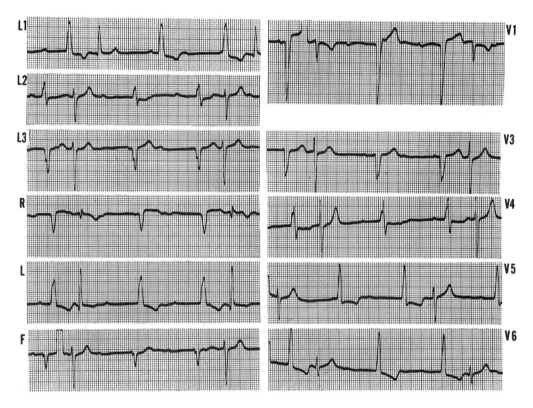

Figure 4-4. VPCs with normal duration QRS. The basic rhythm is AV dissociation with a P-P interval of 760 ms and an R to R interval of 1280 ms. The VPCs are accurately coupled to the preceding idioventricular QRS complex. The duration of the QRS complex is approximately 80 ms and the appearance is that of LAFB. The reason for the normal QRS complex of the VPCs is the fact that the latter originate either high in the septum or in the LPF.

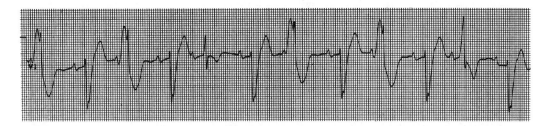

Figure 4-5. Ventricular fusion with normal QRS. The sinus QRS complex manifests LBBB. The VPCs are of RBBB morphology and, thus, originate in the left ventricle, on the side of the LBBB. The VPCs appear fortuitously with sinus impulses. As a result, the two fuse, giving rise to a normal QRS complex (the fifth QRS complex). In other words, while the supraventricular impulse conducts along the right bundle and activates the right ventricle, fortuitously, at the same time, the VPC originating in the left ventricle activates the left ventricle. The two fuse, resulting in a normal QRS complex. The next to the last QRS complex is also a fusion.

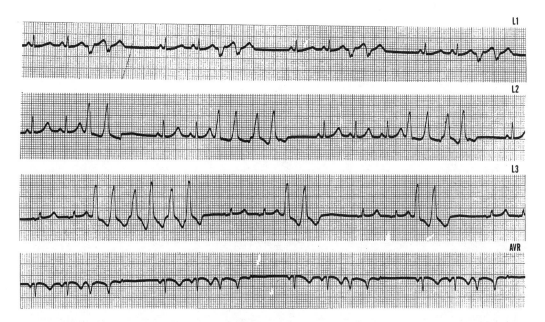

Figure 4-6. Monomorphic paroxysmal VT. The VPCs manifest in the form of couplets and four to six consecutive QRS complexes, constituting VT. Each run is accurately coupled to the preceding sinus impulse, the morphology is identical, and, since the tachycardia lasts less than 30 seconds, it is considered nonsustained.

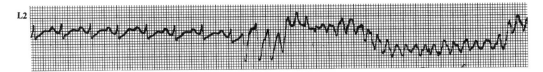

Figure 4-7. Ventricular fibrillation. There is sinus tachycardia at a rate of 125 per minute with a VPC falling on the T (R on T), triggering ventricular fibrillation.

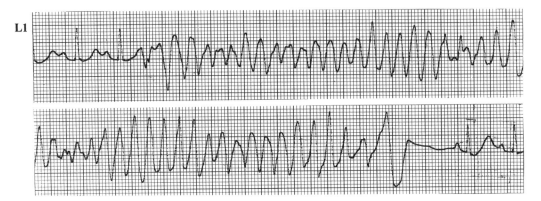

Figure 4-8. Torsades de pointes. Two sinus impulses with a prolonged QT interval are followed by a closely coupled VPC which initiates a run of VT. The axis of the QRS complex rotates almost 180°, characteristic of torsades de pointes. Torsades de pointes is a variant of polymorphic VT.

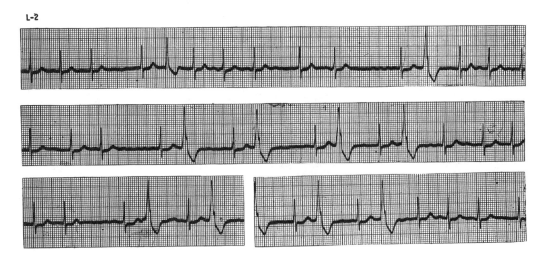

Figure 4-9. Rule of bigeminy. The basic rhythm is atrial fibrillation with varying R-R intervals. The long R-R intervals are followed by accurately coupled VPCs. In the middle and bottom tracings, each compensatory pause is followed by a VPC. Acceleration of the ventricular rate interrupts the bigeminal rhythm. From Mericle JE, Fisch C. The rule of bigeminy. *J Indiana State Med Assoc* 1969;62:172–174.

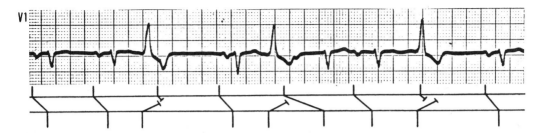

Figure 4-10. Interpolated VPCs. The second VPC is interpolated and is followed by a prolonged P-R interval and a shorter R-R interval, shorter by the difference in the P-R prolongation. The P-R prolongation following the interpolated VPC is due to concealed conduction. The VPC enters the AV node and prolongs the subsequent P-R interval. The attempted retrograde conduction of the VPC is recognized by the unexpected prolongation of the P-R interval.

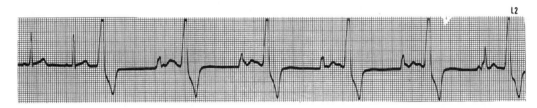

Figure 4-11. Idioventricular rhythm with ventricular bigeminy. Following the first two sinus impulses, the rhythm is idioventricular. The ventricular origin is confirmed by the last QRS complex, which is a fusion between the sinus and the idioventricular complex. The coupling and configuration of the VPCs is constant, thus, unifocal.

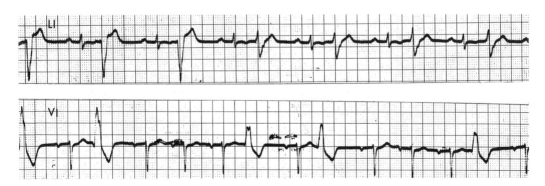

Figure 4-12. Multifocal VPCs (leads L1, V_1). The first three VPCs of the ventricular bigeminy in lead II differ in configuration from the next four. Similarly, their coupling differs. In lead V_1 the first two VPCs differ from the remaining three VPCs. The varying coupling and configuration indicate a multifocal origin of the VPCs.

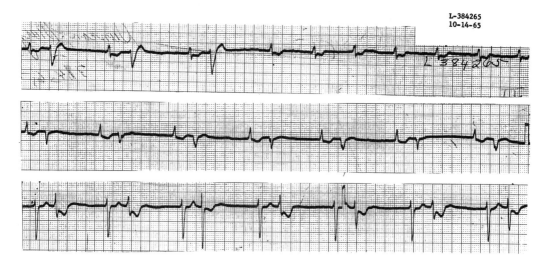

Figure 4-13. NPJT and ventricular bigeminy. The VPCs are accurately coupled, with varying configuration, indicating a unifocal origin with varying direction of exit into the ventricle. Since the R-R of the supraventricular complexes remain constant, the most likely mechanism is persistent junctional tachycardia interrupted by the ventricular bigeminy. From Fisch C, Knoebel SB. Recognition and therapy of digitalis toxicity. *Prog Cardiovasc Dis* 1970;13:71–96.

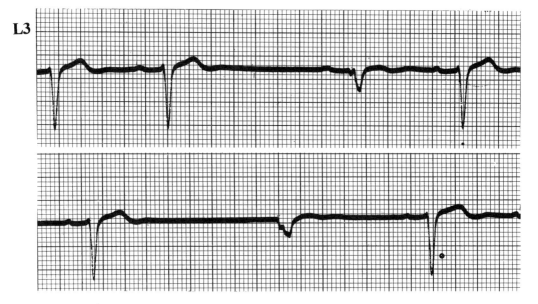

Figure 4-14. Ventricular escape. The long pause due to sinus arrest is terminated by a ventricular complex (ventricular escape).

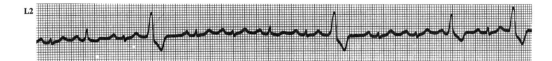

Figure 4-15. Ventricular parasystole. Coupling of the parasystolic impulse to the preceding sinus impulse varies. The interectopic interval is constant at an R-R of 1060 ms. The first and fourth parasystolic impulses are fusions. The failure to record a QRS complex when expected is due to physiological refractoriness of the ventricle.

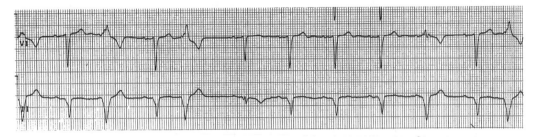

Figure 4-16. Ventricular parasystole. The ectopic impulses exhibit varying coupling to the preceding sinus impulse. There is a fixed interectopic interval of 1400 ms. Failure of the ectopic impulse to appear when expected is due to physiological refractoriness of the myocardium. The fourth parasystolic impulse in leads V_1 and II are fusions.

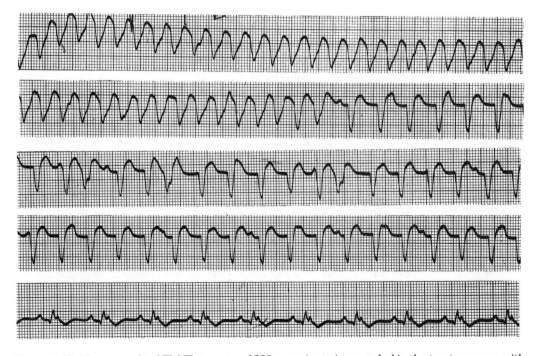

Figure 4-17. Monomorphic VT. VT at a rate of 200 per minute is recorded in the top two rows, with the rate slowing to 136 per minute in row 2. In row 3 the VT is interrupted by VPCs. VPCs do not disturb the rhythmicity of the VT because these are blocked from entering the ectopic focus, largely due to refractoriness of the surrounding tissue. The bottom row shows a return to sinus rhythm at a rate of 75 per minute. Since the arrhythmia lasts more than 30 seconds, it is considered sustained. Independent P waves are noted with slowing of the rate.

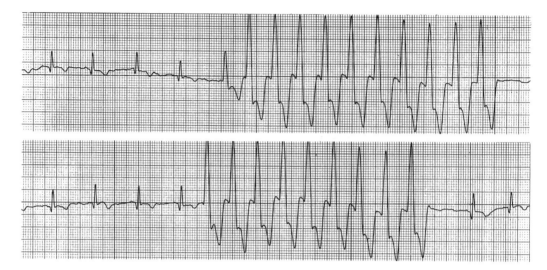

Figure 4-18. Paroxysmal VT. The basic rhythm is atrial fibrillation with recurrent nonsustained monomorphic VT. The first complex of the tachycardia in the top row is a fusion, supporting the diagnosis of VT.

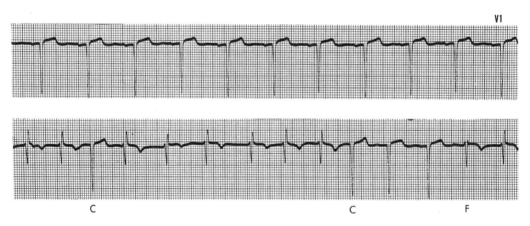

Figure 4-19. Fascicular VT. The top tracing is the control tracing. In the bottom tracing, the sinus rhythm is interrupted by an ectopic tachycardia with an RBBB pattern but with a QRS duration of 80 ms. The letter C indicates captures and the letter F indicates fusion. This is a fascicular VT manifest by RBBB-like pattern and normal duration of the QRS complex. The diagnosis of VT is confirmed by captures and fusions.

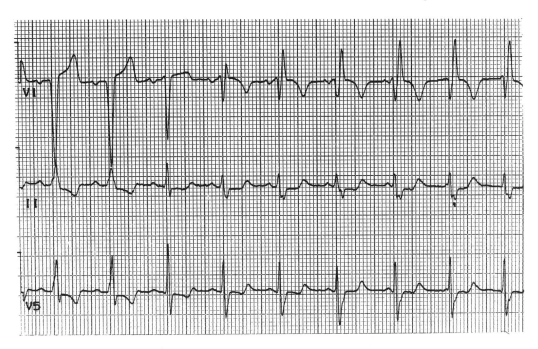

Figure 4-20. Fascicular VT. The first two complexes are sinus in origin. The third, fourth, and fifth complexes are fusions between the sinus and the VT complexes, with an RBBB and QRS duration of 120 ms. Fusion complexes attest to the ventricular origin of the tachycardia.

ID: 70264396   10-APR-1999

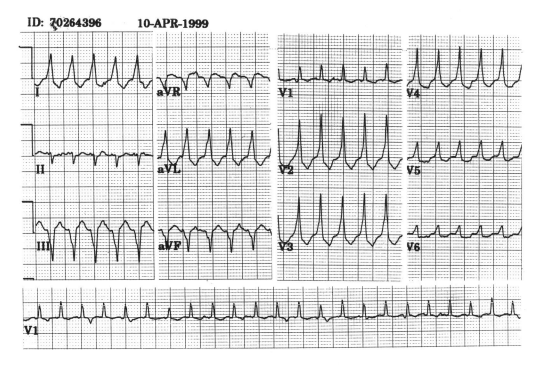

Figure 4-21. Narrow QRS VT. The rate is 215 per minute with AV dissociation, QRS of 110 ms, and positive concordance. Septal origin of the VT explains the narrow QRS complexes.

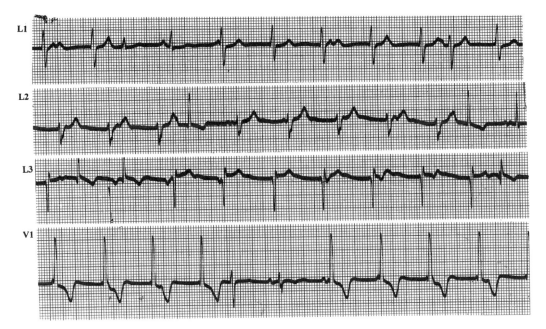

Figure 4-22. Accelerated idioventricular fascicular rhythm. The ventricular rate is 75 per minute with AV dissociation. The configuration is that of RBBB and LAFB. The QRS duration is approximately 100 ms, indicating fascicular origin. Captures and fusions indicate a ventricular origin of the ectopic tachycardia. Examples of captures are the fourth and fifth QRS complexes in L2 and V_1, respectively. An example of fusion is the sixth QRS complex in lead V_1.

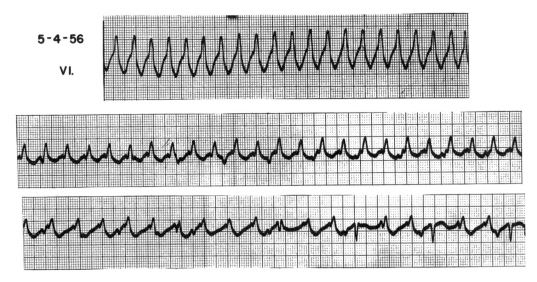

Figure 4-23. Ventricular Tachycardia. The configuration in the top strip is that of RBBB and the rate is 188 per minute. In the middle and the bottom tracings, the rate is slowed and an independent atrial rhythm at a P-P interval of 400 ms is recorded. In the bottom tracing, fusion (i.e., tenth ventricular complex) and captures are present. From Fisch C, Pinsky ST. Diagnosis of ventricular tachycardia. *J Indiana State Med Assoc* 1957;50:184–193.

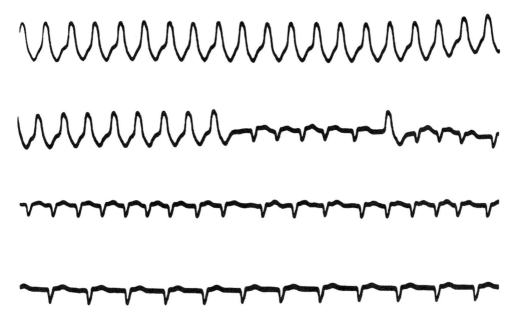

Figure 4-24. Ventricular tachycardia. Wide QRS tachycardia is recorded in the top two rows, with atrial fibrillation in the second and third rows. Fibrillation with NPJT is present in the bottom row. In the second and third rows, the R-R of the normally conducted QRS complex is shorter than the R-R of the bizarre complexes. This indicates absence of preexisting BBB and aberration and, thus, a VT. With aberration, the R-R of the aberrant QRS complex is shorter than the R-R of the normal complexes. From Knoebel SB, Fisch C. Concealed conduction. *Cardiovasc Clin* 1973;5:21–34.

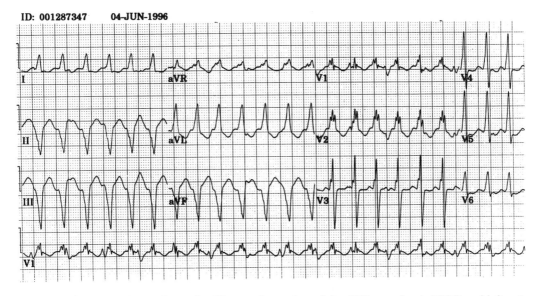

Figure 4-25. Ventricular tachycardia. The configuration of the QRS complex is RBBB and left axis with a duration of 160 ms. AV dissociation with an independent atrial rhythm at a P-P interval of 300 per minute is recorded in the bottom strip. The dissociation is highly diagnostic of VT.

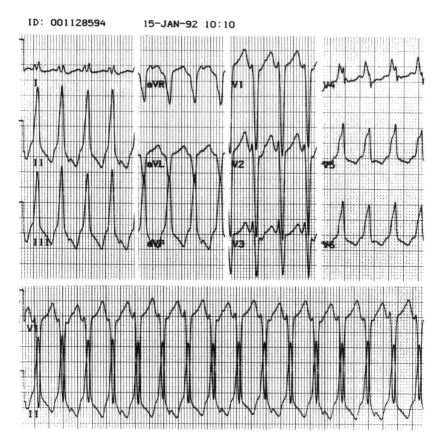

Figure 4-26. VT with 2:1 retrograde conduction. The basic rhythm is VT with retrograde conduction clearly seen in leads II, III, and AVF where every other QRS complex is followed by a retrograde, negative P wave. The QRS configuration is that of LBBB with an inferiorly oriented QRS axis.

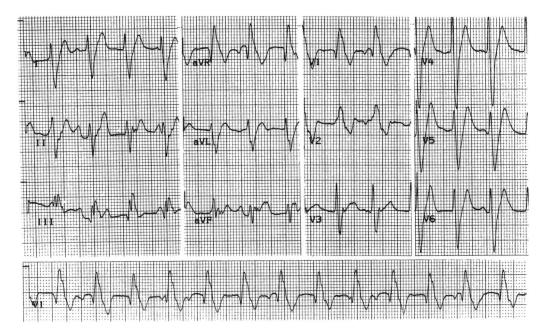

Figure 4-27. Ventricular tachycardia. The QRS morphology is that of RBBB. The duration of the QRS complex is 160 ms and the R/S ratio in V_5 and V_6 is less than 1. AV dissociation with a P-P interval of 360 ms is noted in lead V_1.

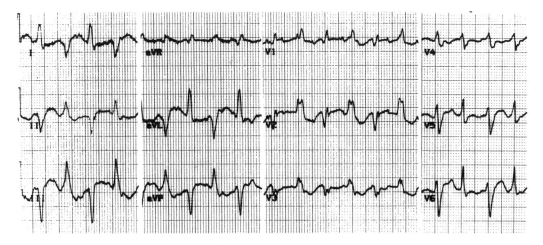

Figure 4-28. Bidirectional VT. The basic rhythm is atrial flutter at a rate of 300 per minute with AV dissociation (lead V_1). The configuration of the QRS complex is that of RBBB with alternating LAFB and LPFB. Such tracings were once considered to be junctional tachycardia with RBBB and alternating LAFB and LPFB. More recently, however, electrophysiological studies have shown that the arrhythmia is a VT originating in the fascicles.

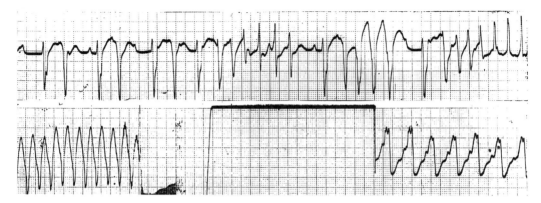

Figure 4-29. Polymorphic VT. The polymorphic VT is characterized by the changing pattern, amplitude, and polarity of the QRS complex. The rate is approximately 125 to 200 per minute. In the bottom row, the pattern is that of VT or flutter with an R-R interval of 240 ms. Cardioversion resulted in a monophasic VT. From Knoebel SB, Konecke LL, Fisch C. Pacing in myocardial infarction. In *Atherosclerosis and Coronary Artery Disease*. New York: Grune and Stratton; 1972:412–421.

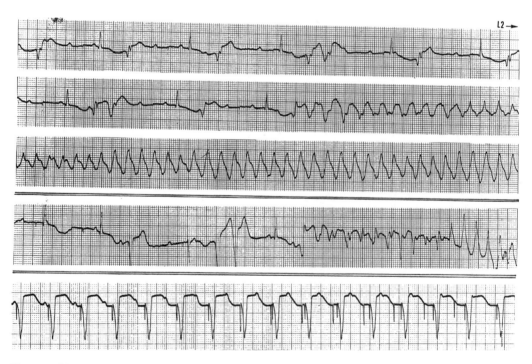

Figure 4-30. Ventricular tachycardia. The basic rhythm is sinus with complete A-V block, ventricular bigeminy, and VT. The QT is greatly prolonged. Polymorphic VT is present in the top and middle panels. In the bottom panel, pacing suppresses the ventricular arrhythmia.

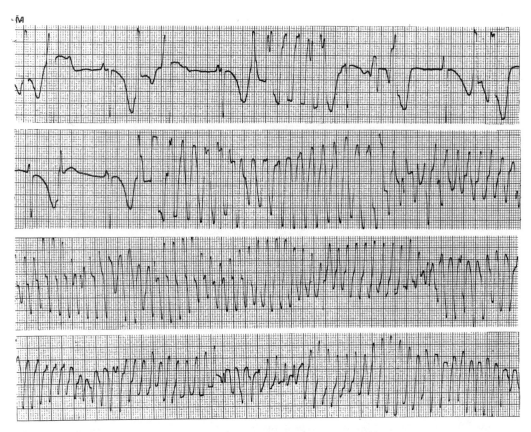

Figure 4-31. Torsades de pointes. AV dissociation with a markedly prolonged QT interval, VPCs, and a short run of VT is recorded in the top row. In the second, third, and fourth rows, the VT is present at a rate of approximately 300 per minute with 180° rotation of the QRS vector, features characteristic of torsades de pointes.

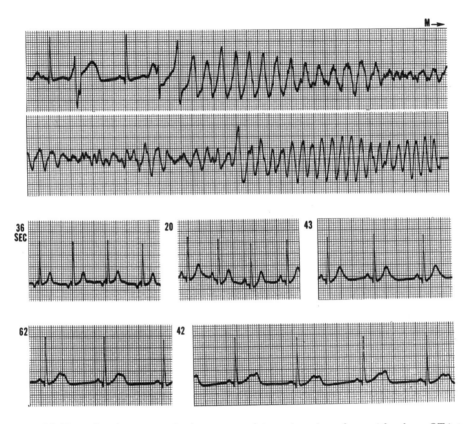

Figure 4-32. Torsades de pointes. In the top panel, two sinus impulses with a long QT interval are interrupted by R on T. This is followed by torsades de pointes and ventricular fibrillation. The middle and bottom rows show a junctional tachycardia followed by sinus tachycardia with gradual slowing of the sinus rate. The QT remains prolonged with a notched T wave.

ID: 001098639   20-APR-91 08:49

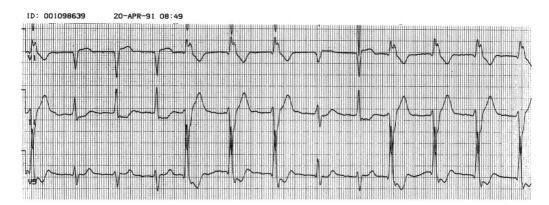

Figure 4-33. Accelerated idioventricular rhythm. The basic rhythm is atrial fibrillation with runs of an accelerated ventricular rhythm at an R-R interval of 800 ms. The QRS complex following the first sequence of idioventricular rhythm is a fusion. The next QRS complex is a capture. Both fusion and capture indicate a ventricular origin of the accelerated rhythm.

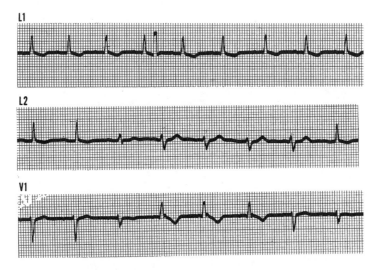

Figure 4-34. Fascicular VT. The basic rhythm is sinus with a rate of 100 per minute. The first QRS complex of the VT in leads L2 and V_1 are fusions. The configuration of the QRS complex is that of RBBB with LAFB. In lead V_1, the third and the last two QRS complexes are fusions.

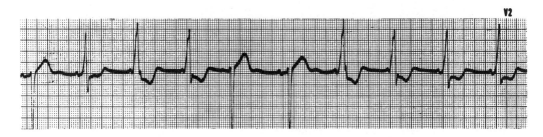

Figure 4-35. Accelerated idioventricular rhythm. The ventricular rate is approximately 60 per minute. The first and the last three QRS complexes of the ectopic rhythm appear to be fusions, indicating a ventricular origin of the aberrant complexes. WPW is difficult to exclude.

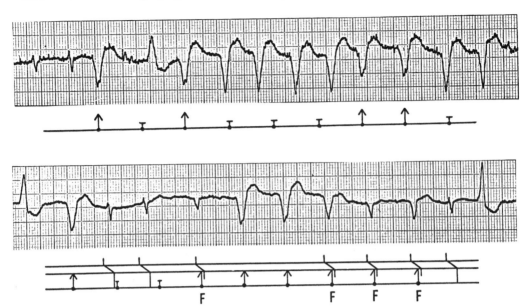

Figure 4-36. Parasystolic VT. The interectopic interval is 880 ms. The manifest parasystolic complexes are indicated with a dot and an arrow. The failure of the parasystolic impulses to manifest is due to physiological refractoriness of the surrounding myocardium induced by a short run of VT. In the bottom row, the parasystolic impulses are indicated with a dot. The arrow indicates manifest parasystolic complexes. The QRS complexes identified with the letter F are fusions of supraventricular and parasystolic impulses. There are three pure supraventricular complexes, namely 3, 4, and 11 in the bottom row.

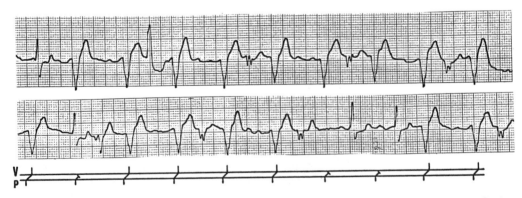

Figure 4-37. Parasystolic VT. The Lewis diagram illustrates conduction of the parasystolic impulse from the Purkinje fiber (P) to the ventricular myocardium (V). There are a number of VPCs, some interpolated between two parasystolic impulses. These do not disturb the parasystolic rhythmicity. In the bottom tracing, failure of the second parasystolic impulse to manifest is due to refractoriness of the surrounding myocardium. Failure of parasystolic impulses 7 and 8 is most likely due to exit block, as this late in diastole the myocardium should no longer be refractory.

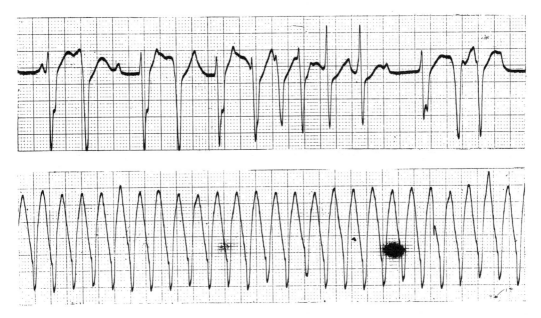

Figure 4-38. Polymorphic VT and ventricular flutter. The polymorphic VT is manifest by varying R-R intervals, QRS amplitude, and configuration. In the bottom row, ventricular flutter is indicated by the absence of discrete ECG components, namely, the QRS complex, ST, and T wave. The QRS rate is 250 per minute.

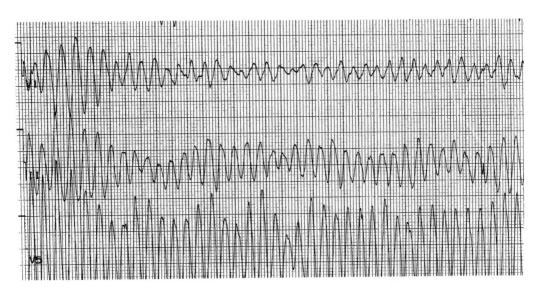

Figure 4-39. Ventricular flutter. The rate of the flutter is greater than 300 per minute. The different components of the QRS-T are not recognizable. A less likely diagnosis is VT with torsades de pointes.

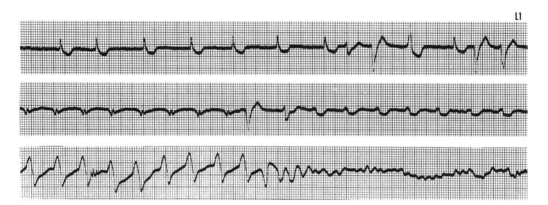

Figure 4-40. VT and fibrillation. In the bottom row, the VT with an R/T deteriorates into ventricular fibrillation. There are four different forms of VT, two in the top row and one each in the middle and bottom rows. Occasional VPCs are also noted.

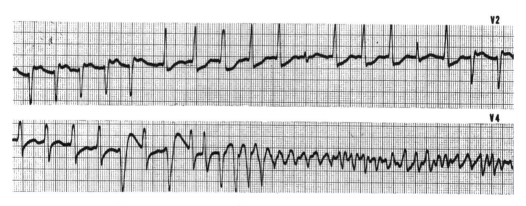

Figure 4-41. NPJT, polymorphic VT, ventricular fibrillation. The first four complexes in V_4 are supraventricular, most likely NPJT. This is followed by two VPCs and a polymorphic VT that deteriorates into ventricular fibrillation.

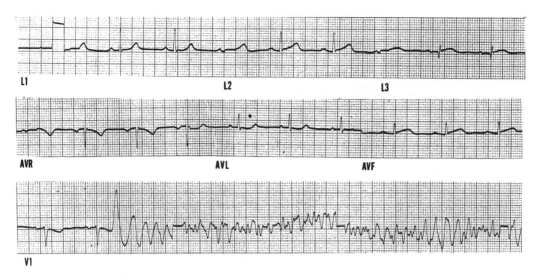

Figure 4-42. Ventricular fibrillation. The ST segment is elevated in leads L2, L3, and AVF. Reciprocal depression is present in AVL. In lead V_1, the two sinus impulses are followed by an R/T deteriorating into ventricular fibrillation.

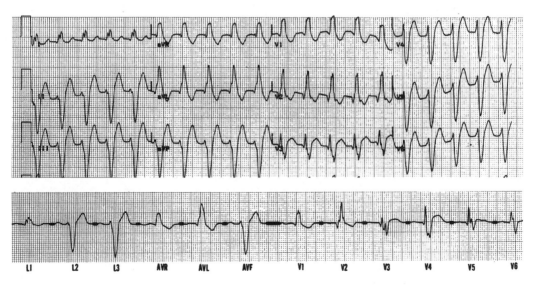

Figure 4-43. NPJT with RBBB. The marked left axis deviation, the monomorphic RBBB, and an R/S ratio smaller than 1 in V_4, V_5, and V_6 all suggest VT. However, the control tracing on the bottom reveals a preexisting RBBB. The rhythm is thus supraventricular with RBBB and LAFB, rather than VT.

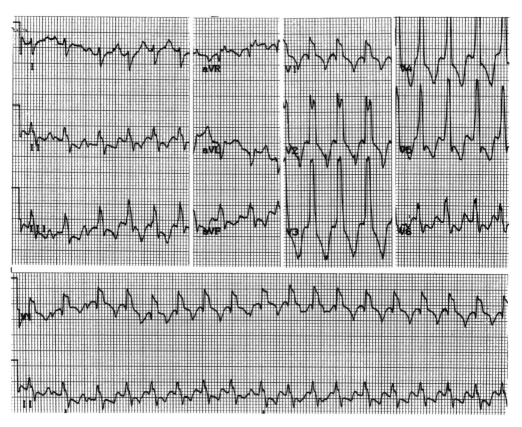

Figure 4-44. SVT with RBBB aberration. The monomorphic RBBB suggests VT. However, the first three complexes in leads V_1 and II are sinus with RBBB. Beginning with the third QRS complex, the retrograde P waves suggest an atypical AVNRT. The diagnosis is therefore SVT with RBBB aberration.

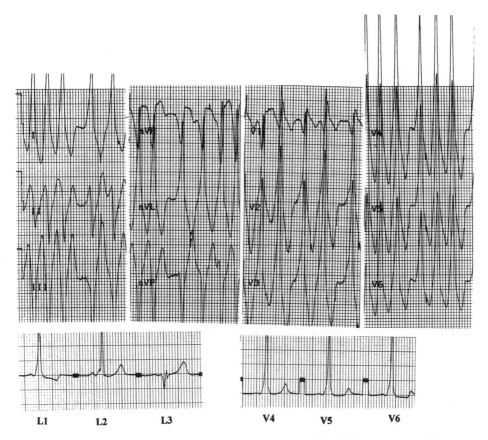

Figure 4-45. WPW with atrial fibrillation. WPW is recorded in the bottom row. The bizarre and irregularly spaced QRS complexes are due to anterograde conduction through the bypass (antidromic). The marked aberration of the QRS complex suggests that the entire QRS complex is a delta wave with total activation of the ventricle through the bypass.

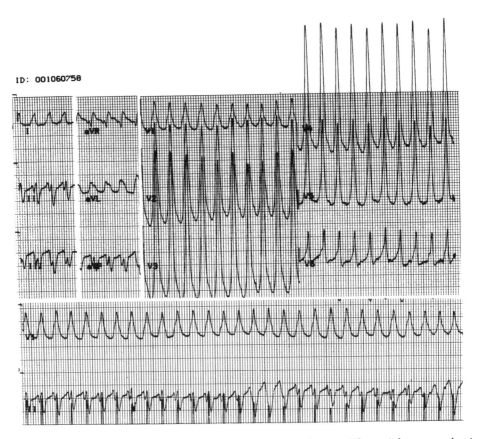

Figure 4-46. Wide QRS tachycardia. The positive concordance with upright monophasic QRS complexes in leads V_1 and V_6 are diagnostic of VT.

ID: 001055972

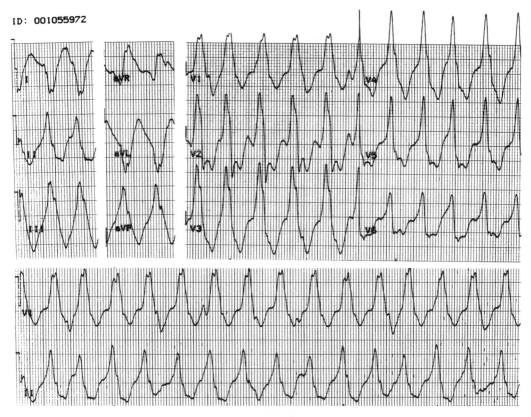

Figure 4-47. Wide QRS tachycardia. The feature indicative of VT is the monophasic RBBB config-uration in V_1 with a positive concordance. In addition, other markers of VT include a marked pro-longation of the QRS complex and an independent atrial rhythm at a rate of 100 per minute, noted in lead V_1.

ID: 001042384

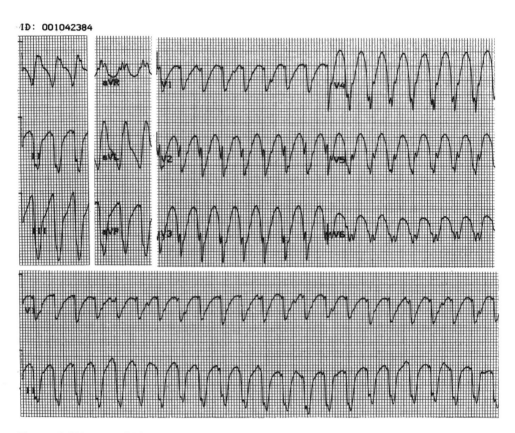

Figure 4-47A. Wide QRS tachycardia. The negative concordance with the QRS complex being negative in V_1 and V_6 indicates that the arrhythmia is most likely a VT.

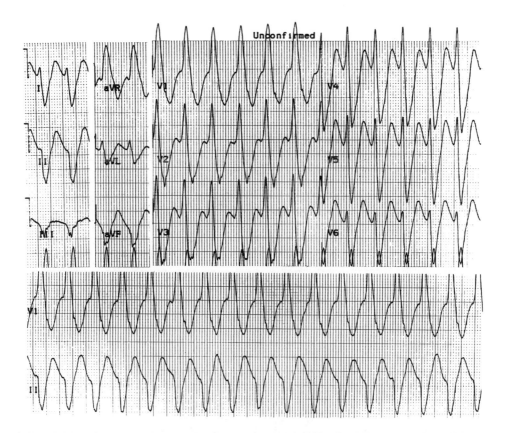

Figure 4-48. Wide QRS tachycardia. The ventricular rate is 150 per minute. The QRS duration is 170 to 180 ms. The configuration is that of a monophasic RBBB in V_1 with an R/S ratio in V_6 of less than 1. These features suggest that the wide QRS tachycardia is a VT.

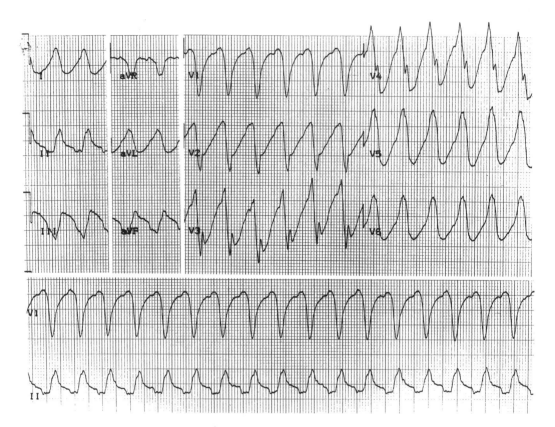

Figure 4-49. Wide QRS tachycardia. The ventricular rate is 150 per minute. The QRS duration is 200 ms. The configuration is that of LBBB. In lead V_1, the duration of the R wave is greater than 30 ms and the time from the onset of the R to the nadir of the S exceeds 70 ms. These features indicate that the "LBBB" QRS tachycardia is ventricular in origin.

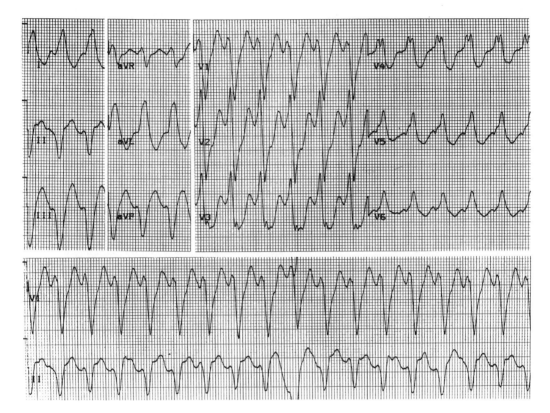

Figure 4-50. Wide QRS tachycardia. The ventricular rate is approximately 150 per minute. There is a marked left axis deviation and significant prolongation of the QRS complex. The duration of the R wave in V_1 is greater than 30 ms and the time from the onset of the R wave to the nadir of the QRS complex exceeds 70 ms. These features indicate that the wide "LBBB" QRS tachycardia is ventricular in origin.

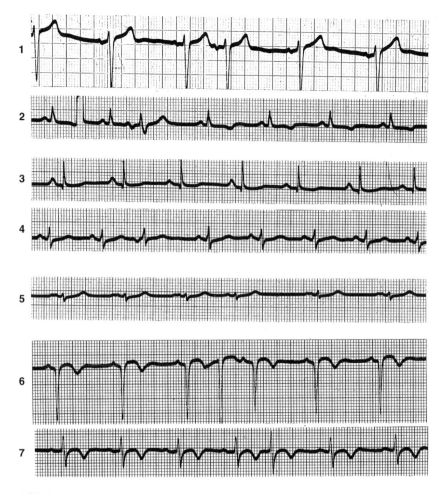

Figure 4-51. Compensatory pause (return cycle) following an APC. In the panel 1, the sinus P-P interval measures 1080 ms. The coupling interval of the APC is 600 ms and the return cycle terminated by a sinus P wave is 1040 ms. The APC discharges the sinus node promptly, there is little or no SA delay, and the return cycle equals a sinus cycle. In panel 2, the sinus P-P interval measures 880 ms. The coupling of the APC is 400 ms and the return cycle terminated by a sinus P wave is 1040 ms. The return cycle, which is longer than expected, includes conduction of the APC to the SAN and from the SAN to the atrium. As a result, the return cycle is longer than the basic sinus cycle. Panels 3 and 4 were recorded from the same patient. In panel 3, the first cycle reflects the basic P-P interval of 880 ms. An atrial bigeminy with a coupling of the APC to sinus P wave by 840 ms follows. The return cycle equals the basic sinus cycle length, indicating reset of the SAN but without suppression. In panel 4, the basic P-P interval is 780 ms with a 680-ms coupling of the APC and a return cycle of 880 ms. The sum of the coupling and return cycles of 680 and 880 ms equals 1560 ms, twice the normal basic cycle length. The return cycle is thus fully compensatory. A full compensatory pause following an APC is present in approximately 40% to 50% of APCs, and is thus an unreliable differential point between JPC, VPC, and APC. The full compensatory pause is fortuitous. In panel 5, the basic SAN rhythm with a P-P interval of 880 ms is interrupted by an APC with a coupling interval of 720 ms and a return cycle of 1200 ms, longer than the SAN cycle. The P-P interval that follows the return cycle measures 1040 ms, is longer than the basic SAN cycle, and indicates suppression of the SAN by the APC with a gradual "warming up" of the SAN. Panels 6 and 7 were recorded from the same patient. In panel 6 the dominant P-P interval of 960 ms is interrupted by an APC with a coupling of 440 ms. The return cycle measures 530 ms and is terminated by a P wave with a configuration identical to that of the sinus P wave. The interval between the two sinus P waves encompassing the APC is 970 ms or 40 ms longer than the P-R interval of the SAN P wave. The most likely explanation for the short return cycle is interpolation of the APC with SAN entrance block preventing discharge of the sinus pacemaker. An alternate but unlikely explanation suggests that APC reenters the atrium, using the SAN as part of the reentrant pathway inscribing two consecutive APCs. In panel 7, the coupling of the APC is 520 or 80 ms longer than in panel 6, the APC finds the perinodal tissue no longer refractory and discharges the SAN.

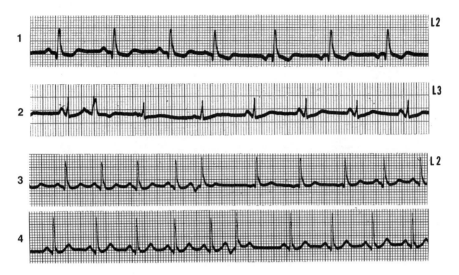

Figure 4-52. Compensatory pause. This figure illustrates displacement of the atrial pacemaker, atrial escape, postextrasystolic P wave aberration, and a full compensatory pause following an APC. In panel 1, the basic P-P interval is 860 ms. The APC is followed by a return cycle of 920 ms and an inverted P wave with a P-P interval of 860 ms identical to the sinus (SAN) interval. The latter is most likely fortuitous. In panel 2, the basic P-P interval is 800 ms. The aberrantly conducted APC is followed by a return cycle of 800 ms, which is the same as the SAN cycle. This suggests that the P wave terminating the return cycle is sinus in origin despite the fact that its configuration is different from the dominant sinus P wave. The P wave aberration is an example of postextrasystolic P wave aberration, a common finding. The exact mechanism of the aberration is unclear. In panel 3, the basic P-P interval is 560 ms. The APC is followed by a return cycle of 840 ms and three negative P waves representing an escape, either atrial or junctional, with a P-P interval of 680 ms. The return cycle of 840 ms, longer than the dominant cycle of 560 ms, indicates suppression of the SAN pacemaker by the APC. In panel 4, the basic P-P intervals vary from 560 to 660 ms. The pause following the APC is compensatory, with the interval between the two sinus P waves encompassing the APC of 1240 ms, twice the basic sinus cycle. The fact that the compensatory pause is full is fortuitous. The return cycle is longer than an SAN cycle and includes conduction from the APC to the SAN, from SAN to the atrium, and often suppression of the SAN. It has been suggested that the difference between the return cycle and the dominant cycle, divided by two, estimates the exit time from the sinus node. This, however, assumes equal retrograde and anterograde conduction to and from the SAN, an assumption that is difficult to prove. Furthermore, this formula does not consider the possible suppression of the SAN by the ectopic impulse.

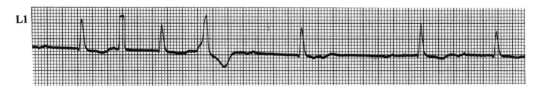

Figure 4-53. "Postponed" compensatory pause. The basic rhythm is sinus with a P-P of 920 ms and a P-R interval of 520 ms. The rhythm is interrupted by an interpolated VPC. The next P wave conducts with a P-R interval of 600 ms. The P that follows, with an R-P interval of 280 ms, is blocked. The compensatory pause is thus postponed.

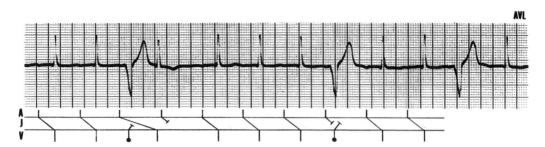

Figure 4-54. "Postponed" compensatory pause. The basic rhythm is sinus with a P-P interval of 630 ms interrupted by three VPCs, each with a coupling interval of 560 ms. The second VPC is followed by a full compensatory pause. The first VPC is interpolated with prolongation of the P-R interval from 280 to 600 ms and block of the subsequent P wave. Thus, the compensatory pause is postponed. The P wave that under ordinary circumstances would conduct to the ventricle, is blocked, postponing the compensatory pause. The slight aberration of the QRS complex following the interpolated VPC is caused by the shorter R-R interval.

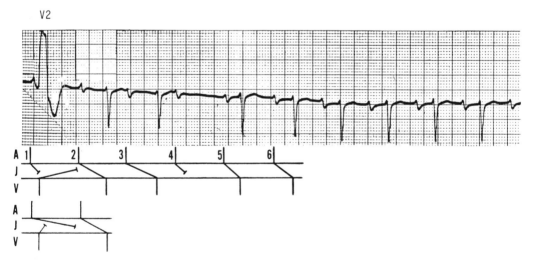

Figure 4-55. Pseudo Type I A-V block with a "postponed" compensatory pause. The PVC conceals into the AV node, delaying the P-R interval to 400 and 460 ms. The fourth P wave is blocked and is followed by the postponed compensatory pause.

5

Atrioventricular Conduction Abnormalities

First Degree Atrioventricular Block
Second Degree Atrioventricular Block
 Type I—Typical (Wenckebach)
   Atypical
 Type II—Mobitz
2:1 Second Degree Atrioventricular Block
High Degree (Advanced)
Paroxysmal Atrioventricular Block
Complete (Third Degree) Atrioventricular Block
Dual Atrioventricular Conduction
Atrioventricular Dissociation

A brief statement regarding His bundle electrocardiography (HBE) is pertinent at this point, because of the major contribution of the His recording to our understanding of A-V conduction and its various manifestations.

A multipolar electrode catheter is introduced percutaneously and positioned near the AV node. The His potential is recorded as a well defined spike between low atrial (A) and ventricular (V) electrograms. The interval between the earliest inscription of the P wave and the low atrial deflection is a measure of intraatrial conduction. The interval between A and H (A-H) estimates conduction across the AV node and measures 50 to 120 ms. The H-V interval is an estimate of His-Purkinje conduction, and is measured from His potential to the earliest ventricular deflection in any surface lead. The H-V interval is fairly constant, measuring 30 to 55 ms (Figure 5-1).

As indicated, our understanding of A-V conduction has been enhanced by the advent of HBE. A prolonged P-R interval may be due to delay of the P-A, A-H, or H-V intervals or a combination of the above. Most often, however, a prolonged P-R interval is due to a prolonged AV nodal conduction indicated by a prolonged A-H interval. HBE confirmed the fact that in the presence of a normal QRS complex, the block is usually at the level of the A-H or nodal site (Figure 5-1). On the other hand, with a prolonged QRS complex, the block can be either at A-H or H-V level. In the absence of preexisting BBB or aberration, an abnormal QRS complex indicates an infra-His block. Second degree, Wenckebach Type I block is nearly always at the level of the AV node, while Mobitz II Type II block, is nearly always infra-His. On rare occasions the block may be intra-His, resulting in Mobitz Type II with a normal QRS complex.

First Degree Atrioventricular Block

The P-R interval is a measure of A-V conduction time, the component of which includes intraatrial, A-H, and H-V conduction. Any one or all of the above may contribute to P-R interval prolongation. As a rule, however, P-R reflects intranodal (A-H) delay. The ECG diagnosis of first degree A-V block is based on a P-R interval longer than 200 ms. Occasionally, especially in the presence of slow rates, a P-R interval of 220 ms may be normal. Although the P-R interval may be prolonged to 600 or even 1000 ms, the usual range of first degree A-V block varies from 210 to 400 ms (Figure 5-2).

Second Degree Atrioventricular Block

The two types of second degree A-V block, namely Type I or Wenckebach and Type II or Mobitz, are characterized by block of some but not all of the P waves.

Wenckebach block is characterized by progressive prolongation of the P-R interval with gradual shortening of the R-P interval until a P wave is blocked. In the typical Wenckebach, the greatest P-R prolongation increment follows the second P of the Wenckebach sequence. The P-R interval increases but, importantly, with a decreasing increment thereafter. As a result, there is a gradual shortening of R-R interval. The P-R interval following the pause is normal. This, coupled with the fact that the longest P-R interval is before the block of the P wave and the shortest after the block results in the long pause being less than the sum of two preceding basic cycles (Figures 5-3, 5-4, and 5-5) (see Chapter 16). In Type I A-V block, the first P-R of a sequence may be normal or prolonged.

On occasion, the Wenckebach sequence can be terminated by an APC or a retrograde P wave (Figures 5-6 and 5-7), and the long pause by a junctional escape or escape rhythm (Figure 5-8).

In atypical Type I A-V block, the P-R and R-R intervals terminating the Wenckebach sequence are longer than expected and, in fact, may be the longest of the sequence. Other findings indicative of atypical Wenckebach block include consecutive P-R intervals of the same duration, an unexpected decrease in P-R, or failure of the second P-R interval to manifest the greatest increment in P-R. The longer the Wenckebach sequence, the more likely that the Wenckebach will be atypical. The prevalence of atypical forms exceeds 50% (Figure 5-9).

Rarely, the P-R interval may be longer than the P-P interval and the P wave may be "skipped" by the long P-R interval (Figure 5-10).

Since the A-V block is at the level of the AV node and above the bifurcation of the bundle of His, the QRS complex in Type I A-V block is normal unless there is a preexisting BBB or rate-related aberration.

In Type II A-V block, the P-R interval is constant and does not change prior to the block. Type II block is below the bundle of His; thus, the QRS complex is abnormal, with the most common abnormality being RBBB with LAFB (Figures 5-11, 5-12, and 5-13). When the block is within the bundle of His (a rare finding) the QRS complex is normal.

2:1 Second Degree Atrioventricular Block

As stated above 2:1 A-V block may be either Type I or Type II (Figure 5-14). In the absence of two consecutive sinus impulses, it is difficult if not impossible to differentiate the two. Certain findings may be helpful. If the P-R interval is prolonged and the QRS complex normal, the block is most likely Type I. If the P-R interval is normal and the QRS complex abnormal, the block is most likely Type II (Figure 5-14). On the other hand, if the P-R interval is prolonged with a BBB or if the P-R interval is normal with a normal QRS complex, the differential between Type I and Type II A-V block is confounded.

High Degree (Advanced) Atrioventricular Block

High degree Type I, but more often Type II, A-V block is characterized by two or more consecutive blocked P waves. The block may be interrupted by isolated junctional or ventricular escape or by intermittent AV dissociation with ventricular captures (Figures 5-15, 5-16, and 5-17).

Paroxysmal Atrioventricular Block

This form of A-V block is characterized by an abrupt and persistent A-V block in the presence of otherwise normal A-V conduction. The block may be initiated by a conducted or blocked APC or VPC or acceleration or slowing of the sinus rhythm. Once the block is initiated, it persists until terminated by an escape, usually ventricular, with a predictable relationship of the escape to the following conducting P wave. The block is most likely infra-His or subnodal and due to bilateral BBB (Figure 5-18), although the exact mechanism is unclear.

Complete (Third Degree) Atrioventricular Block

Complete A-V block is characterized by failure of all P waves to reach the ventricle. The subsidiary pacemaker discharges regularly, at a rate of 40 to 50 per minute if junctional, and on occasion at a rate of 30 per minute or lower if the impulse originates in the Purkinje fibers.

In the absence of preexisting BBB or aberration, the QRS complex is normal when the subsidiary pacemaker is junctional. The QRS complex is wide if the pacemaker site is ventricular (Figures 5-19, 5-20, and 5-21).

Dual Atrioventricular Conduction

Dual AV conduction is most likely a variant of normal AV conduction with two pathways that have differing refractory periods and conduction. The two pathways may be distinct anatomical structures or they may be functionally distinct.

On the surface ECG, the most common manifestation of dual AV conduction is AVNRT with anterograde slow and retrograde fast pathway conduction. In the presence of sinus rhythm, the dual conduction may manifest as an abrupt change in P-R interval, P-R alternans (Figure 5-22), or, rarely, dual ventricular response to a single supraventricular stimulus (see Chapter 17).

Atrioventricular Dissociation

With AV dissociation, the atria are under the control of the SAN, an atrial ectopic focus, or, rarely, a junctional focus, while the ventricles are driven by an independent usually junctional or, occasionally, ventricular focus. Dissociation occurs when the dominant rate slows allowing the subsidiary pacemaker to escape (Figures 5-23 and 5-24) or when a pathologically accelerated subsidiary pacemaker usurps the control of the heart (Figures 5-25 and 5-26). Dissociation is maintained because the P wave arrives at the junction at a time when the latter is refractory following the immediately preceding junctional discharge. It is therefore apparent that in the case of slow junctional rhythms, AV dissociation can exist only if the sinus and junctional rates are approximately the same. A faster sinus rhythm will sooner or later arrive after recovery of the junction, capturing control of the ventricles for one or more cycles. This type of AV dissociation, due to a physiological interference between two pacemakers with almost identical rates, has been referred to as isorhythmic dissociation (Figures 5-25 and 5-26). If such is present for a short period of time, it is occasionally referred to as "accrochage" and, if present for longer periods, "synchronization."

With depressed A-V conduction, either anterograde or retrograde, AV dissociation can be maintained with greater ease.

A rare form of AV dissociation may occur when two independent foci exist in the junction, one activating the atria with inverted P to II, III, and AVF, and the second activating the ventricles. There may be an occasional ventricular capture by the upper focus. This type of rhythm, "double" junctional rhythm, is differentiated from junctional rhythm with reentry by: 1) the lack of a fixed relationship between the P wave and the QRS complex and 2) the atria and ventricles both exhibiting a regular rhythm but at different rates (Figures 5-27 and 5-28).

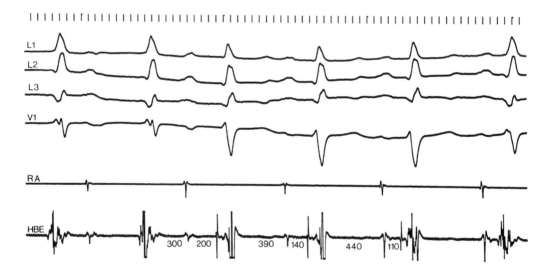

Figure 5-1. The R-P to P-R relationship. The leads include L1, L2, L3, V_1, right atrial (RA), and HBE. The first two and the last QRS complexes are ventricular in origin as indicated by lack of a His potential. The R-P following the three sinus-conducted impulses measure 300, 390, and 440, and the respective P-R measure 200, 140, and 110 ms. The figure illustrates the inverse relationship of the R-P and the P-R. This relationship of R-P and P-R is one of the basic principles of A-V conduction.

ID: 001033620

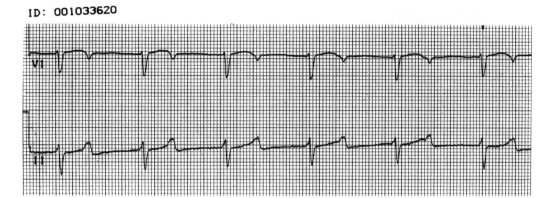

Figure 5-2. First degree A-V block. The diagnosis is indicated by the prolonged P-R interval of approximately 640 ms.

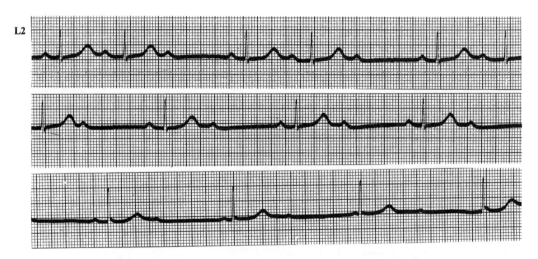

Figure 5-3. Wenckebach Type I A-V block. The top row illustrates a 3:2 Wenckebach A-V block presenting as a bigeminal rhythm. A bigeminal rhythm in the absence of premature ectopic impulses is nearly always a 3:2 Wenckebach. In the middle tracing, the rhythm is sinus with a 2:1 A-V block. In the bottom tracing, the block is complete with a regular R-R interval of 1800 ms and a P-P of 920 ms.

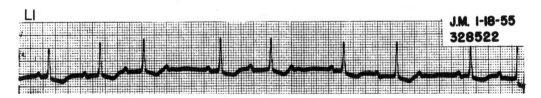

Figure 5-4. Wenckebach Type I A-V block. The basic rhythm is sinus with a P-P interval of 720 ms. There is a gradual prolongation of the P-R interval from 240 ms to 340 ms and block of the third P wave. The long pause is less than the sum of two preceding R-R intervals, a classic pattern of Wenckebach conduction.

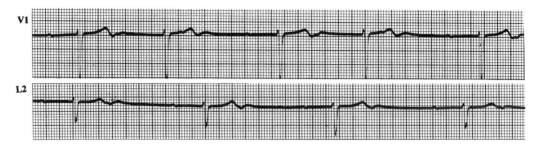

Figure 5-5. Wenckebach Type I A-V block. In lead V_1, the rhythm is bigeminal. The P-R interval lengthens from 490 ms to 640 ms before the P wave is blocked. In L2, the A-V conduction is 2:1 with a P-R interval of the conducted P of 480 ms.

ID: 001061621

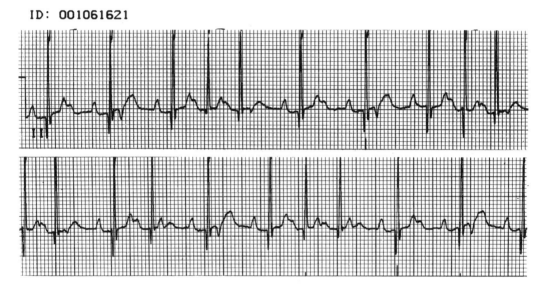

Figure 5-6. Wenckebach Type A-V block. An example of the Wenckebach sequence is recorded in the middle of the bottom row. Beginning with the sixth sinus P wave, the P-R interval increases gradually from 180 ms to 240 ms until a sinus P wave is blocked. In the remainder, the Wenckebach sequence is terminated by a negative, retrograde, reentrant P wave.

ID: 001074507

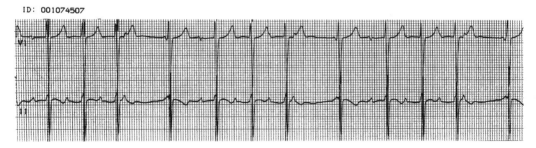

Figure 5-7. Wenckebach Type I A-V block. The Wenckebach sequence is terminated by an APC and a junctional escape.

L2

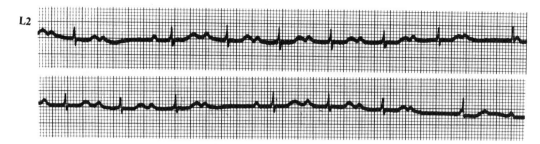

Figure 5-8. Atypical Wenckebach Type I A-V block. A 7:6 A-V block is illustrated in the top row and a 4:3 block in the bottom row. The long pause is followed by a junctional escape. The R-R does not shorten, as expected, indicating an atypical form of Wenckebach block.

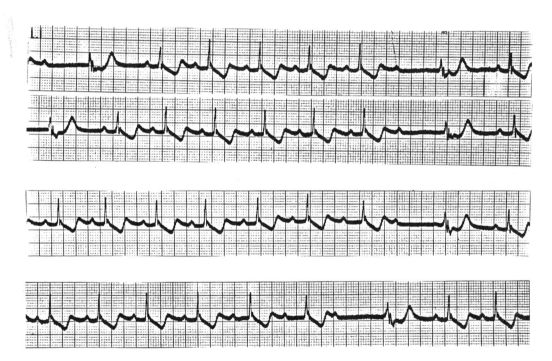

Figure 5-9. Atypical Wenckebach Type I A-V block. The four tracings are part of a continuous record. In the top two rows, the P-R interval is constant at approximately 240 ms with sudden block of a P wave. In the third and the fourth rows, there is a gradual prolongation of the P-R interval from 240 to 340 and 360 ms, respectively. Each pause is terminated by a ventricular escape. In the top two tracings, the sudden block of the P wave without antecedent prolongation of the P-R interval suggests Mobitz Type II A-V block. However, the gradual prolongation of the P-R interval in the third and fourth tracings indicate a Type I A-V block. One can assume an attempted Type I A-V block in the top two tracings. The maximal increment of the P-R just before the block in the third and fourth rows and the failure of the last R-R to shorten indicate an atypical Wenckebach block. From Knoebel SB, Konecke LL, Fisch C. Pacing in myocardial infarction. In: *Atherosclerosis and Coronary Artery Disease.* New York: Grune and Stratton; 1972:412–421.

VI

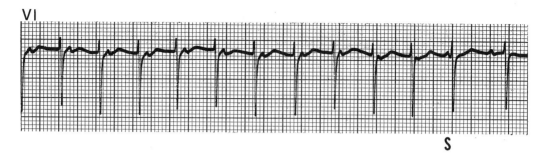

Figure 5-10. Wenckebach Type I A-V block with "skipped" P waves. The basic rhythm is an atrial tachycardia with an R-R of 400 ms. The first P-R interval measures 320 ms. Gradual minimal prolongation of the P-R interval continues until the P-R reaches 360 ms. The third P wave from the end, partially "buried" in the QRS complex, conducts to the ventricle "skipping" the second from the end sinus P wave. This is possible because the P-R interval is longer than the P-P interval. A sinus impulse follows the tachycardia.

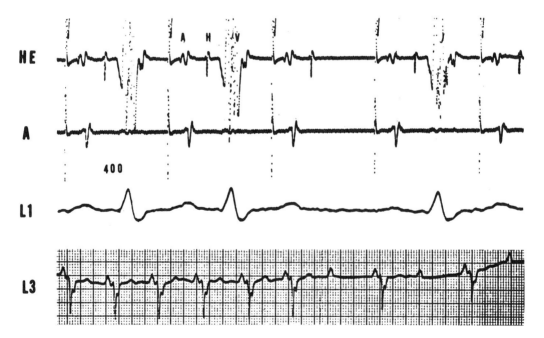

Figure 5-11. Mobitz Type II block. The heart is paced. The first two A-H and H-V intervals are constant, the third paced atrial complex is blocked below the His bundle. In the surface ECG, the QRS complex exhibits RBBB and LAFB. In L3 of the surface ECG, the P-R interval is constant with an abrupt block of a P wave, a feature characteristic of Mobitz Type II A-V block.

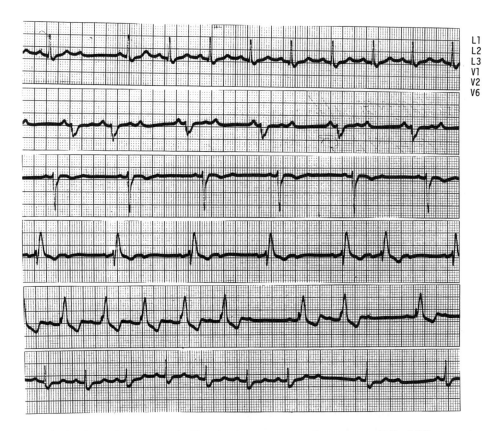

Figure 5-12. Mobitz Type II block. The rhythm is sinus with a constant P-R of 200 ms with an abrupt block of a P wave. The QRS morphology is that of RBBB with LAFB, a common pattern seen with Mobitz Type II block.

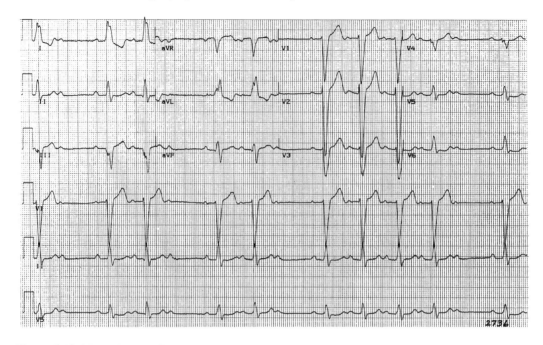

Figure 5-13. Mobitz Type II A-V block. The basic rhythm is sinus, with a constant P-R of 240 ms with an abrupt block of a P wave. The QRS morphology is that of LBBB. Failure of the P-R interval to lengthen coupled QRS complexes with LBBB are indicative of Mobitz Type II A-V block.

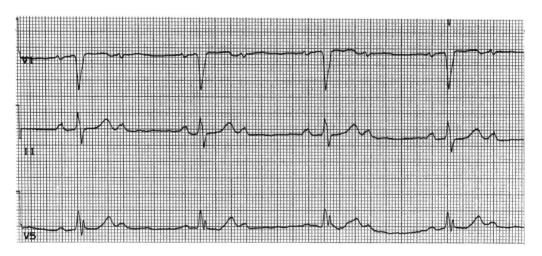

Figure 5-14. Second degree A-V block. The basic rhythm is sinus at a rate of 75 per minute, a P-R interval of 240 ms, a QRS duration of 120 ms, and a 2:1 A-V block. A 2:1 A-V block is difficult to differentiate between Type I and Type II. In this instance, the P-R interval is only slightly longer than normal, and the QRS complex abnormal, suggesting Mobitz Type II block.

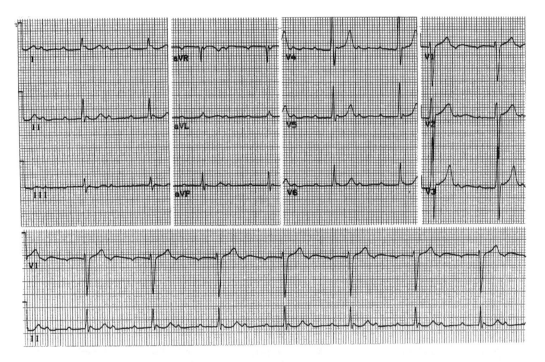

Figure 5-15. Advanced (high degree) A-V block. The basic rhythm is sinus or an atrial tachycardia at a rate of 167 per minute. There is a 3:1 A-V block with a P-P of 360 ms, a P-R interval of 320 ms, and a normal QRS complex. The prolonged P-R interval and a normal QRS complex suggest that the block is at the AV nodal level.

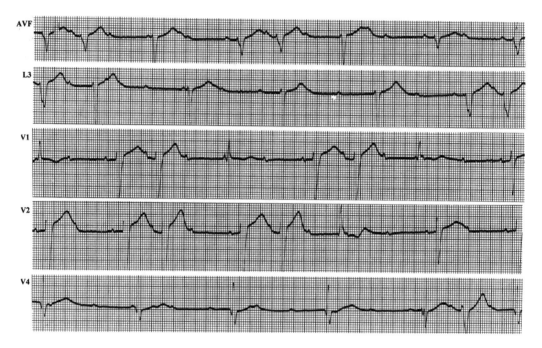

Figure 5-16. Advanced (high degree) A-V block. The basic rhythm is sinus with a P-P interval of 720 ms and a constant P-R of 220 ms. The ventricular configuration is that of LBBB. In leads L3 and V$_4$, the return cycle following the blocked P wave is terminated by a junctional escape rhythm. Normalization of the QRS complex following a prolonged cycle indicates that the LBBB is acceleration-dependent aberration.

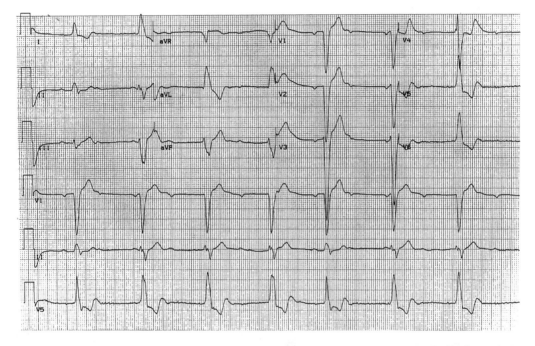

Figure 5-17. Advanced (high degree) A-V block. The basic rhythm is sinus with AV dissociation with a P-P interval of 800 ms and an R-R interval of 1320 ms. The idioventricular complexes are of LBBB configuration. That this is not a complete heart block is indicated by two captures (first and fifth QRS complexes) in II with a P-R interval of 260 ms.

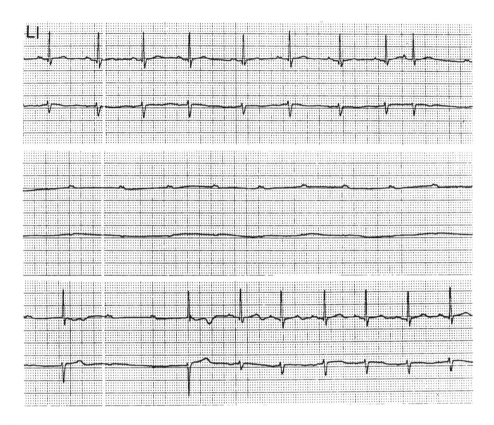

Figure 5-18. Paroxysmal A-V block. The basic rhythm is sinus with a P-P of 720 ms, and a normal P-R interval and QRS complex. Complete A-V block with a ventricular standstill terminated by a junctional QRS complex is followed by sinus rhythm. While most likely the block is infra-His, the exact mechanism is unclear.

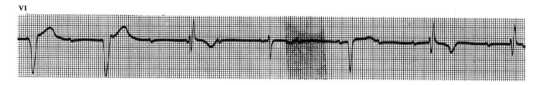

Figure 5-19. Complete A-V block with fusions. The basic rhythm is sinus with a P-P of 800 ms and complete A-V block. The first two idioventricular impulses originate in the right ventricle, and the third, sixth, and seventh originate in the left ventricle. The fourth and fifth complexes are fusions. The fusion is the result of simultaneous activation of both chambers by the respective ectopic impulses.

ID: 001033570

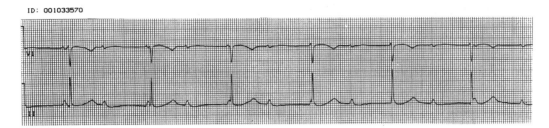

Figure 5-20. Complete A-V block. The basic rhythm is sinus with a P-P interval of 800 ms. The QRS complexes are normal and the R-R intervals regular at 1600 ms. The site of origin of the ventricular rhythm is in the AV junction.

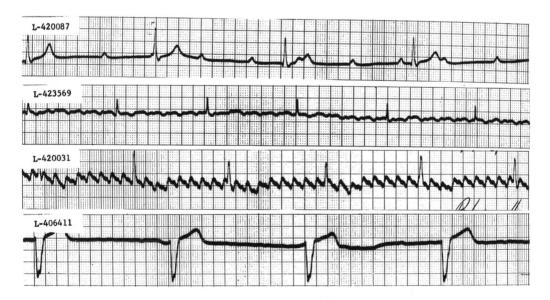

Figure 5-21. Complete A-V block. The complete A-V block is associated with sinus rhythm (top row), atrial tachycardia (second row), atrial flutter (third row), and atrial fibrillation (bottom row).

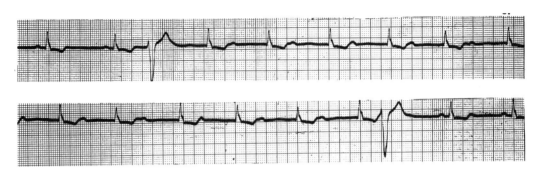

Figure 5-22. Dual AV nodal conduction. Following the first interpolated VPC, the R-P interval shortens from 1320 to 480 ms and the P-R interval lengthens from 180 to 720 ms. The second VPC is followed by normal A-V conduction. The first interpolated VPC blocks the fast pathway and forces the impulse down the slow pathway. Repetitive concealed conduction from the slow pathway to the fast pathway blocks conduction in the latter and contributes to the perpetuation of the long P-R interval. The second VPC blocks the slow pathway, with conduction along the fast pathway and normal A-V conduction (see Chapter 17).

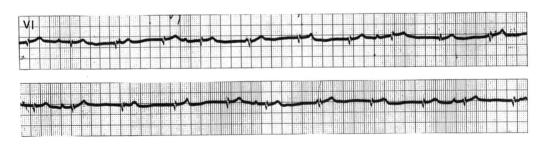

Figure 5-23. AV dissociation. The basic rhythm is sinus bradycardia with a P-P interval of 1200 ms. The QRS complexes are junctional with an R-R of 1050 ms. An occasional sinus impulse conducts to the ventricle (capture), ruling out A-V block. The P-R of the captures is inversely related to the respective R-P interval.

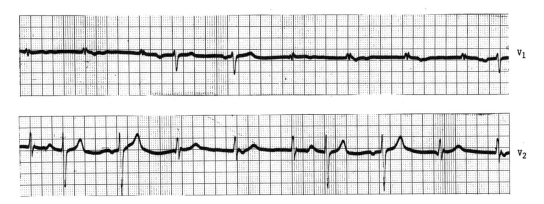

Figure 5-24. AV dissociation. The basic rhythm is sinus with a P-P of approximately 600 ms and an escape rhythm either junctional, fascicular, or ventricular with an R-R of 1040 ms. The escape rhythm is interrupted on three occasions by sinus impulses with a P-R that is inversely related to the R-P interval. The sinus conduction with a normal P-R rules out A-V block. From Zipes DP, Fisch C. Atrioventricular dissociation. *Arch Intern Med* 1973;131:593–595.

ID: 001099014

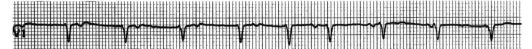

Figure 5-25. AV dissociation. There are two independent rhythms with an R-R of 720 ms and a P-P of 760 ms. In the middle of the tracing, two P waves with R-P intervals of 220 and 320 ms, respectively, capture the ventricles, ruling out A-V block. The AV dissociation is due to the fact that the more rapid ventricular rhythm usurps control of the heart. However, since the two rates differ, the P wave will ultimately fall outside the refractory period of the AV node, and will capture the ventricle. This type of physiological AV dissociation with almost identical pacemaker rates is referred to as "isorhythmic dissociation."

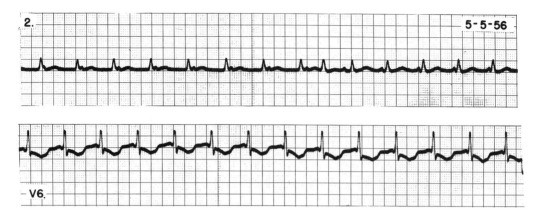

Figure 5-26. AV dissociation. The P-P and the R-R intervals measure approximately 600 ms. Although the difference is minimal and difficult to detect, the junctional rhythm must be slightly faster than the atrial, as indicated by the gradual prolongation of the R-P interval and ultimate capture of the ventricle by the sinus P waves. The eighth and ninth P wave in lead II conduct to the ventricles with P-R intervals of 320 ms and 160 ms, respectively. Conduction of the P wave to the ventricles with a normal P-R interval indicates that the AV dissociation is functional and due to physiological refractoriness.

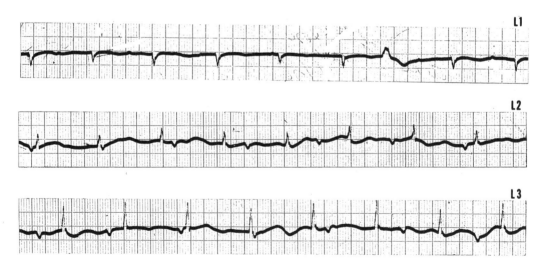

Figure 5-27. "Double" AV nodal rhythm. The P waves are nearly isoelectric in lead I, and negative in L2 and L3. The P-P interval is regular at 1100 ms. The R-R interval is also regular at 960 ms. Since none of the P waves capture the ventricles, the dual AV nodal rhythm is associated with complete A-V block.

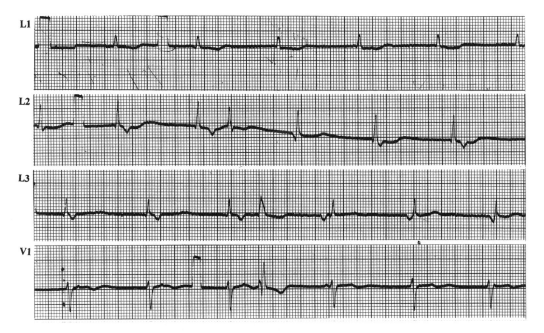

Figure 5-28. "Double" AV nodal rhythm. The P waves are isoelectric in lead I and inverted in L2 and L3 with a regular P-P interval of 1200 ms. The fourth complexes in L2, L3, and V$_1$ are sinus captures with an appropriate P-R interval. Two rhythms, each regular but at a different rate, indicate AV dissociation. In this instance, both pacemakers, the atrial and the ventricular, are located in the AV node; thus, a double nodal rhythm.

Section II

Complex Arrhythmias Diagnosis and Mechanisms Based Primarily on Deductive Analysis

---

6

Concealed Conduction

Concealed conduction is manifest by incomplete conduction of an impulse that results in an unexpected, "unphysiological," response of the subsequent impulse (Figure 6-1).

Historical Perspective

Recognition of concealed conduction antedates the advent of the ECG. In 1894, some 9 years before Einthoven introduced the ECG, Engelmann,[1] working with a hanging heart preparation, wrote, " . . . *every effective atrial contraction, even if it does not elicit a ventricular systole it prolongs the subsequent AV interval.*" Although Engelmann did not study impulse conduction or the concept of concealed conduction per se, he noted that atrial activity, even if it does not conduct to the ventricle, may influence subsequent transmission of an atrial impulse. This observation set the stage for recognition of concealed conduction as a mechanism for altered, albeit "silent," electrophysiological events on the surface ECG.

Concealed conduction of sinus impulses at the level of the AV node was documented independently in dogs in 1925 by Lewis and Master,[2] Drury,[3] and Scherf and Shookhoff .[4] In 1925, Ashman[5] noted concealed conduction in compressed turtle hearts. Beginning some 20 years later, Langendorf, Pick, and Katz[6–9] published a series of papers expanding the concept and applying it to humans. Subsequent studies in animals and humans showed that the concept of concealed conduction is applicable to the atria, the SA perinodal tissue, the SAN, the intraventricular conducting tissues, and the His-Purkinje system.[10–12]

General Concepts

As stated above, the basis for the diagnosis of concealed conduction is incomplete (concealed) penetration of an impulse resulting in an unexpected behavior of the subsequent impulse (Figure 6-2). The effect on subsequent events is an important part of the definition of concealed conduction because it differentiates the concept of concealed conduction from other forms of incomplete conduction, such as conduction blocks (Figure 6-3). It should be recalled that although the ECG reflects the electrophysiological properties of the myocardium, alterations of conduction more often reflect electrophysiological changes in the specialized tissues, the activity of which is not recorded on the surface ECG. The diagnosis of concealed conduction is therefore based on deductive analysis, much as was Engelmann's on the effect of atrial conduction on the timing of ventricular contraction.

A diagnosis of concealed conduction ideally should be supported, if possible, by evidence that an impulse that is blocked at times will, given the opportunity and the proper physiological setting, conduct fully (Figures 6-4, 6-5, and 6-6). Such stringent evidence cannot always be satisfied, however, nor is it absolutely essential for the diagnosis of concealed conduction. For example, even though it is certain that prolongation of the P-R interval following an interpolated VPC is the result of retrograde concealed conduction of the ventricular impulse, instances of complete retrograde conduction of a VPC may not always be demonstrable (Figure 6-7).

Electrocardiography of Concealed Conduction

Because of variations of the site of impulse formation, the different effects of the anatomical site, the direction of the concealment, and the changing electrophysiological milieu at the time of the concealment (e.g., the heart rate, automatic tone, drugs, or electrolyte balance), the manifestations of concealed conduction are numerous and are listed in Table 6-1.

The most common forms of concealment are at the level of the AV node and the bundle branches, and include: 1) alteration of anterograde conduction, 2) alteration of retrograde (ventriculoatrial [V-A]) conduction, 3) displacement of a junctional pacemaker, 4) enhancement of A-V conduction, 5) effects on His bundle potentials, and 6) alteration of His-Purkinje conduction.

Effects on Conduction at the Level of the Atrioventricular Node

At the level of the AV node, anterograde A-V concealment may be manifest by: 1) delay of A-V conduction (Figure 6-4); 2) block of A-V conduction (Figure 6-2); 3) delay and block of A-V conduction (Figure 6-8); 4) block of retrograde (V-A) conduction (Figure 6-9); and 5) slowing of the ventricular response to atrial fibrillation (Figure 6-10).

Table 6-1

Manifestations of Concealed Conduction

Anterograde A-V concealment manifested by
    Delay of A-V conduction
    Block of A-V conduction
    Continued delay or block of A-V conduction
    Block of retrograde (V-A) conduction
    Slowing of ventricular rate due to concealment of atrial fibrillatory waves
Retrograde (V-A) concealment manifested by
    Delay of A-V conduction
    Block of A-V conduction
    Delay and block of A-V conduction
    Initiation and termination of A-V junctional tachycardia
Displacement of a junctional pacemaker by concealment of
    An anterograde conducting impulse
    An anterograde conducting impulse during the supernormal period
    Concealed reentry
    Retrograde (V-A) conduction
Enhancement of A-V conduction
Concealed junctional (His) impulse manifested by
    Isolated P-R prolongation
    Pseudo type I A-V block
    Pseudo type II A-V block
    Exit block of a nonparoxysmal junctional tachycardia impulse
Concealed conduction in the His-Purkinje tissue

Retrograde (V-A) concealment may be manifest by delay of A-V conduction, delay and block of A-V conduction, and initiation and termination of AV junctional tachycardia (Figure 6-12).

Displacement of Junctional Pacemaker

Displacement of a junctional pacemaker may be due to a concealed anterograde conducting impulse (Figures 6-11 and 6-13), a concealed anterograde conduction during the supernormal period (Figure 6-14), concealed anterograde reentry (Figure 6-15), and retrograde (V-A) conduction.

A concealed junctional (His bundle) impulse may be manifest by: 1) block of P wave (Figure 6-16); 2) isolated P-R prolongation (Figure 6-17); 3) Type I A-V block (Figure 6-18); 4) Type II A-V block (Figure 6-19; 5) 2:1 A-V block (Figure 6-20); 6) NPJT with exit block (Figure 6-21; and 7) concealed VPC (Figure 6-22).

Aberration

Concealed conduction as a cause of aberration is discussed in Chapter 7 (see aberration).

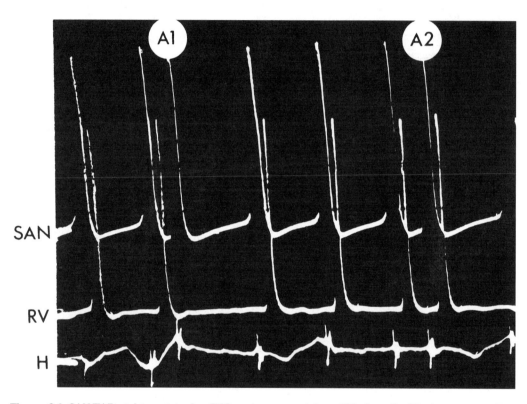

Figure 6-1. SAN TAP, right ventricular (RV) action potential, and His bundle (H) electrogram. The automatic sinus impulse conducts to the H and the RV. It is interrupted by two premature stimuli (A1 and A2). A2 conducts to the H and RV while A1 activates the H but fails to reach the RV. This tracing demonstrates incomplete conduction of A2 with block at the level of the His bundle. This record confirms the validity of the concept of concealed conduction by documenting incomplete conduction at the cellular level. From Knoebel SB, Fisch C. Concealed conduction. In Fisch C (ed): Complex Electrocardiography *I.* Philadelphia: FA Davis; 1973:22.

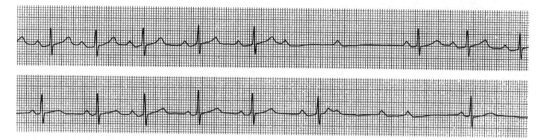

Figure 6-2. Concealed conduction and block of atrial conduction. Following the APC, the sinus P wave fails to conduct. In the bottom row, the APC is followed by a couplet of sinus P waves, neither of which reaches the ventricle. The unexpected block of the P waves is due to concealed conduction of the APCs to the level of the AV node.

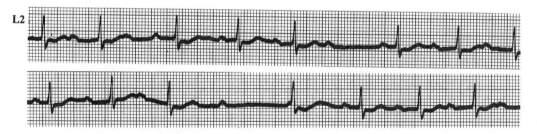

Figure 6-3. Concealed conduction with block of atrial conduction. The basic rhythm is sinus with APCs and Wenckebach A-V block. In the bottom row, the P-R interval prolongs gradually. This Wenckebach sequence is interrupted by a nonconducted APC (superimposed on third T), which blocks the subsequent P wave. The return cycle is terminated by a junctional escape, following which a Wenckebach sequence resumes. The failure of the APC to conduct is due to prematurity. Block of the P wave that follows is unexpected, as the sufficiently long R-P interval would allow conduction. The failure of the P wave to conduct in the presence of a sufficiently long R-P interval is due to concealed conduction of the blocked premature APC to the level of the AV node.

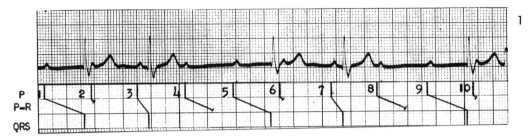

Figure 6-4. Concealed conduction, sinus rhythm, 2:1 A-V block. The mechanism responsible for the unexpectedly long P-R interval of 520 ms following P5 and P9 is concealed conduction of P4 and P8, respectively. P2 and P6, because of a short R-P interval, are blocked high in the AV node and, thus, do not interfere with conduction of P3 and P7, the latter conducting with a P-R interval of 140 ms. It is possible that P4 and P8 block conduction of P5 and P9 and that the QRS complexes that follow represent junctional escapes. In either event, the mechanism responsible for abnormal prolongation of the P-R interval or for A-V block with escape is concealed conduction of P4 and P8. From Knoebel SB, Fisch C. Concealed conduction. In Fisch C (ed): *Complex Electrocardiography I.* Philadelphia: FA Davis; 1973:22.

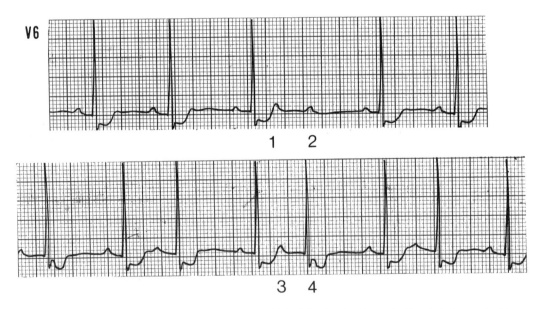

Figure 6-5. Concealed conduction and block of APCs. The basic sinus rhythm is interrupted by a couplet of APCs. In the upper tracing, the second APC (2) is blocked by concealed conduction of the first APC (1). The assumption of concealed conduction of the first APC to the level of the AV node is supported by the fact that a "similar" APC (3) in the bottom tracing, after a slightly longer R-P interval, conducts to the ventricle. From Fisch C. Concealed Conduction. In Zipes DP (ed): *Symposium on Arrhythmias I. Cardiac Clinics.* Philadelphia: W.B. Saunders; 1983:63.

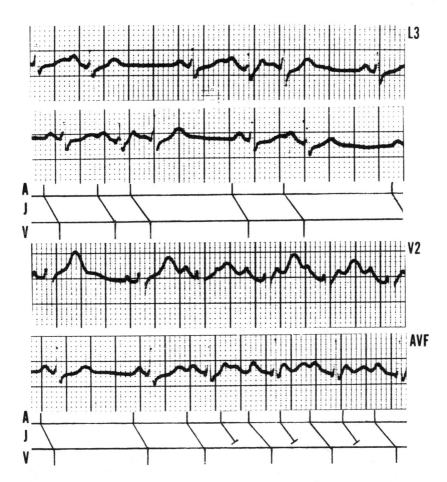

Figure 6-6. Concealed conduction and atrial tachycardia with 2:1 A-V block. The records are sections of a continuous tracing. The first cycles in leads V$_2$ and AVF are the last of the basic sinus rhythm and are followed by an APC and atrial tachycardia with 2:1 A-V block. The P-R interval of the conducted P waves of the atrial tachycardia lengthens from 60 to 180 ms. The paradoxical or unexpected prolongation of the P-R interval of the conducted P from 120 to 180 ms with the onset of atrial tachycardia is due to concealed conduction of the blocked P wave. This assumption is supported by the fact that the second APC of the couplet in lead III, at a slightly longer R-P interval than the R-P interval of the blocked P wave in leads V$_2$ and AVF, conducts to the ventricle. From Fisch C. Concealed Conduction—85 years after engelmann. In Befeler B (ed): *Selected Topics in Cardiac Arrhythmias.* Mount Kisco: Futura Publishing Co., Inc.; 1980:359.

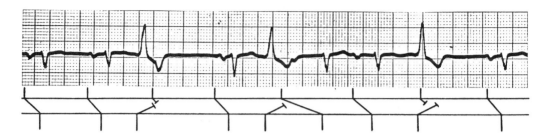

Figure 6-7. VPCs with concealed retrograde conduction. Block or delay of A-V conduction depends on the proximity of the P wave to the preceding QRS complex. The two blocked sinus P waves reach the AV junction during its absolute refractory period induced by concealed retrograde conduction of the VPC and thus fail to conduct. The sinus P wave following the interpolated VPC (second premature) reaches the AV node during its relative refractory period induced by concealed retrograde conduction of the VPC, and conducts with a prolonged P-R interval of 400 ms; the R-P interval of the subsequent sinus P wave is lengthened. The P wave falls during the relative refractory period of the AV junction and conducts with a prolonged P-R interval of 320 ms.

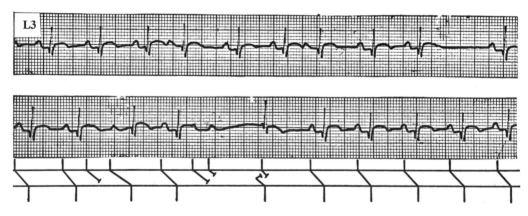

Figure 6-8. APCs with concealed conduction. Conducted and blocked APCs are recorded in the top tracing. The R-P and P-R intervals of the conducted APCs are 300 and 200 ms, respectively. Two premature atrial couplets are recorded in the bottom tracing. The second premature of the first couplet with an R-P interval of 490 ms conducts with a P-R interval of 280 ms. The second premature of the second couplet, with an R-P interval of 440 ms, is blocked. The APCs suppress the sinus node, and the pause is terminated by a junctional escape. Delay and failure of conduction of the second premature of the respective couplets is due to concealed conduction of the first P wave of the couplet. This assumption is supported by fact that the first APC in the top tracing, with a slightly longer R-P interval than the R-P interval of the first APC of the couplet in the bottom tracing, conducts to the ventricle. From Knoebel SB, Fisch C. Concealed conduction. In Fisch C (ed): *Complex Electrocardiography I.* Philadelphia: FA Davis; 1973:22.

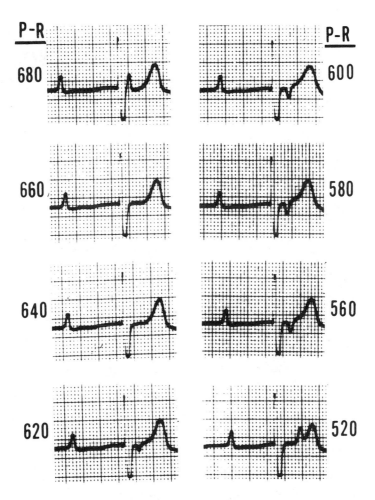

Figure 6-9. Concealed anterograde conduction blocking V-A conduction. The sections are a part of a continuous record illustrating the temporal relationship of the sinus P wave, the QRS complex, and V-A conduction. In the right panel, at a "P-R" interval of 600, 580, and 560 ms, the atria are activated retrogradely. At a "P-R" interval of 520 ms, concealed anterograde conduction of the sinus P wave blocks retrograde conduction. In the left panel, at a "P-R" interval of 680 ms, a normal sinus wave follows the QRS complex. At "P-R" intervals of 660, 640, and 620 ms, the retrograde and the sinus impulses collide, resulting in atrial fusions.

V-1

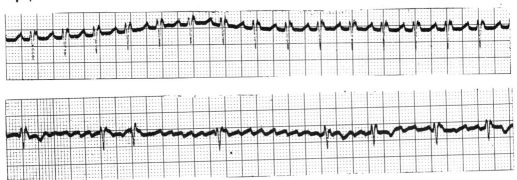

Figure 6-10. Atrial flutter, atrial fibrillation, and concealed conduction. With atrial fibrillation, the numerous atrial impulses and consequently the potential for concealed conduction is greatly increased. The concealed conduction is random with regard to rate and depth of junctional penetration. Repetitive concealment of successive atrial impulses may result in relatively long R-R intervals. Since the "strength" of the atrial impulse, depth of penetration, speed of conduction, duration of the refractory periods, and number of successive concealed impulses are random, the ventricular response during atrial fibrillation is also random. On the other hand, atrial flutter with regular atrial activity and thus a uniform duration of the refractory period results in a regular ventricular rhythm with the rate depending on the degree of A-V block. From Knoebel SB, Fisch C. Concealed conduction. In Fisch C (ed): *Complex Electrocardiography I.* Philadelphia: FA Davis; 1973:22.

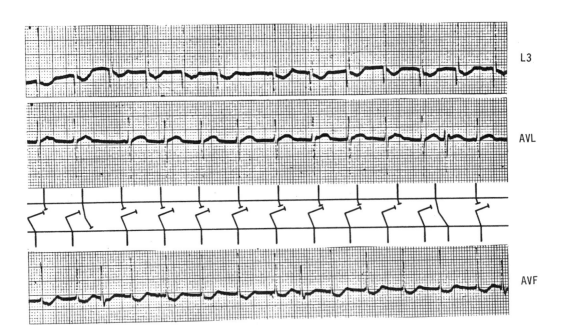

L3

AVL

AVF

Figure 6-11. Concealed conduction with reset of the junctional pacemaker. The figure illustrates AV dissociation with a NPJT with an R-R interval of 560 ms. The unexpected prolongation of the R-R interval to 820 ms is caused by concealed conduction of the sinus P wave into the AV node with discharge and displacement of the junctional pacemaker. This is supported by captures with a slightly longer R-P interval. Similarly, the longer R-R equals the R-R enclosing a sinus capture. From Knoebel SB, Fisch C. Concealed conduction. In Fisch C (ed): *Complex Electrocardiography I.* Philadelphia: FA Davis; 1973:22.

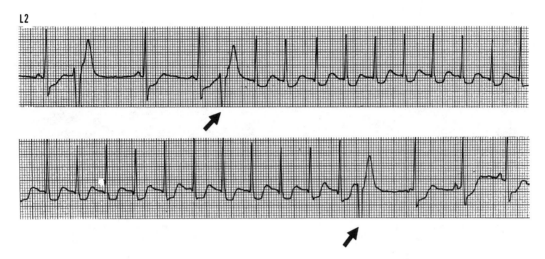

Figure 6-12. Initiation and termination of reentrant junctional tachycardia by concealed conduction of VPCs. The second VPC (arrow) conducts retrogradely to the atrium and initiates a reentrant junctional tachycardia. Evidence for V-A conduction is the retrograde P wave recorded on the upstroke of the T wave and the absence of the sinus P wave where expected. The junctional tachycardia is terminated by concealed retrograde conduction of a VPC (second arrow). The latter reaches the reentrant pathway and interrupts the circus movement.

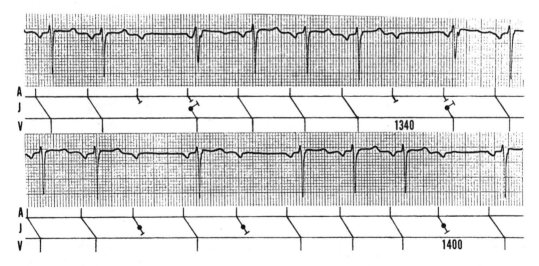

Figure 6-13. Displacement of an escape pacemaker by a concealed sinus impulse. In the bottom tracing, the sinus rhythm with a P-R interval of 180 ms is interrupted by what appears to be Type II A-V block. The R-R intervals encompassing the blocked P wave measure 1400 ms. In the top tracing, the long R-R cycles encompassing the blocked P wave measure 1340 ms, and are terminated by an escape. Failure of an escape in the bottom tracing, despite an R-R interval of 1400 ms, is due to concealed conduction of the blocked P wave to the level of the junctional pacemaker discharging and resetting the escape pacemaker, thus allowing sufficient time for the next sinus P wave to conduct to the ventricle. In the top tracing, the P wave was blocked above the site of the escape pacemaker. Otherwise the junctional pacemaker would have been reset, as in the bottom tracing, and a normal sinus impulse conduction would have followed.

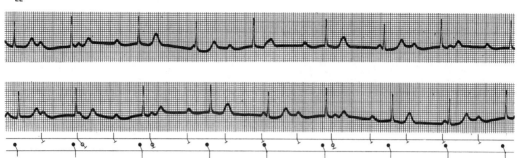

Figure 6-14. Concealed conduction during the supernormal period. The P-P interval measures 740 ms, and the basic R-R interval measures 1200 ms. Five R-R cycles are longer than the basic R-R cycles, varying in duration from 1360 to 1480 ms. Each encompasses an early P wave with an R-P interval that varies from 120 to 160 ms. The normal QRS configuration indicates that the site of origin is above the bifurcation of the bundle of His. The P wave with an R-P interval that varies from 120 to 160 ms reaches the junction during the supernormal phase of recovery and resets the pacemaker, accounting for the unexpectedly long R-R intervals. From Fisch C. Concealed conduction— 85 years after Engelmann. In Befeler B (ed:) *Selected Topics in Cardiac Arrhythmias.* Mount Kisco:

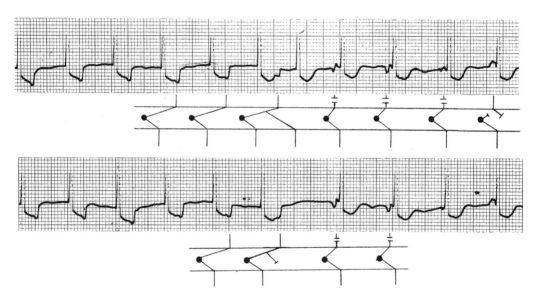

Figure 6-15. NPJT with retrograde Wenckebach conduction and concealed ventricular reentry. In the top tracing, the junctional QRS complexes, at an R-R of 600 ms, are followed by retrograde P waves with a progressively lengthening R-P interval. The sixth junctional complex with the longest R-P interval is followed by ventricular reentry with an R-R interval of 480 ms. The next three P waves are fusions between retrograde and sinus P waves. The last P wave is sinus. A similar sequence of retrograde conduction is present in the bottom tracing, with the exception that the longest R-P interval is followed by an unexpectedly long R-R interval of 960 ms. The unexpectedly longer R-R interval in the bottom tracing is due to concealed, attempted ventricular reentry. The concealed impulse reaches the site of junctional impulse formation, discharges, and resets the pacemaker but fails to reach the ventricle. The interval between the two junctional impulses encompassing the manifest reentry in the top tracing measures 1000 ms, approximately the same as the long R-R encompassing the concealed reentry in the bottom tracing. Similar R-R intervals, encompassing the concealed and manifest reentry, support concealed reentry as a mechanism of the long R-R in the bottom tracing.

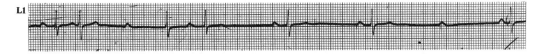

Figure 6-16. A-V block due to concealed conduction. The first sinus impulse is followed by a JPC, and this by a long P-R interval of 720 ms and a normal QRS complex. The next QRS complex is a JPC followed by sinus P wave with a P-R interval of 240 ms and normal QRS complex. The next P wave is blocked due to concealed discharge of a JPC.

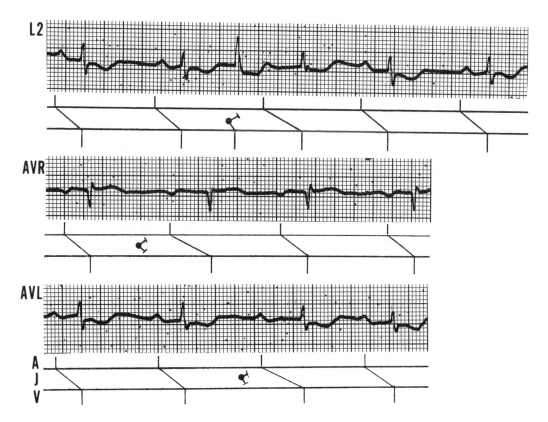

Figure 6-17. Concealed junctional (His) discharge with unexpected prolongation of the P-R interval. In L2, the sinus rhythm with a P-R interval of 280 ms is interrupted by an interpolated JPC, and a P-R interval of 400 ms follows. The second P in lead AVR and the third in lead AVL conduct with the P-R intervals of 440 and 480 ms, respectively. The QRS complex following the prolonged P-R interval is slightly aberrant. The mechanism responsible for the unexpected prolongation of the P-R interval is concealed junctional discharge. The assumption of concealed discharge is supported by a manifest JPC in L2, and by the facts that 1) the prolonged P-R intervals are similar in duration whether or not preceded by an interpolated JPC, and 2) the R-R intervals encompassing the unexpectedly long P-R interval without a JPC (leads AVR and AVL) are approximately the same in duration as those encompassing the JPC in L2, each measuring approximately 1240 ms. The minor aberration of the QRS complex following the prolonged P-R interval in L2 and AVL is due to the shorter R-R interval and, more specifically, to incomplete recovery of the His-Purkinje system. From Fisch C, Zipes DP, McHenry PL. Electrocardiographic manifestations of concealed junctional ectopic impulses. *Circulation* 1976;53:217–233. By permission of the American Heart Association, Inc.

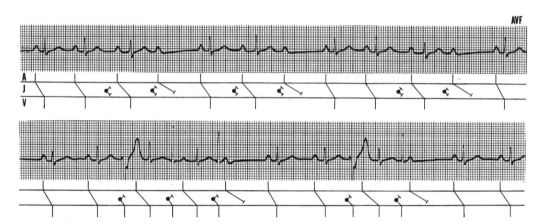

Figure 6-18. Pseudo Type I A-V block caused by concealed junctional impulses. In the top tracing, blocked P waves are preceded by gradual prolongation of the P-R interval, suggesting Type I A-V block. However, the gradual prolongation of the P-R interval is due to concealed interpolated junctional impulses. In the bottom tracing, the first two P waves are sinus in origin, with a P-R interval of 200 ms. The third QRS complex is an interpolated JPC conducting with aberration. The P-R interval that follows is prolonged. The second interpolated JPC is followed by further prolongation of the P-R interval. The third JPC blocks conduction of the next P wave. This sequence is repetitive. By disregarding the interpolated JPC in the bottom tracing, the sequence of gradual prolongation of the P-R interval and block of the P wave is identical to the one in the top tracing. Therefore, based on the findings in the bottom tracing, the A-V delay and block in the top tracing can be assumed to be due to concealed junctional (His) impulses. The aberration of the JPCs in the bottom trace is due to the Ashman phenomenon. From Fisch C, Zipes DP, McHenry PL. Electrocardiographic manifestations of concealed junctional ectopic impulses. *Circulation* 1976;53:217–223. By permission of the American Heart Association, Inc.

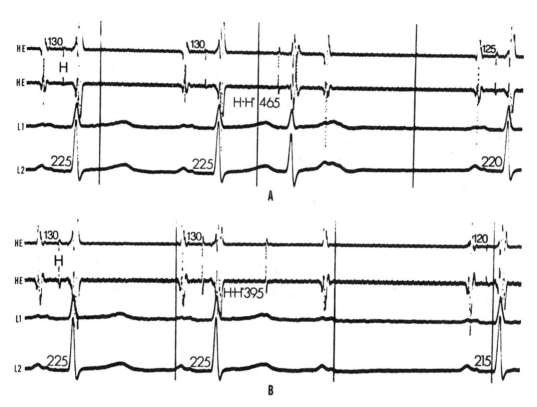

Figure 6-19. Premature concealed His bundle impulses (H′) with pseudo Type II A-V block. A. The H′ preceded by an H-H′ of 465 ms conducts to the ventricle. B. The H-H′ of 395 ms is followed by a blocked A (P) wave simulating Mobitz Type II A-V block. In B, the H′ follows a shorter H-H′ of 395 ms and thus fails to reach the ventricle. However, the nonconducted impulse induces local re-fractoriness and blocks the subsequent sinus P (A) wave. The P (A) wave blocks without any an-tecedent prolongation of the P-R (A-H) interval, and suggests Type II A-V block. In reality, the block is caused by a concealed His bundle discharge H′, and therefore is a pseudo Type II A-V block. From Fisch C, Zipes DP, McHenry PL. Electrocardiographic manifestations of concealed junctional ectopic impulses. *Circulation* 1976;53:217–223. By permission of the American Heart Association, Inc.

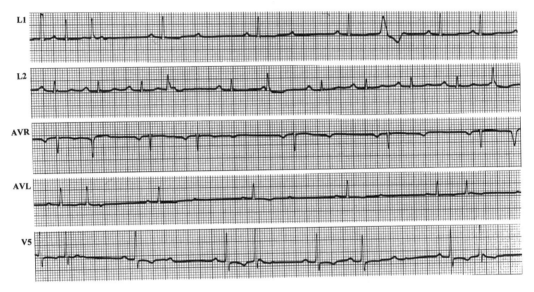

Figure 6-20. Concealed junctional (His) discharge. The basic rhythm is sinus with a P-P of 800 ms and a normal P-R interval. JPCs are present in leads L1, L2, AVR, AVL, and V$_5$. Leads AVR and AVL register a 2:1 A-V block. The 2:1 A-V block is due to concealed junctional (His) His discharge. The R-R interval with 2:1 A-V block without encompassing a manifest JPC equals the R-R encompassing a manifest JPC, thus supporting the diagnosis of concealed junctional (His) discharge.

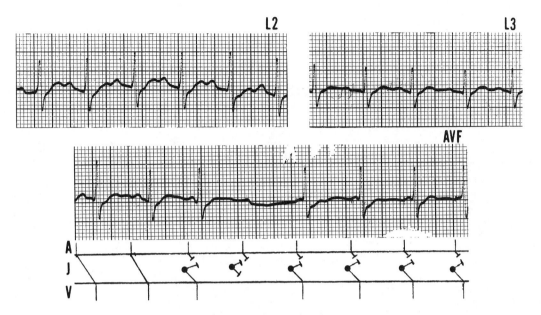

Figure 6-21. NPJT with exit block due to concealed junctional (His) discharge. Sinus tachycardia is recorded in leads L2 and L3. In lead AVF, the first two QRS complexes, sinus in origin, are followed by NPJT at a rate of approximately 100 per minute with AV dissociation. The long R-R cycle, following the third QRS complex and encompassing the blocked P wave, is approximately twice that of the basic junctional cycle. The unexpected block of the P wave is due to a nonconducted junctional discharge that, although failing to conduct to the ventricle, induces local refractoriness and blocks A-V conduction. This record suggests that exit block from the ectopic focus reflects failure of impulse propagation rather than failure of impulse formation. Were it the latter, the P wave would not have been registered. From Fisch C. Concealed conduction. In Zipes DP (ed:) *Symposium on Arrhythmias I. Cardiology Clinics.* Philadelphia: W.B. Saunders; 1983:63.

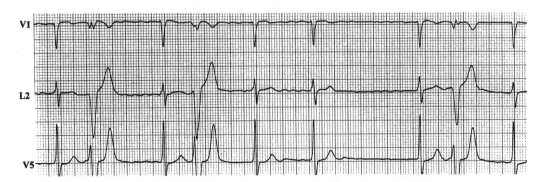

Figure 6-22. Concealed Purkinje discharge. The basic rhythm is atrial fibrillation with accurately coupled VPCs. The two R-R intervals encompassing the second and third VPCs are equal and measure 1480 ms. The long cycle equals the R-R encompassing the second and third VPCs. This relation of the R-R intervals suggests that the long cycle is due to concealed discharge from a Purkinje focus (concealed VPC).

References

1. Engelmann TW. Beobachtungen and Versuche am Suspendierten Herzem. *Pflugers Arch* 1894;56:149.
2. Lewis T, Master AM. Observations upon conduction in the mammalian heart. A-V conduction. *Heart* 1925;12:209.
3. Drury AN. Further observations upon intraauricular block produced by pressure or cooling. *Heart* 1925;12:143.
4. Scherf D, Shookhoff C. Reizleitungsstorungen im Bundel. I Mittelung. Uber Veranderungen des atrioventrkularen Rhythms durch Extrasystolen. *Wein Arch Finn Med* 1925;10:978.
5. Ashman R. Conductivity in compressed cardiac muscle. I. The recovery of conductivity following impulse transmission in compressed auricular muscle of the turtle heart. *Am J Physiol* 1925;74:121.
6. Langendorf R. Concealed A-V conduction: The effect of blocked impulses on the formation and conduction of subsequent impulses. *Am Heart J* 1948;35:542.
7. Langendorf R, Mehlman JS. Blocked (nonconducted) A-V nodal premature systoles imitating first and second degree A-V block. *Am Heart J* 1947;34:500.
8. Langendorf R, Pick A. Concealed conduction. Further evaluation of a fundamental aspect of propagation of the cardiac impulse. *Circulation* 1956;13:381.
9. Langendorf R, Pick A, Katz LN. Ventricular response in atrial fibrillation: Role of concealed conduction in the A-V junction. *Circulation* 1965;32:69.
10. Langendorf R, Pick A. Concealed intraventricular conduction in the human heart. Recent advances in ventricular conduction. *Adv Cardiol* 1975;14:40.
11. Sung RJ, Myerburg RJ, Castellanos A. Electrophysiological demonstration of concealed conduction in the human atrium. *Circulation* 1978;58:940.
12. Rosen KM, Rahimtoola SH, Gunnar RM. Pseudo A-V block secondary to premature non-propagate His bundle depolarization. Documentation by His bundle electrocardiography. *Circulation* 1970;42:367.

7

Aberration

Isolated supraventricular impulses or sustained supraventricular rhythms may, at times, have wide and bizarre QRS complexes as a manifestation of aberration (Figures 7-1 and 7-2). Aberration may be the result of a changing heart rate, be it acceleration or deceleration. It does not, however, include QRS abnormalities due to preexisting BBB, accessory pathway (WPW) conduction, or the effect of drugs.

Historical Perspective

The earliest reference to abnormal intraventricular conduction of supraventricular impulses can be found in a paper published in 1910 entitled, *Paroxysmal Tachycardia, the Result of Ectopic Impulse Formation.* In this paper, Sir Thomas Lewis[1] described APCs with "three separate types of ventricular electrocardiogram." In the same paper, he illustrated five consecutive APCs. The first QRS complex of the sequence, the one preceded by a sinus cycle, was abnormal and bizarre. In a subsequent writing in 1911, Lewis[2] suggested that the

> *"abnormal ventricular electrocardiograms . . . are due to disturbances of conduction in the smaller branches of this system and it is held that definite branches are affected in this manner, though these branches cannot be identified at the present time. It is proposed that the phenomena discussed should be termed 'aberration of supraventricular impulses' or simply 'aberration'; the anomalous beats may be conveniently spoken of as 'aberrant beats' or aberrant ventricular conduction."*

Electrocardiography of Aberration

The suggestion that abnormal intraventricular conduction, more specifically asynchrony of conduction, results in aberration has been confirmed, and the sites of the disturbed conduction have been localized to the bundle branches, their divisions, Purkinje fibers, the Purkinje-myocardial "gates," or combinations of the above, and, perhaps, to preferential A-V conduction.

Some of the more common and easily identifiable factors that may result in aberration include changes in heart rate, the rate of change of the heart rate, concealed conduction, autonomic influences, and metabolic disturbances.

The pattern of aberration varies including RBBB, LBBB, LAFB, LPFB, and/or a combination of the above. The most common form of aberration is RBBB, which is seen in more than 80% of patients with aberration; LBBB is present in less than 10%. In fact, in the normal heart, the prevalence of RBBB aberration may approach 100% percent. The most common combination of aberration is RBBB and LAFB (Figure 7-3).[3,4] In experimentally induced aberration, the pattern is nearly always that of RBBB. The block occurs high the bundle during anterograde conduction and low in the bundle during retrograde conduction. The reason for the prevalence of RBBB is the longer TAP of the right bundle and, thus, its refractoriness. It has also been suggested that the RBB, being a long, narrow wire-like structure, is more prone to slowing of conduction.

Mechanisms of Aberration

In general, the mechanisms of aberration include: 1) premature excitation; 2) acceleration of the heart rate; 3) concealed transseptal conduction; and 4) deceleration of the heart rate.

Aberration Caused by Premature Excitation

In the normal heart, aberration following an APC is, with rare exception, caused by attempted excitation prior to full recovery of the TAP, namely during the period of the so-called voltage-dependent refractoriness, and the aberration is nearly always in the form of RBBB (Figures 7-1 and 7-3).[3–5]

Occasionally, and most often in the abnormal heart, aberration may be that of the right and left bundle. LBBB occurs at shorter cycles than RBBB and is largely independent of the duration of the preceding cycles, the duration of the refractory periods of the two bundles being "crossed over"[6]: at short cycles, the refractory period of the LBB is longer than that of the RBB, and at longer cycles the refractory period of the RBB is longer than that of the LBB (Figure 7-4). However, the refractory periods alone may not be the reasons for the failure of bundle branch conduction.

The coupling interval at which the conduction of a premature impulse is either delayed, blocked, or conducted aberrantly depends not only on its prematurity but also on the dominant heart rate. With acceleration of the heart rate, the refractory period shortens and, consequently, a shorter coupling is necessary to evoke aberration.[7] The opposite is also true, namely that prolongation of the basic cycle length results in a longer refractory period, and aberration may occur at longer coupling intervals.

With increasing heart rate, the occasional normalization of a previously aberrant QRS complex may be explained by the greater shortening of the refractory period of the bundle branches than that of the AV node. Similarly, aberration initiated by an abrupt acceleration of the heart rate, such as in SVTs, may disappear with persistence of the tachycardia, a phenomenon occasionally referred to as "restitution." This may be a result of time-dependent gradual shortening of the refractory period of the affected bundle (Figure 7-5).

Because of the directional relationship of the refractory period and the heart rate, aberration of a premature complex can be induced in the presence of fixed coupling by prolonging the immediately preceding basic cycle. This mechanism of aberration was first noted by Lewis[1] and subsequently emphasized by Langendorf[8]; it is commonly referred to as the Ashman phenomenon (Figure 7-6).[9,10] Interestingly, aberration caused by the Ashman phenomenon may persist for a number of cycles. The persistence might reflect a time-dependent adjustment of refractoriness of the bundle branch to an abrupt change in cycle length, or it might be the result of concealed transseptal activation, as detailed below.[5,11]

On occasion, such as with rapid pacing or vagal stimulation, the refractory period of the AV node may exceed that of the bundles. Aberration is not possible when this happens, as the delay in the AV node allows sufficient time for recovery of the bundles.

Aberration Caused by Acceleration of Heart Rate

Acceleration-dependent aberration is a result of failure of the refractory period to shorten, or in some cases to lengthen, in response to acceleration of the rate (Figures 7-7 and 7-8). Acceleration-dependent aberration differs in many respects from aberration in the normal heart.[12] The aberration appears at relatively slow heart rates (frequently below 70 beats per minute), often displays LBBB, and may appear with a gradual rather than abrupt acceleration of the rate and frequently at cycle length shortening of 5 ms or less (Figure 7-9). Aberration may appear after a number of cycles of accelerated but regular rate, rarely disappears with acceleration of the heart rate, and is nearly always a marker of some form of cardiac abnormality, the latter not necessarily clinically evident at the time the record is made. Because of the small changes in duration of the cycle length that may initiate aberration ("critical cycle"), recognition of acceleration-dependent aberration may require a long record documenting the gradual, and at times minimal, shortening of the R-R intervals (Figure 7-10).

Four features of acceleration-dependent aberration are of particular interest. These include the slow heart rate at which aberration may appear, the frequent inverse relationship of the refractory period and the cycle length (i.e., lengthening of the refractory period with tachycardia), the persistence of aberration at cycles longer than the critical cycle (Figures 7-9, 7-10, and 7-11), and the appearance of aberration only after a number of cycles of an accelerated but regular rate (Figure 7-12).[12] Mechanisms that may explain the above include prolongation of the voltage- or time-dependent refractoriness, failure of the refractory period to shorten or, in fact, prolong, changing electrophysiological determinants of conduction, namely reduction of resting membrane potential or shift of membrane responsiveness to the right, geometry of the bundle branch lesion and its relation to the impulse, "fatigue,"[13] overdrive suppression,[12] and concealed transseptal conduction.[5,11,14,15]

Acceleration-dependent aberration appearing at rapid rates may be due to failure of the action potential (voltage-dependent refractoriness) to shorten or, in fact, paradoxically, it may lengthen. However, acceleration-dependent aberration may occur at relatively long cycles, occasionally exceeding 1000 ms. In such instances simple prolongation of the action potential duration will not account for the aberration (Figure 7-13).

Evidence also suggests that with a change in the heart rate, attainment of the new steady state of conduction is time-dependent, requiring a number of cycles. Although time-dependent refractoriness is a major cause of aberration (Figures 7-13 and 7-14), some have suggested that the geometry of the bundle branch lesion coupled with a change in current strength may contribute to aberration. In the presence of such an "impedance mismatch," when a few fibers carry the current, small changes in intensity and strength of input may result in slowing or failure of conduction. Such a mismatch may be partly caused by changes in the determinants of conduction.

Aberration Caused by Concealed Transseptal Conduction

During slowing of the heart rate, intraventricular conduction often fails to normalize at the critical cycle length (cycle length at which it first appeared) and aberration persists at cycles longer than the critical cycle that initiated the aberration.[13] This paradox is most commonly ascribed to concealed conduction from the contralateral or conducting bundle branch, across the septum with delayed activation of the blocked bundle (Figures 7-9 and 7-15). Such concealed transseptal activation results in a bundle branch-to-bundle branch interval that is shorter than the manifest QRS cycle, and explains the unexpected persistence of acceleration-dependent aberration. However, unexpected delay of normalization of conduction cannot always be explained solely by concealed transseptal activation. In some cases, for example, the conduction normalizes with slowing of the heart rate only to recur at cycles that are still longer than the critical cycle. Such a sequence excludes transseptal concealment as the mechanism of recurrence of the aberration. Similarly, when the discrepancy between the critical cycle and the cycle at which normalization finally occurs is long, as, for example, 210 ms, transseptal concealment alone cannot explain the delay. The duration of transseptal conduction in healthy humans has been estimated to be approximately 60 ms, and in diseased states it may reach 100 ms.[16] Fatigue and overdrive suppression have been suggested as possible mechanisms of the delay of normalization of conduction. Overdrive suppression is, in some respects, similar to the overdrive suppression recorded in the sinus node, the AV node, and accessory bundles. The duration of suppression of conduction depends on the rate; the more rapid the rate, the longer the recovery time.

Overdrive Suppression

In humans, overdrive suppression is indicated by the fact that with cessation of rapid ventricular rhythms, the BBB disappears gradually in face of acceleration of the heart rate (Figure 7-16).[17] Although fatigue may not explain the persistence of BBB after a single short cycle, overdrive suppression may. The fatigue and overdrive suppression mechanisms of aberration have been demonstrated experimentally.[18]

Fatigue and overdrive suppression may be partly responsible for the time-dependent adjustment of conduction. When exaggerated, such time-dependent adjustment of conduction, with rare exception, indicates an abnormal state.

It is evident from the above that, as a rule, the manifestations and mechanisms of aberration in the normal heart and of acceleration-dependent aberration encountered in the abnormal heart differ significantly.

Concealed Transseptal Conduction with Alternation of Aberration

Alternation of aberration of an APC during atrial bigeminy was first observed in 1922 by Stenstrom.[19] The alternation may be between a normal QRS complex and BBB or between right and left bundle blocks. The bigeminal rhythm may be caused by atrial bigeminy, 3:2 A-V block, or atrial flutter with alternating 2:1 and 4:1 A-V block. When the alternation is between a normal QRS complex and RBBB, the following events are assumed (Figure 7-17): after normal conduction, the bundle branch-to-bundle branch interval is relatively "long" with a relatively "longer" refractory period of the RBB and, thus, the RBBB. In the presence of RBBB, the impulse is conducted along the LBB and across the septum, activating the RBB after some delay and thus shortening the RBB-to-RBB interval as well as its refractory period. As a result, the next early QRS complex is normal.[20] The same phenomenon, namely, the concealed transseptal conduction with an obligatory change in duration of its refractory period, explains alternating RBBB and LBBB (Figure 7-18). In the presence of RBBB, transseptal concealed conduction from the LBB to the RBB shortens the RBB-to-RBB interval relative to the now longer LBB-to-LBB interval. As a result, the refractory period of the LBB is longer and conduction in the LBB fails. In the presence of LBBB, conduction proceeds along the RBB. The delayed transseptal activation of the LBB shortens the LBB-to-LBB interval. The refractory period of the RBB is now relatively longer, as the RBB conduction is blocked.

Aberration Caused by Deceleration of the Heart Rate

In 1934, Drury and Mackenzie[21] noted that injury to either the RBB or LBB accompanied by slowing of the heart by vagal stimulation resulted in ventricular aberration. They also observed that, while the aberration was dependent on deceleration of the heart rate and bundle branch injury, the duration of aberration was directionally related to the severity of bundle branch damage. Noting that the slowing of the heart rate by interventions other than vagal stimulation did not cause aberration, they suggested that factors other than mere slowing of the heart rate contributed to the aberration. They proposed that the vagal action altered the "quality" of the impulse at the level of the AV node, resulting in, for example, decremental conduction, and they proposed that the altered impulse was of insufficient strength to traverse the site of injury. Interestingly, they suggested that, "*in the human subject as a result of deficient arterial supply or other factors, local impairment occurs and vagal action on the impulse in the upper part of the junctional tissue in these conditions produces aberrant beats.*" Subsequent studies using a similar experimental design confirmed these early observations (Figures 7-19 and 7-20).[22]

The most widely accepted mechanism of deceleration-dependent aberration is a gradual spontaneous reduction of phase 4 of the TAP in an abnormal cell or group of cells. It is suggested that, as a result of the spontaneous depolarization made possible by a prolonged cycle, the cell is activated from a less negative potential, resulting in impaired conduction. Demonstration of incomplete LBBB terminating cycles shorter than those terminated by complete LBBB, and escape complexes with a QRS configuration opposite that of the deceleration-dependent QRS aberration, supports, at least in humans, diastolic depolarization as the mechanism of deceleration-dependent aberration (Figures 7-21, 7-22, and 7-23).[22,23] Since the full width of the bundle branch must be affected in order to slow or block conduction, the thickness of the LBB argues against this hypothesis. However, such an objection may not be pertinent, because in a diseased bundle there is a great likelihood that the number of conducting fibers is reduced. Also, diastolic depolarization may actually enhance conduction by bringing the resting potential closer to TP. To circumvent this argument, it has been proposed that generalized reduction of the resting potential, gradual spontaneous depolarization, and a shift of the TP all play a role.[22]

L1
V6

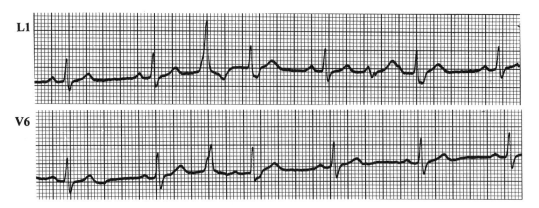

Figure 7-1. Aberration due to premature excitation. The interpolated VPC is followed by a prolonged P-R interval and RBBB aberration. Ventricular aberration following an interpolated VPC is relatively common and should not be confused with a ventricular couplet. Aberrations are caused by attempted conduction during the refractory period of the His-Purkinje system.

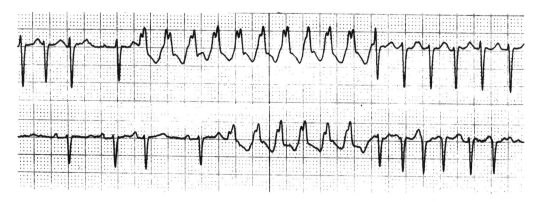

Figure 7-2. Normalization of intraventricular conduction without change in heart rate. The tracing is continuous. In the top tracing, an APC and SVT with aberration follow the sinus impulse, and with an R-P interval of approximately 240 ms. The intraventricular conduction normalizes without any change in the heart rate. The aberration is the result of acceleration of the rate. The most plausible explanation for normalization of intraventricular conduction is a gradual shortening of the bundle branch refractory period in response to tachycardia, a physiological phenomenon. A likely mechanism maintaining the aberration is transseptal concealed conduction blocking conduction in the contralateral bundle. With dissipation of the transseptal conduction, the QRS complex normalizes. Other possible mechanisms of normalization, although less likely, include acceleration of conduction in the blocked bundle secondary to catecholamine release, or a uniform delay of conduction in both bundles.

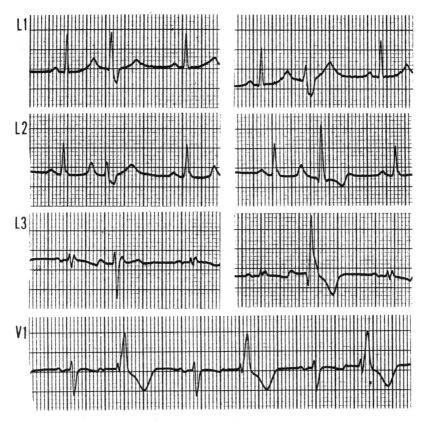

Figure 7-3. Aberration due to premature excitation. The aberration manifest by RBBB with LAFB and LPFB are recorded in the left and right panels, respectively. RBBB with LAFB is the most common combination of fascicular blocks.

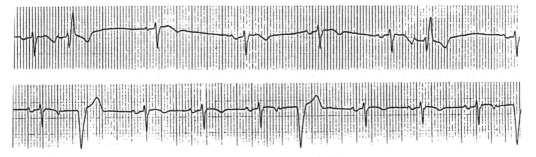

Figure 7-4. Cross-over of the refractory periods of the bundles. Although the most common form of aberration is RBBB, on occasion shortening of coupling of an APC may result in LBBB aberration. This is the so-called cross-over phenomenon, in that in short cycles the refractory period of the LBBB is longer than that of the RBBB.

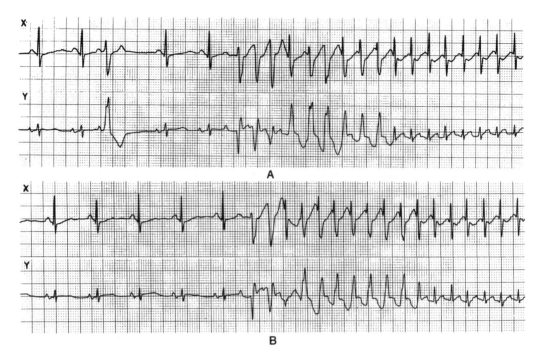

Figure 7-5. SVT with aberration and normalization of the QRS complex without change in the rate. In panels A and B, the APC initiates an SVT with aberration. The aberration ceases spontaneously without change in the heart rate. The aberration is the result of acceleration of the heart rate. The normalization of the QRS complex is due to a gradual shortening of the bundle branch refractory period in response to the tachycardia, a physiological phenomenon. Other possible mechanisms are noted in Figure 7-2.

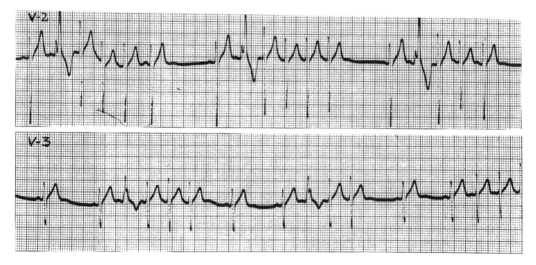

Figure 7-6. Aberration due to the Ashman phenomenon. The basic rhythm is a repetitive atrial tachycardia. The second QRS complex of each run of tachycardia is aberrant with RBBB. The latter follows a long preceding cycle. The QRS complex following short R-R intervals conducts normally. The long R-R interval is followed by a prolonged refractory period of the RBB and, thus, RBBB. The subsequent R-R is short, refractory periods are also short, and, thus, there is normal conduction. This is the Ashman phenomenon. The reason for the high prevalence of RBBB is that the refractory period of the RBB is normally longer than that of the LBB.

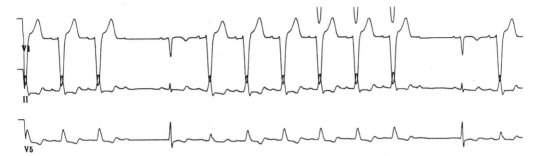

Figure 7-7. Acceleration-dependent aberration. The basic rhythm is sinus with a Mobitz Type II A-V block. During 1:1 A-V conduction, the sinus complex conducts with LBBB. The blocked P wave is followed by a prolonged return cycle which terminates with a normal QRS complex. The LBBB is due to failure of the refractory period to shorten during a 1:1 conduction. The pause following block of the P wave is sufficiently long to allow the LBB to recover and conduct normally.

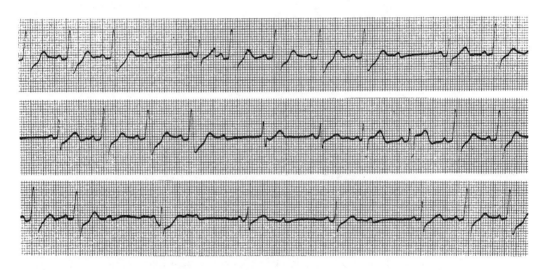

Figure 7-8. Acceleration-dependent aberration. The basic rhythm is sinus with a Mobitz Type II A-V block. With 1:1 AV conduction, the QRS complex is prolonged. The long pause following the blocked P wave allows for recovery of the His-Purkinje tissue and, thus, the normal QRS complex. The mechanism of aberration is failure of the refractory period to shorten with acceleration of the rate.

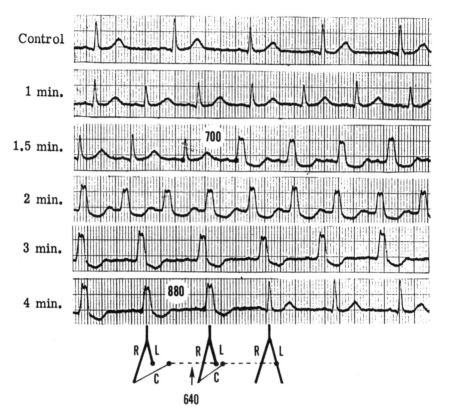

Figure 7-9. Mechanisms of persistence of the LBB at cycles longer than the critical R-R cycle. We assume that concealed transseptal conduction from RBB to LBB shortens the LBB-to-LBB interval to 700 ms or less, resulting in acceleration-dependent LBBB. This figure stresses the fact that the LBB-to-LBB interval and not the manifest QRS-to-QRS interval determines whether the conduction will be normal or aberrant. An alternate mechanism that could explain persistence of LBBB at R-R intervals of 880 ms is "fatigue" caused by the tachycardia with delayed recovery of conduction in the LBB. It is likely that both concealed transseptal activation and fatigue contribute to the unexplained persistence of LBBB. To assume that concealed transseptal activation alone is responsible for the paradoxical persistence of LBBB, one must assume a transseptal conduction time of 180 ms (880 − 700 = 180). This is considerably longer than would be suggested from studies in animals and humans. From Fisch C, Zipes DP, McHenry PL. Rate dependent aberrancy. *Circulation* 1973;48:714. By permission of the American Heart Association, Inc.

ID: 000687771

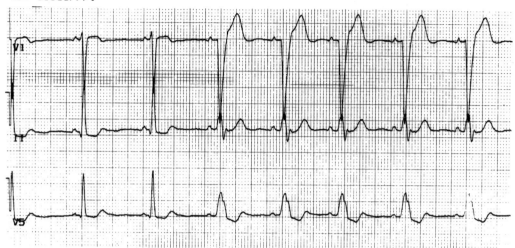

Figure 7-10. Acceleration-dependent aberration. This tracing emphasizes the small changes in rate that may result in acceleration-dependent aberration. In this tracing, the aberration is LBBB at a cycle length of 800 ms, long for usual aberration. The LBBB aberration and the slow rate are strongly suggestive of an abnormality of the conduction system.

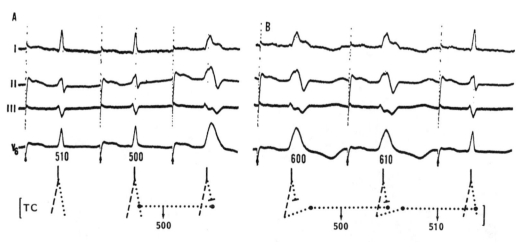

Figure 7-11. Aberration caused by concealed transseptal conduction or "fatigue" or both. Panels A and B are part of a continuous record. Each pacing cycle is changed by 10 ms. A change in cycle length from 510 to 500 results in LBBB. Similarly, with gradual slowing of the pacing interval, a prolongation of the cycle length from 600 to 610 ms is associated with a normal QRS complex. This tracing emphasizes that small changes in cycle length, some not recognizable in the surface ECG, may determine whether an impulse will conduct or be blocked. Persistence of LBBB at cycles longer than the critical cycles at which block occurs is thought to be due to concealed transseptal conduction from RBB to the LBB. In B, delayed transseptal concealment from the RBB shortens the LBB-to-LBB interval to an arbitrary length of 500 ms and thus results in persistence of LBBB. With prolongation of the R-R interval to 610 ms, the LBB-to-LBB cycle is lengthened to 510 ms, 10 ms longer than the critical cycle of 500, and the QRS complex normalizes. From Fisch C, Zipes DP, McHenry PL. Rate dependent aberrancy. *Circulation* 1973;48:714. By permission of the American Heart Association, Inc.

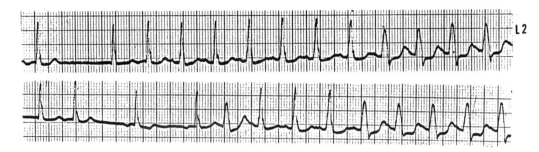

Figure 7-12. Acceleration-dependent LBBB due to "fatigue." The top tracing illustrates a junctional escape followed by atrial tachycardia with an R-R interval of 440 ms and progressive prolongation of LBBB conduction. In the bottom tracing, the first QRS complex of the atrial tachycardia conducts with LBBB, and the next three conduct with incomplete LBBB progressing to complete LBBB. Aberration without any demonstrable changes in the heart rate suggests fatigue as the mechanism. In the bottom tracing, the first aberrant QRS complex of the atrial tachycardia caused by the Ashman phenomenon is followed by a normal QRS complex with gradually increasing LBBB aberration. The appearance of the aberration without any demonstrable change in cycle length suggests that fatigue is the dominant mechanism. The fatigue may be the result of an inappropriate restitution of ions across the membrane resulting in a gradual prolongation of time-dependent refractoriness of the LBB. From Fisch C, Zipes DP, McHenry PL. Rate dependent aberrancy. *Circulation* 1973;48:714. By permission of the American Heart Association, Inc.

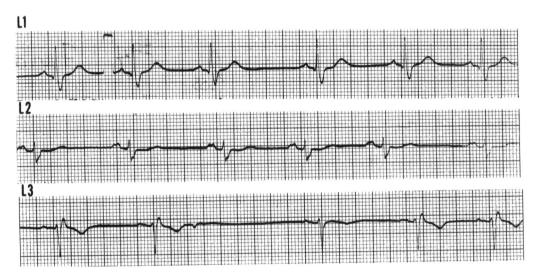

Figure 7-13. Acceleration-dependent aberration at slow heart rates. The aberration persists at an R-R interval of 920 to 1250 ms. In L3, the APC with a return cycle longer than any of the sinus cycles is terminated by a normal QRS complex. The aberration at extremely low rates is probably a result of a significant prolongation of the time-dependent refractory period of the RBB and a sign of an abnormality in the Purkinje system.

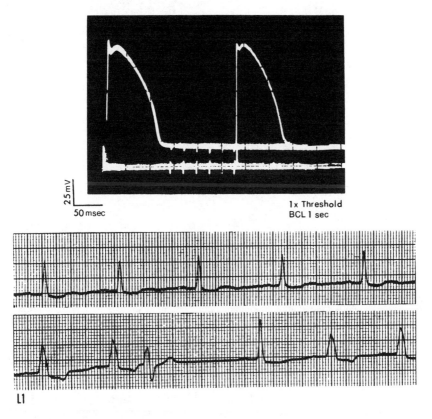

Figure 7-14. Time-dependent refractoriness, a mechanism of acceleration-dependant aberration. The QRS complex is normal at cycle lengths longer than 1000 ms, and LBBB appears at cycle lengths of 1000 ms or shorter. Because of the length of the R-R at which aberration is recorded, it is unlikely that TAP duration alone is responsible. Time-dependent refractoriness is more likely responsible for the LBBB. The TAP was recorded from a Purkinje fiber paced at a basic cycle length of 1 second with a threshold strength stimulus. Despite recovery of the TAP, the stimulus fails to generate an action potential for an additional 125 ms. This 125-ms period is the time-dependent refractoriness.

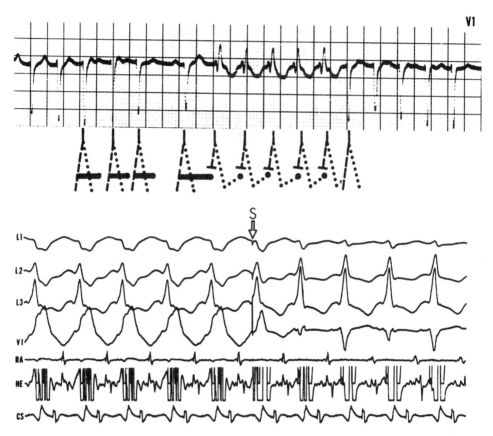

Figure 7-15. Aberration due to the Ashman phenomenon and concealed transseptal conduction. The basic rhythm is an atrial tachycardia with Type I A-V block. The solid horizontal bars represent the refractory period, and the dashed and dotted lines represent the RBB and LBB, respectively. The refractory period is prolonged after the pause and this is followed by RBBB (Ashman phenomenon) with the BBB perpetuated by concealed transseptal conduction. The atrial impulse conducts along the LBB, traverses the septum, enters the RBB, and blocks conduction of the subsequent impulse in the RBB, thus perpetuating the RBBB. The constant rate, fixed temporal relationship between the concealed transseptal conduction, and the anterograde conduction of the atrial impulse are essential for the aberration to persist. The transseptal conduction was confirmed by recording directly from the heart. The bottom panel is a recording of a stimulus-initiated AVRT with RBBB aberration. The ECG leads including I, L2, L3, V_1, and right atrial (RA) are recorded. Atrial activation is retrograde, as indicated by the fact that the atrial electrogram is first recorded in the coronary sinus. Preexcitation(s) of the right ventricle shortly before expected activation by the transseptal impulse terminates the concealed transseptal conduction, and the intraventricular conduction normalizes. From Fisch C. Electrocardiography of arrhythmias: From deductive reasoning to laboratory confirmation. 25 Years of progress. *J Am Coll Cardiol* 1983;1:306. Reprinted with permission.

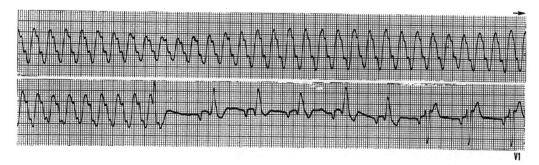

VI

Figure 7-16. Overdrive suppression of the RBB. Following the VT, five sinus impulses conduct with RBBB with the last three QRS complexes normal. The P-P and R-R intervals shorten gradually from 880 to 800 ms with normalization of intraventricular conduction. The mechanism of the RBBB is probably rapid and repetitive depolarization of the RBB by the VT, resulting in the overdrive suppression or "fatigue" of the RBB. From Fisch C. Bundle branch block after ventricular tachycardia: A manifestation of fatigue or overdrive suppression. *J Am Coll Cardiol* 1984;3:1562. Reprinted with permission.

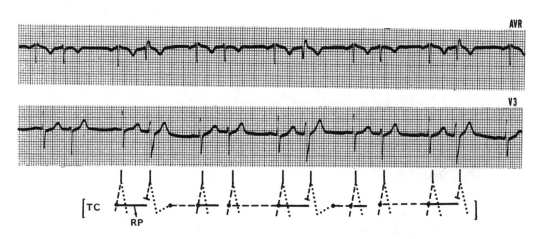

Figure 7-17. Atrial bigeminy with alternating normal QRS complexes and RBBB caused by concealed transseptal conduction. Diagram: concealed transseptal conduction, LBBB (dots), RBBB (interrupted line). The horizontal bar indicates the refractory period. The first sinus impulse is followed by a normally conducted APC and, therefore, a "longer" RBB-to-RBB interval with a resultant longer refractory period of the RBB. The next APC finds the RBBB refractory period prolonged, and RBB is recorded. Concealed transseptal conduction from the normally conducting LBB activates the RBB after some delay and shortens the RBB-to-RBB interval as well as the refractory period of the RBB. As a result of the shortening of the R-R, the next APC conducts normally. From Wen-Heng QT, Fisch C. Concealed transseptal conduction. *Chin Med J* 1985;98:271.

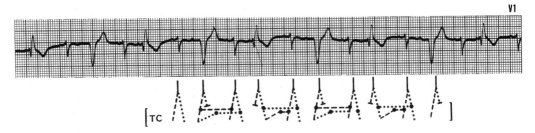

Figure 7-18. Atrial bigeminy with alternating RBBB and LBBB caused by concealed transseptal conduction. The RBB and the RBB-to-RBB cycles are identified by the interrupted line. The LBB and LBB intervals are identified by the dots. The first sinus impulse indicated by the Lewis diagram conducts normally. The first APC conducts with LBBB. The impulse proceeds along the RBB, traverses the septum and, with some delay, activates the LBB. As a result, the LBB-to-LBB interval is shorter than the RBB-to-RBB interval. The refractory period of the RBB is therefore relatively longer and, thus, the next APC conducts with RBBB (Ashman phenomenon). Because of the RBBB, the impulse conducts along the LBB and engages the RBB after a delay. This results in a relatively shorter RBB-to-RBB interval, a longer LBB-to-LBB interval, and longer refractory period of the LBB. As a result, the next APC conducts with an LBBB. This sequence repeats itself throughout the tracing. From Wen-Heng QT, Fisch C. Concealed transseptal conduction. *Chin Med J* 1985;98:271.

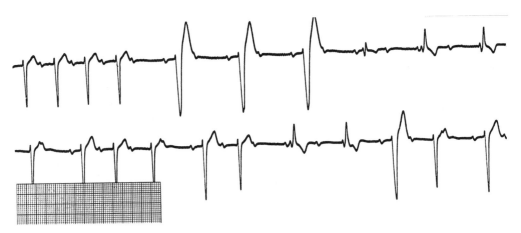

Figure 7-19. Deceleration-dependent LBBB. The basic rhythm is sinus with Type I A-V block. In general, the short cycles with 1:1 conduction of approximately 720 ms are terminated by a normal QRS complex. Intermediate R-R cycles from 1080 to 1200 ms are terminated by incomplete LBBB, and the long cycles of 1240 to 1320 ms are terminated by LBBB. The last P-R interval of the Wenckebach periodicity shows the largest increment, indicating an "atypical" Wenckebach block. The QRS complex with RBBB pattern is idioventricular in origin, as indicated by the fusion in the top tracing. The mechanism of aberration at slow rates is thought to be due to a gradual decline in the phase 4 of the TAP. A supraventricular impulse reaches phase 4 at a reduced potential, resulting in LBBB. Occasionally, if the gradual depolarization of phase 4 reaches the TP, a pattern of RBBB will be inscribed. The escape due to phase 4 reaching threshold, and the fusion, support the concept of phase 4 depolarization as the mechanism of deceleration-dependent conduction block. From Fisch C. Electrocardiography. In Braunwald E (ed:) *Heart Disease.* 5th ed. Philadelphia: W.B. Saunders; 1997:116–152.

M

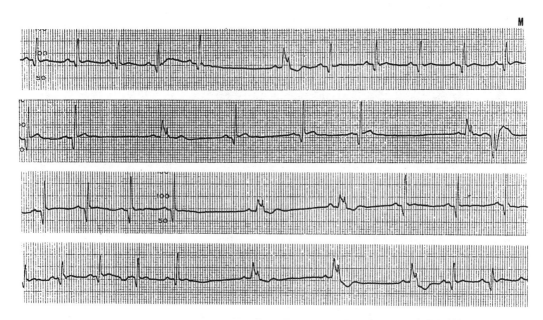

Figure 7-20. Deceleration-dependent LBBB. The basic rhythm is sinus with the long cycles caused by SA block or sinus arrest terminating with LBBB. The LBBB is due to a gradual loss of phase 4 of the transmembrane potential (see Figure 7-19).

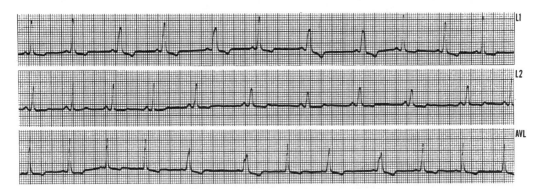

Figure 7-21. Deceleration-induced LBBB. The basic rhythm is sinus arrhythmia with a P-P interval varying from 680 to 1080 ms and a constant P-R interval of 130 ms. The duration of the QRS complex varies from 80 to 130 ms. The shortest R-R cycles are followed by a normal QRS complex, the intermediate R-R cycles by incomplete LBBB, the longest RR cycles by complete LBBB (see Figures 7-22 and 7-23). The progressive delay of LBBB conduction is accompanied by gradually more prominent secondary ST-T changes. In lead I, the first five QRS complexes illustrate the relation of the duration of QRS to heart rate. The first R-R interval measures 740 ms and is terminated by a QRS complex of 80 ms. The third QRS complex with complete LBBB follows an R-R interval of 860 ms. The fourth QRS complex with LBBB follows an R-R interval of 820 ms, intermediate between cycles with a normal QRS complex and complete LBBB. Similarly, the fourth through sixth QRS complex in AVL reveal transition from incomplete LBBB to complete LBBB parallel with lengthening of the R-R interval from 720 to 1040 ms. This directional relationship of the cycle length to the duration of LBBB supports spontaneous diastolic phase 4 depolarization as the likely mechanism of the deceleration-dependent aberration. The longer the R-R, the greater the reduction of phase 4, the lower the take-off potential, and, thus, the LBBB. From Fisch C, Miles WM. Deceleration dependent left bundle branch block: A spectrum of bundle branch conduction delay. *Circulation* 1982;65:1029. By permission of the American Heart Association, Inc.

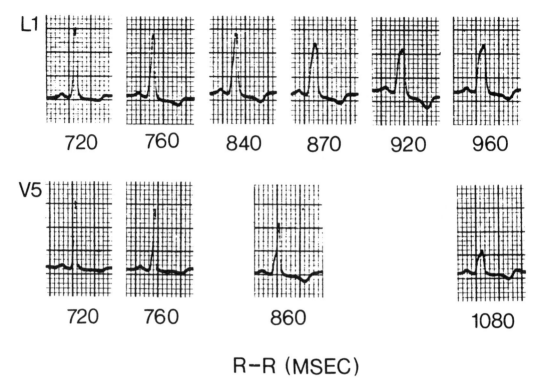

Figure 7-22. Sections from Figure 7-21 relating the duration of the QRS complex to the preceding cycle length. In lead I, the QRS complex changes from normal at R-R cycles of 720 to 740 ms, to incomplete LBBB at R-R cycles of 760 to 870, and to complete LBBB at R-R cycles of 920 and 960. In lead V_5, an increase in the cycle length from 720 to 760 and 860 ms is associated with incomplete LBBB, a decrease of R wave amplitude, and more pronounced secondary ST-T changes. Complete LBBB is recorded at a cycle length of 1080 ms. From Fisch C, Miles WM. Deceleration dependent left bundle branch block: A spectrum of bundle branch conduction delay. *Circulation* 1982;65:1029. By permission of the American Heart Association, Inc.

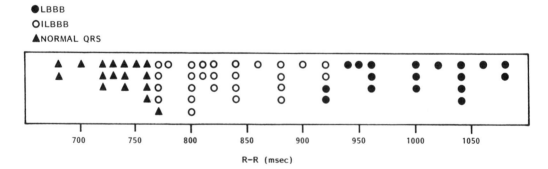

Figure 7-23. A scattergram based on data from Figures 7–21 and 7–22 relating the QRS duration to the R-R cycle. All QRS complexes with an R-R of 760 ms or shorter are normal (triangles). Complete LBBB follows R-R cycles longer than 900 ms (solid circles), while incomplete LBBB terminates cycles from 760 to 920 ms (open circles). As expected, there is some overlap between the normal QRS complex and incomplete LBBB and between incomplete LBBB and complete LBBB. From Fisch C, Miles WM. Deceleration dependent bundle branch block: A spectrum of bundle branch conduction delay. *Circulation* 1982;65:1029. By permission of the American Heart Association, Inc.

References

1. Lewis T. Paroxysmal tachycardia, the result of ectopic impulse formation. *Heart* 1910;1:262.
2. Lewis T. Observations upon disorders of the heart's action. *Heart* 1911/1912;3:279.
3. Cohen SI, Lau SH, Haft JI, Damato AN. Experimental production of aberrant ventricular conduction in man. *Circulation* 1967;36:673.
4. Cohen SI, Lau SH, Stein E, Young MW, Damato AN. Variations of aberrant ventricular conduction in man: Evidence of isolated and combined block within the specialized conduction system. *Circulation* 1968;38:899.
5. Moe GK, Mendez C, Han J. Aberrant A-V impulse propagation in the dog heart: A study of functional bundle branch block. *Circ Res* 1968;16:261.
6. Burchell HB. Sino-auricular block, interference dissociation, and different recovery rates of excitation in the bundle branches. *Br Heart J* 1949;11:230.
7. Schuilenburg RM, Durrer D. Rate dependency of functional block in the human His bundle and bundle branch Purkinje system. *Circulation* 1973;48:526.
8. Langendorf R. Aberrant ventricular conduction. *Am Heart J* 1951;41:700.
9. Ashman R, Byer E. Aberration in the conduction of premature ventricular impulses. *J La State Univ Sch Med* 1946;8:62.
10. Gouaux JL, Ashman R. Auricular fibrillation with aberration simulating ventricular paroxysmal tachycardia. *Am Heart J* 1947;34:366.
11. Glassman RD, Zipes DP. Site of anterograde and retrograde functional right bundle branch in intact canine heart. *Circulation* 1981;64:1277.
12. Fisch C, Zipes DP, McHenry PL. Rate-dependent aberrancy. *Circulation* 1973;48:714.
13. Shearn HA, Rytand DA. Intermittent bundle branch block. Observations with special reference to the critical heart rate. *Arch Intern Med* 1953;91:448.
14. Spurrell RAJ, Krikler DM, Sowton E. Retrograde invasion of the bundle branches producing aberration of the QRS complex during supraventricular tachycardia studied by programmed electrical stimulation. *Circulation* 1974;50:487.
15. Wellens HJJ, Durrer D. Supraventricular tachycardia with left aberrant conduction due to retrograde invasion into the left bundle branch. *Circulation* 1968;38:474.
16. Katz AM, Pick A. The transseptal conduction time in the human heart. An evaluation of fusion beats in ventricular parasystole. *Circulation* 1963;27:1061.
17. Fisch C. Bundle branch block after ventricular tachycardia: A manifestation of "fatigue" or "overdrive suppression." *J Am Coll Cardiol* 1984;3:1562.
18. Scherf D, Schott A. *Extrasystoles and Allied Arrhythmias.* Chicago: Year Book Medical Publishers; 1973:100.
19. Stenstrom N. Contribution to the knowledge of incomplete bundle branch block in man. *Acta Med Scand* 1923;57:385.
20. Cohen SI, Lau HS, Scherlag BJ, Damato AN. Alternate patterns of premature ventricular excitation during induced atrial bigeminy. *Circulation* 1969;39:819.
21. Drury AN, Mackenzie DW. Aberrant ventricular beats in the dog during vagal simulation. *Q J Exp Physiol* 1934;24:237.
22. Elizara MV, Nau GJ, Levi RJ, Lazzari JO, Halpern MS, Rosenbaum MB. Experimental production of rate-dependent bundle branch block in the canine heart. *Circ Res* 1974;34:730.
23. Fisch C, Miles WM. Deceleration-dependent left bundle branch block: A spectrum of bundle branch conduction delay. *Circulation* 1982;65:1029.

8

Fusions and Captures

Fusion

A fusion complex reflects simultaneous activation of the atria (Figures 8-1 and 8-2) or ventricles (Figure 8-3) by two, or rarely more, impulses originating in the same or, more often, in different chambers of the heart. Ventricular fusion was first noted by Lewis[1] in humans in 1913 and in the canine model in 1920.[2]

General Comments

The configuration of a fusion complex varies depending on the relative contribution of the two impulses (Figures 8-4 and 8-5) with the timing of the two impulses, such that both excite the given chamber simultaneously (Figure 8-6).[3,4] For example, in the case of fusion of a supraventricular impulse with a ventricular complex, the P-R interval must be long enough to allow the supraventricular impulse to reach the ventricle early enough to fuse with the ventricular impulse (Figure 8-7).

Atrial Fusion

Fusions of SA impulses with APCs are rare because the sinus node is discharged by the APCs, thus precluding dual excitation of the atria. In addition, the low amplitude of the P wave and a frequent lack of configuration detail make recognition of atrial fusions difficult. More often, atrial fusion is seen with an atrial parasystole and, less often, junctional rhythm (Figure 8-1). Theoretically, atrial fusion could result from collision of two atrial ectopic impulses, but differentiation from multifocal APCs is impossible.

Ventricular Fusion

Ventricular fusions are common and, with rare exception, indicate a ventricular arrhythmia (Figure 8-8).[5,6] A ventricular fusion may result from collision of a ventricular impulse with either a sinus impulse, a supraventricular ectopic impulse, or another ventricular impulse. The latter may be a single late VPC, an idioventricular rhythm (Figure 8-9), a ventricular parasystole, a VT, or a paced ventricular rhythm.

Ventricular fusion may differ from the normal supraventricular QRS complex only slightly, and in such cases, analysis of the T wave may prove helpful (Figure 8-10). In the presence of BBB, fusion of a supraventricular impulse with a VPC or pacing-induced QRS complex originating on the same side as the block (ipsilateral) may result in a normal-appearing QRS complex (Figure 8-11).[7] The QRS complex in WPW is a fusion of a supraventricular impulse, usually an SA nodal impulse, activating the ventricle simultaneously through the accessory pathway and the normal A-V pathway. This is an exception to the stated rule that a fusion results from collision of impulses arising from two different foci. The configuration of the fusion in WPW depends on the relative contribution of the impulses conducting through the two pathways. Fusion between a supraventricular impulse conducting through an accessory pathway and one originating in the AV junction has been recorded and is an exception to the general rule that a ventricular fusion indicates a ventricular arrhythmia (Figures 8-12 and 8-13).

Capture

A capture is a QRS complex initiated by a sinus or ectopic supraventricular impulse that traverses the AV junction when the latter is no longer refractory, and thus "captures" a ventricle that is under primary control of a junctional or ventricular focus (Figures 8-8 and 8-14).

A ventricular capture (QRS) may be normal or aberrant. The capture may or may not discharge and reset the ventricular pacemaker. For example, if a supraventricular impulse reaches an ectopic ventricular pacemaker at the time the latter is discharging, or shortly thereafter, the capture will not affect its rhythmicity. Under these circumstances, failure of the capture to discharge the ectopic pacemaker is the result of physiological refractoriness and is an example of interference.

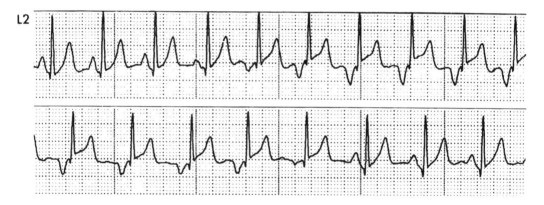

Figure 8-1. Atrial fusion. The third, fourth, and fifth P waves in the top tracing and the fifth P wave in the bottom tracing are fusions. The fusion is between sinus and junctional P waves.

LII

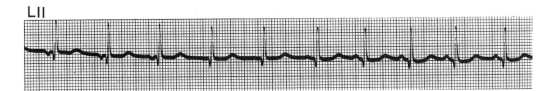

Figure 8-2. Atrial fusion. The initial junctional rhythm with a P-R interval of 120 ms and negative P waves is followed by a normal sinus rhythm with a P-R interval of 160 ms. The fourth, fifth, and sixth P waves are fusions. The fusion complexes are nearly isoelectric.

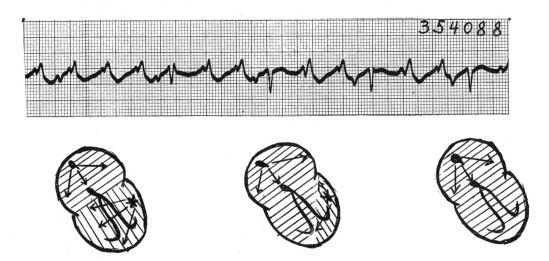

Figure 8-3. VT with fusions and captures. The ECG records a VT at an R-R interval of 440 ms with AV dissociation, a P-P interval of 1280 ms, and a QRS complex with RBBB configuration. The tachycardia is interrupted by captures (QRS 8, 11, 14) and a fusion (QRS 5). The diagram, from left to right, illustrates a ventricular ectopic QRS complex, fusion, and capture. Fusion and captures indicate that the wide QRS tachycardia is ventricular in origin. From Fisch C, Pinsky ST. Diagnosis of ventricular tachycardia. *J Indiana State Med Assoc* 1957;2:184.

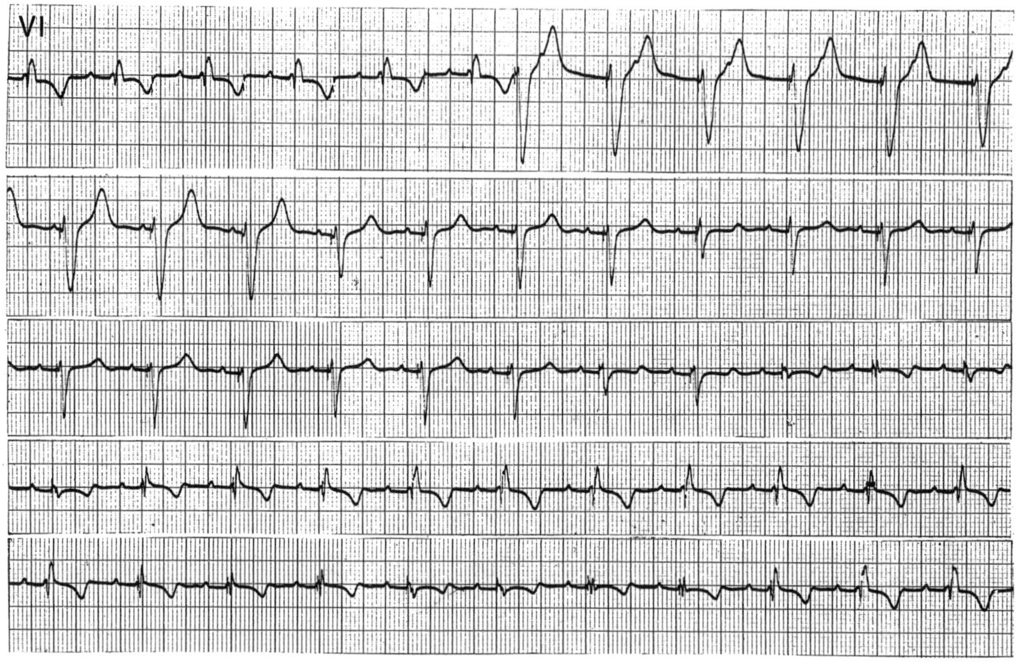

Figure 8-4. A spectrum of ventricular fusions. The basic sinus rhythm with RBBB and a P-P interval of approximately 800 ms is interrupted by a fixed-rate pacemaker with a pacing interval of 820 ms. Beginning with the fourth QRS complex in the second row and continuing through the remainder of the tracing, the QRS complex represents a spectrum of ventricular fusion. Depending on the mass of the ventricle activated by the sinus complex or the pacemaker, the capture will resemble more that of the sinus- or pacemaker-initiated QRS complex. Activation of the right ventricle by the pacemaker and simultaneously that of the left ventricle by the sinus impulse results in a normal QRS complex as shown in the fourth row. From Fisch C. Pacemaker electrocardiography. *J Indiana State Med Assoc* 1968;61:193.

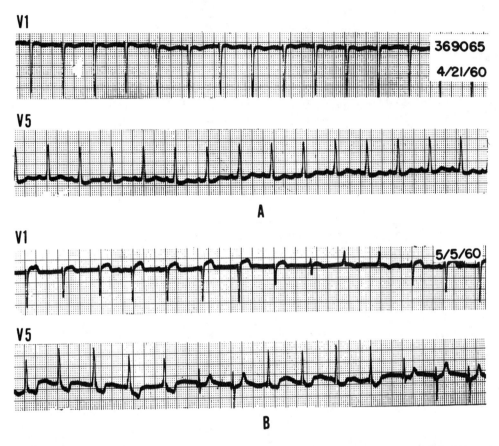

Figure 8-5. Fascicular VT. Panel A, the control tracing, shows rhythm sinus with P-P, P-R, and QRS intervals of 640, 160, and 60 ms, respectively. In panel B there is AV dissociation. In lead V_1 of panel B, three QRS complexes, each of different configuration, represent junctional complexes (i.e., QRS 1), ventricular fusion (i.e., QRS 8), and ventricular complexes (i.e., QRS 10), respectively. All QRS complexes are normal in duration. The ventricular complexes are upright in lead V_1. The R-R interval of the junctional and ventricular complexes is approximately 660 to 680 and 640 ms, respectively. Fusion indicates that the QRS complex is ventricular in origin despite the normal duration, and that the site of origin is in one of the fascicles of the LBB. Fascicular VT recorded in humans and induced in the laboratory is characterized by normal QRS durations, RBBB configuration, and either LAFB or LPFB. From Fisch C, Zipes DP, Noble RJ. Digitalis intoxication: Mechanisms and recognition. In Yu P, Goodwin R (eds): *Progress in Cardiology*. Philadelphia: Lea and Febiger; 1975:37.

L2

V2

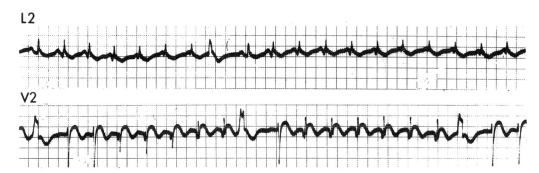

Figure 8-6. Fascicular VT with fusion complexes. AV dissociation with synchronization at a rate of 115 per minute is noted in L2. In lead V_2, the initial complex is a VPC followed by two normal QRS complexes and a series of fusions terminated by a VPC. The next sinus impulse is followed by VT and is terminated by a VPC and two normal QRS complexes. As indicated in Figure 8-5 fascicular VT is characterized by normal-duration QRS complexes, and the diagnosis of VT is indicated by fusions.

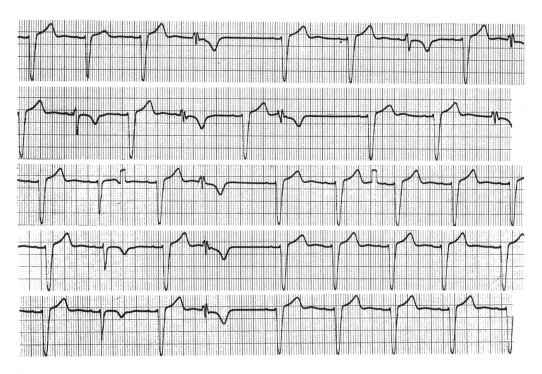

Figure 8-7. Spectrum of ventricular fusions between sinus impulses with LBBB and left ventricular parasystole. The basic rhythm is sinus with a P-P interval of 940 ms, a P-R interval of 180 ms, and LBBB. The parasystolic QRS complex exhibits an RBBB pattern. The second QRS complex in each row is a ventricular fusion. The pattern is intermediate between the RBBB of the parasystole and LBBB of the sinus rhythm. Simultaneous excitation of the ventricles by sinus and parasystolic impulses results in ventricular fusions. The parasystolic impulse activates the left ventricle while the sinus impulse conducts along the RBB and activates the right ventricle. Depending on a temporal relation of the two, a larger or small ventricular mass will be activated by one or the other impulse. In the bottom tracing, the parasystolic impulse activates most of the left ventricle and the sinus impulse via the RBB, the right ventricle. The result is a fusion resembling a normal QRS complex.

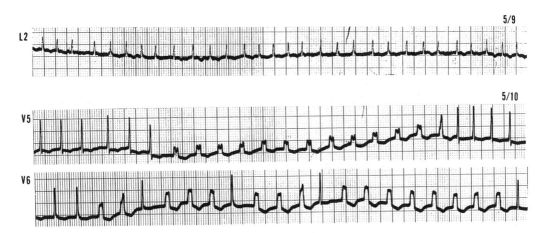

Figure 8-8. Ventricular fusions and captures. The basic rhythm is atrial fibrillation at a rate of approximately 200 per minute. In lead V_5, the fifth from the end is a fusion, as is the fourth QRS complex in lead V_6. In lead V_6, the six normal QRS complexes are captures. The presence of captures and fusions indicates that the tachycardia is ventricular in origin. Similarly, R-R intervals with normal QRS complexes shorter than R-R intervals with a wide QRS complex, by ruling out aberration, indicate VT. From Fisch C, Zipes DP, Noble RJ. Digitalis intoxication: Mechanisms and recognition. In: Yu P, Goodwin R (eds): *Progress in Cardiology.* Philadelphia: Lea and Febiger; 1975:37.

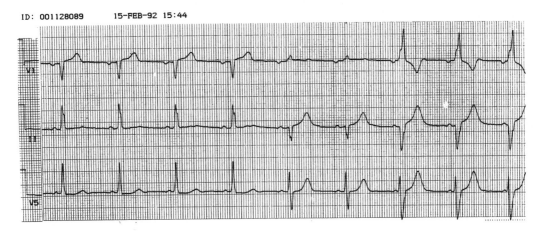

Figure 8-9. Ventricular fusions. Normal sinus rhythm with a P-R interval of 160 ms is followed by an idioventricular rhythm with RBBB configuration. The fifth and sixth QRS complexes are fusions between the sinus and idioventricular complexes.

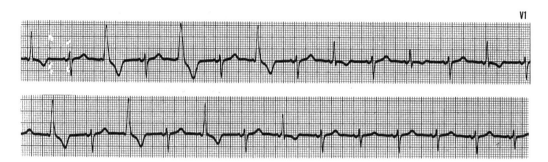

Figure 8-10. Ventricular fusion. The coupling of the VPC to the sinus QRS complex varies from 600 to 680 ms. The third QRS complex in the top tracing represents a "pure" VPC. The remaining VPCs reflect a spectrum of fusions. For example, the last two in the bottom tracing indicate that most of the ventricular mass is activated by sinus impulses, while the second VPC in the top tracing indicates that most of the ventricular mass is activated by the VPC. The spectrum of fusion results from the changing coupling interval of the VPC and, consequently, a changing temporal relation of the P and the VPC. The longer the P-R interval, the more normal the fusion; the shorter the P-R interval, the more bizarre the fusion.

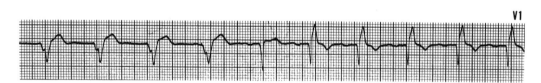

Figure 8-11. Ventricular fusion. The first four QRS complexes with an LBBB configuration are initiated by a subendocardial pacemaker. The last five QRS complexes are sinus in origin, with a P-R interval of 260 ms and RBBB. The normal QRS complex preceded by a P-R interval of 180 ms is a fusion between the sinus impulse with RBBB and the pacemaker impulse with LBBB configuration. The fortuitous, simultaneous activation of the right ventricle by the pacemaker and the left ventricle by the sinus impulse via the LBB results in a normal QRS complex.

ID: 000115487

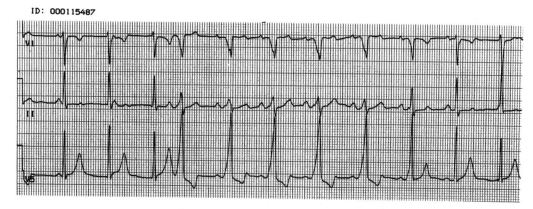

Figure 8-12. WPW, a fusion. The first three QRS complexes are junctional in origin. The third P wave conducts along both the AV node and the accessory pathway, resulting in a fusion. The component activated along the accessory pathway is represented by the initial slurring of the QRS complex, the delta wave. The remainder of the QRS complex is probably the result of conduction along the AV node. The third QRS complex from the end is also a fusion but with less of the myocardium being activated along the accessory pathway and more along the AV node. The next complex reflects normal sinoventricular conduction. The junctional complexes are not fusions and are thus normal.

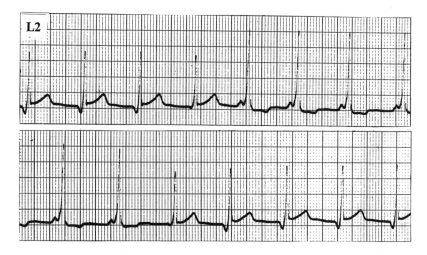

Figure 8-13. WPW and fusions. The basic rhythm is sinus with P-P and P-R intervals of 640 and 80 ms, respectively. In the top panel, the first four QRS complexes and P waves are junctional in origin. The R-R interval of the junctional tachycardia is 720 ms. The fourth P wave in the top row and third in the second row are fusions. These are shallow and intermediate between a fully retrograde negative P wave and a sinus P wave. The fourth QRS complex in the top row and the third in the bottom row are ventricular fusions. The QRS complexes are lower in amplitude with secondary ST-T changes, which differ from the ST-T of the WPW and the junctional complexes. The atrial fusion is the result of simultaneous activation of the atria by the sinus and junctional impulses. The ventricular fusion is the result of simultaneous activation of the ventricles by a junctional impulse and a sinus impulse reaching the ventricles along the accessory pathway.

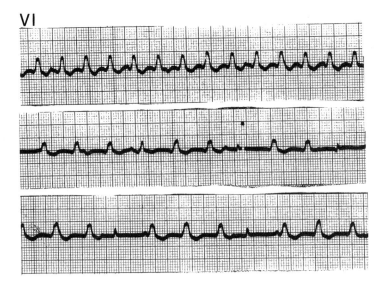

Figure 8-14. VT with captures and fusions. AV dissociation is recorded in the top tracing, with a P-P interval of 650 ms and a wide QRS tachycardia with an R-R interval of 400 ms. In the middle and bottom tracings, the P-P and R-R lengthen to 800 and 560 ms, respectively, with the appearance of captures and fusions. The fusion is represented by the fourth QRS complex in the middle row. Captures are illustrated by the seventh and tenth QRS complexes in the middle row and fourth and eighth in the bottom row. From Fisch C, Pinsky ST. Diagnosis of ventricular tachycardia. *J Indiana State Med Assoc* 1957;2:184.

References

1. Lewis T. *Clinical Electrocardiography.* London: Shaw and Sons; 1918:58.
2. Lewis T. *The Mechanisms and Graphic Registration of the Heart Beat.* London: Shaw and Sons; 1920:216.
3. Malinow MR, Langendorf R. Different mechanisms of fusion beats. *Am Heart J* 1948;35:448.
4. Dressler W, Roesler H. Occurrence in paroxysmal ventricular tachycardia of ventricular complexes transitional in shape to sinoauricular beats. *Am Heart J* 1952;44:485.
5. Bisteni A, Sodi-Pallares D, Medrano GA, Pileggi F. A new approach for the recognition of ventricular premature beats. *Am J Cardiol* 1969;5:358.
6. Marriott HJL, Schwartz NL, Bix HH. Ventricular fusion beats. *Circulation* 1962;26:880.
7. Schamroth L, Chesler E. Simulated 2:1 left bundle branch block. Normalization of the left bundle branch block pattern by ventricular extrasystoles. *Circulation* 1962;25:395.

9

Parasystole

General Features

Parasystole, with some exceptions, is a protected, independent, automatic, regular ectopic rhythm.

The classic electrocardiographic features of parasystole include: 1) variable coupling of the parasystolic impulse to the dominant rhythm; 2) a common parasystolic interval; 3) fusion between the parasystolic and the nonparasystolic complexes; and 4) failure of the parasystolic complex to manifest at times because of physiological refractoriness of the surrounding myocardium.

Parasystolic protection is evidenced by failure of extraneous impulses to disrupt the rhythmicity of the parasystolic pacemaker (Figures 9-1 and 9-2). The mechanism of the protection is not clear. The two prevailing theories are: 1) unidirectional block: the impulse is able to exit but is unable to "enter" the parasystolic focus,[1-5] and 2) the parasystolic focus discharges rapidly and maintains an area of physiological refractoriness about its site, thus preventing entry and discharge by other impulses (Figure 9-3).[3-6]

A diagnosis of parasystole requires evidence of protection of the parasystolic pacemaker. Protection can be assumed when an extraneous impulse that should discharge the pacemaker fails to do so. To satisfy this criterion, the impulses must reach the parasystolic focus after full recovery of the surrounding tissue; otherwise the failure of the ectopic parasystolic focus to discharge may be due to physiological interference rather than unidirectional block. An example of physiological interference is failure of sinus or other extraneous impulses to affect the site of the parasystolic focus because of the rapid rate of the parasystole (Figure 9-3).[7]

Irregular Parasystolic Rhythm

Although classic parasystolic impulses manifest a regular rate with variation of the interectopic interval of no more than 40 to 50 ms,[8] more recent data suggest that a much wider variation of the parasystolic rate, namely from 40 to 270 ms, is possible. As a rule, however, the variation is less than 180 ms.[9] The mechanism responsible for the irregularity of the interectopic interval varies. For example, when parasystolic impulses enclose a sinus impulse, the interectopic intervals are shorter than the interval between two consecutive parasystolic impulses without an intervening sinus impulse.[10] Variation of the parasystolic rate may be due to a changing slope of phase 4 of the TAP secondary to sympathetic and parasympathetic influences.[10] The irregular rhythm may also be the result of electronic modulation,[11,12] the effect of drugs, or of changing myocardial milieu surrounding the parasystolic focus. Based on experimental in vitro models, it has been shown that if the sinus impulse is close to the preceding parasystolic impulse, the effect of the electronic modulation is prolongation of the manifest ectopic cycle. On the other hand, the effect of electrotonus late during the parasystolic cycle is a shortening of the interectopic interval.[13]

The parasystolic impulse may fail to manifest when it would be expected to, that is, when the heart is no longer refractory. This phenomenon, first noted by Kaufmann and Rothberger[1] in 1920, was termed "exit block" (Figure 9-4). If the parasystolic interval is a multiple of the basic parasystolic cycle, the exit block is Type II. If, however, the interectopic interval shortens gradually with the long interval being less than the sum of two preceding parasystolic cycles, the exit block is Type I or Wenckebach. When the long interval is neither a multiple of the basic cycle nor associated with Wenckebach periodicity, the parasystole is intermittent (Figures 9-5 and 9-6).

In the presence of regular sinus rhythm, each intermittent parasystolic sequence begins with a fixed coupling to the preceding sinus impulse. The time of penetration of the parasystolic focus is estimated by measuring back one parasystolic interval from the first manifest parasystolic impulse. This will identify the point of interruption of the parasystole (Figures 9-5 and 9-6).

Fixed Coupling

As indicated, one of the diagnostic features of parasystole is a variable coupling of the ectopic impulse to the preceding dominant impulse, usually sinus. Occasionally, however, the coupling is constant (Figure 9-7). This may be the result of a simple mathematic relationship between the parasystole and the dominant rhythm when the rates of both are equal and regular and each protected against the other.

Fixed coupling also may be the result of "linkage" where the parasystolic impulse regularly discharges and resets the dominant pacemaker. Since the dominant pacemaker, i.e., sinus, also discharges at a constant interval, the two maintain a fixed relationship.[14-16] Such linkage is frequent with atrial parasystole (Figure 9-7).[17] Linkage is also possible in the presence of a regular sinus rhythm and a ventricular parasystole with retrograde atrial activation, the latter discharging the sinus pacemaker.

Specific Forms of Parasystole

The general features outlined earlier apply to all forms of parasystole; however, some forms of parasystole exhibit their own specific characteristics.

Sinus Parasystole

Sinus parasystole is rare and implies continuous protection of the SAN against atrial and retrograde junctional or ventricular impulses (Figure 9-8).[18]

Atrial Parasystole

Atrial parasystole is relatively rare, and the rate is slow (Figure 9-9). Because of the linkage described earlier, an atrial parasystole will most often manifest as an atrial bigeminy and thus the parasystole is unrecognized (Figures 9-6 and 9-7). The parasystole becomes manifest only when the bigeminal rhythm is disrupted, as, for example, when the sinus impulse is discharged by an extraneous impulse other than the atrial parasystole, leaving the latter undisturbed (Figure 9-7). Similarly, exit block from the parasystolic focus may disturb the parasystolic sinus relationship sufficiently to unmask the atrial parasystole.

Atrial fusions are rare, largely because of resetting of the sinus rhythm by the parasystole and because the configuration of the P wave makes recognition of fusions difficult (Figures 9-7 and 9-9).[19]

In the presence of a regular sinus rhythm, the postparasystolic interval is longer than the sinus P-P interval because of delayed arrival of the parasystolic impulse at the SAN, suppression of the SAN, delay of exit from the SAN, or a combination of the above. If the postparasystolic cycle equals the dominant sinus P-P interval, then prompt discharge of the sinus node by the parasystolic impulse has taken place. If the postparasystolic cycle is shorter than the sinus P-P interval, interpolation of the parasystolic impulse is assumed. The postectopic sinus impulse may, however, be delayed in its exit from the sinus node so that the postparasystolic sinus P-P interval is longer than the dominant sinus P-P. It has been estimated that the delay of exit may vary from 80 to 340 ms.[20] Furthermore, because the postectopic sinus P is delayed, the subsequent sinus P-P interval is shorter than expected.

Junctional Parasystole

A junctional parasystolic interval may vary by as much as 120 ms or more.[2,6] The parasystolic rhythm may parallel the sinus rate. In approximately one half of cases, the parasystole activates the atria retrogradely. If the retrograde atrial activation precedes the QRS complex, differentiation of junctional parasystole from low atrial or coronary sinus parasystole is difficult or impossible. Similarly, in the presence of aberration, differentiation between junctional and ventricular parasystole is difficult.

Ventricular Parasystole

Because the sinus rhythm and the ventricular parasystole originate in different chambers and because the ventricular parasystole rarely activates the atria retrogradely, the two rhythms coexist without interference (Figure 9-10). This allows the ventricular parasystole to manifest the four classic features of a parasystole stated above (Figures 9-10 and 9-11). It is also possible, as indicated, for a ventricular parasystole with retrograde atrial conduction, through linkage, to manifest fixed coupling to the preceding sinus impulse. Rarely, a ventricular parasystole may, by conducting retrogradely, induce ventricular reentry (Figure 9-12). Similarly, a ventricular parasystole may manifest as a ventricular bigeminy with fixed coupling.

Double ventricular parasystoles (both ectopic or one due to an artificial pacemaker) exist but are rare. Multiple, namely more than two, simultaneous parasystolic rhythms have been reported.[7,9,21]

Concealed parasystole is a rare form of parasystole that is recognized by an unexpected disturbance of A-V conduction that is not otherwise explainable.

Parasystolic Ventricular Tachycardia

The rate of this parasystole is 100 per minute or greater. Extraneous impulses, including sinus impulses, fail to alter the rhythmicity of the tachycardia (Figures 9-13 and 9-14). The mechanism of the parasystole may be twofold: 1) a rapidly discharging parasystolic pacemaker induces an area of refractoriness, thus protecting the ectopic impulse site, a form of dissociation (Figure 9-3), and 2) unidirectional block.

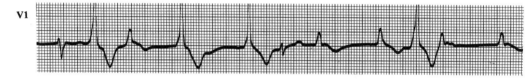

Figure 9-1. Ventricular parasystole. There are three different QRS complexes. The narrow QRS complex with a deep S wave is the normal supraventricular impulse. Of the two ectopic ventricular complexes, the one of lower amplitude is the parasystolic QRS complex. The coupling of the parasystolic QRS complex to the preceding impulse varies. The interectopic parasystolic interval is constant and measures 900 ms. The parasystolic impulse fails to manifest when falling during the refractory period induced by the preceding QRS complex.

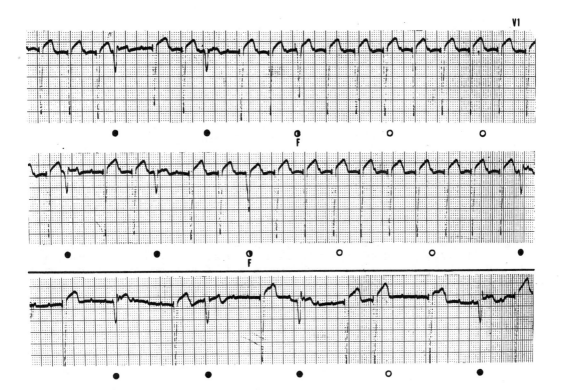

Figure 9-2. Ventricular parasystole, atrial tachycardia, and the effect of vagal stimulation. The parasystolic complexes are identified with the solid circles, failure to manifest by open circles, and fusions by half solid circles and the letter F. In the top tracing, the basic rhythm is an atrial flutter. The coupling of the parasystolic impulse to the preceding supraventricular QRS complex varies. The interectopic interval is constant at 1640 ms. The parasystolic impulse fails to manifest during refractoriness of the surrounding myocardium. The black line in the bottom tracing indicates carotid sinus pressure resulting in an increased A-V block but without any change in the interectopic parasystolic interval. The response to the vagal stimulation suggests that the vagus has no effect on the parasystolic pacemaker. From Fisch C, Knoebel SB. Digitalis toxicity. *J Am Coll Cardiol* 1985;5:91A. Reprinted with permission.

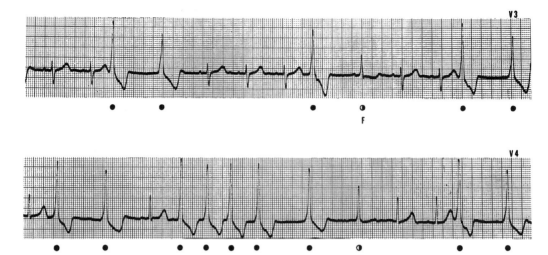

Figure 9-3. Parasystolic VT with Type II exit block. The basic rhythm is sinus. The parasystolic complexes are identified with a solid circle and fusions by a half solid circle and the letter F. The basic interectopic interval is 500 to 510 ms, with the longer interectopic cycles being a multiple of the basic interval. Failure of the sinus impulses to disrupt the regularity of the ectopic rhythm indicates a protected parasystolic pacemaker. The longer pauses, a multiple of the basic interectopic cycle length of 500 to 510 ms, indicate Type II exit block. This tracing suggests a possible mechanism of parasystolic protection, namely interference caused by the rapidly discharging pacemaker. The rapidly discharging pacemaker induces a continuous local refractoriness that results in protection of the parasystolic pacemaker. A rapidly discharging pacemaker, when accompanied by exit block, will falsely suggest a slower rate of the parasystole.

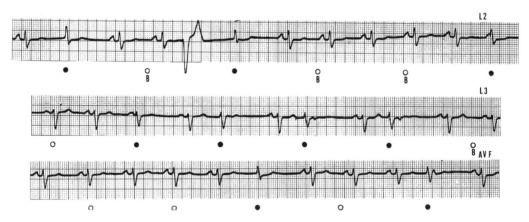

Figure 9-4. Junctional parasystole with exit block. The basic rhythm is sinus with a P-P interval of approximately 920 ms and a single VPC in lead L2. The parasystolic interectopic interval is approximately 1760 ms or multiple of this basic interval. The manifest parasystolic junctional impulses are identified with a solid circle. In lead L3, the parasystolic complexes conduct retrogradely to the atria. Impulses that fail to manifest because of physiological refractoriness are identified with open circles, and impulses that fail to manifest because of an exit block are identified by an open circle and the letter B. A constant interectopic interval, varying coupling and failure of sinus impulse to disturb the rhythmicity of the ectopic rhythm, indicates a parasystole. Failure to manifest when the ventricle is no longer refractory indicates an exit block.

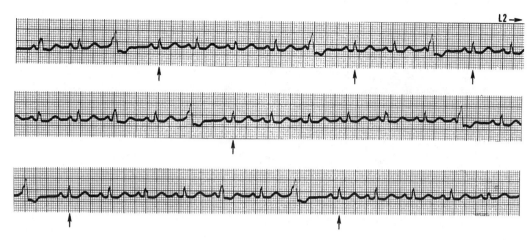

Figure 9-5. Intermittent ventricular parasystole. The tracing is continuous. The basic rhythm is sinus with a P-P interval of 680 ms interrupted by an intermittent ventricular parasystole. The time of resetting of the parasystole is indicated by an arrow. Each parasystolic sequence bears a constant relationship to the resetting sinus complex, identified by an arrow. It is likely that at this point, that the parasystolic pacemaker is not protected, and is penetrated and discharged and reset. The interval from the last parasystolic QRS complex to the moment of penetration of the parasystolic pacemaker by the sinus impulse is 800 ms. It is possible that as phase 4 of the transmembrane potential of the parasystolic pacemaker nears the TP, it loses its protection, and the sinus impulse, sufficiently strong, brings the transmembrane potential to threshold, discharging the parasystolic pacemaker.

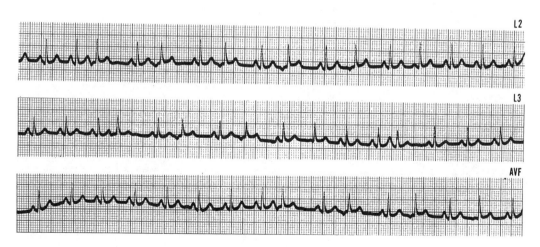

Figure 9-6. Intermittent atrial or junctional parasystole. The dominant rhythm is a sinus tachycardia with a P-P interval of 540 ms. Parasystolic P waves are inverted in leads L2, L3, and AVF. The interectopic interval is regular at 1120 ms and the coupling varies. Fusions are present and the parasystolic impulse fails to excite the atrium because of surrounding myocardial refractoriness. Upright APCs are recorded in lead L3. The intermittent nature of the parasystole is indicated by a fixed coupling of the first parasystolic P of each parasystolic sequence.

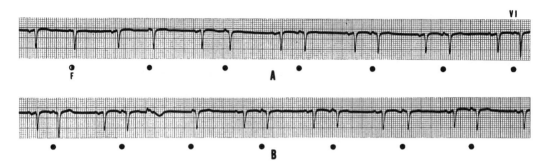

Figure 9-7. Atrial parasystole manifesting as an atrial bigeminy. The parasystole is identified with a solid dot, the fusion by a half solid dot with the letter F. The parasystole is manifest as an atrial bigeminy. In panel B, following the first two parasystolic complexes, a VPC with retrograde conduction discharges the sinus node. The compensatory pause is terminated by an atrial parasystolic impulse. Were it not for the VPC with retrograde conduction the parasystole would not have been recognized. The parasystole discharges the SAN. The compensatory pause terminated each time by the regularly discharging sinus impulse results in a constant, fixed relationship of sinus node to the parasystole.

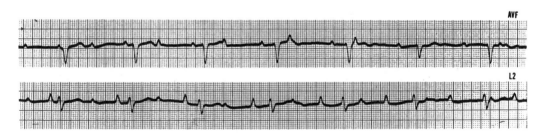

Figure 9-8. Atrial and sinus or dual atrial parasystole. Two P waves differing in amplitude are noted. The first two P waves in lead AVF identify one parasystole with an interval of 720 ms. The fifth and seventh P waves identify the second parasystole with an interval of 1460 ms. The distance between the two different P waves ranges from 500 to 700 ms. Varying relation of two regular rhythms, each with a constant interectopic interval, a different common denominator, and failure to be reset indicate two protected pacemakers, a sinus and atrial or dual atrial parasystole.

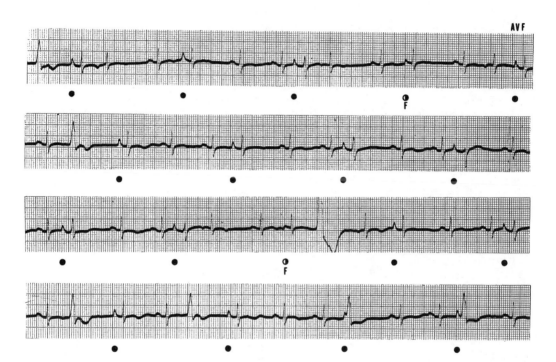

Figure 9-9. Atrial parasystole and APCs. The dominant rhythm is sinus with a P-P interval of 760 ms. The parasystolic P waves are identified with a solid circle. The negative P waves are APCs. The P waves following the longer cycles are the sinus P waves. The half solid circles with the letter F indicate fusions between the parasystolic P and the APCs. The varying coupling of the parasystolic P wave, a fixed interectopic interval at a cycle length of 2260 ms, and fusions indicate an atrial parasystole.

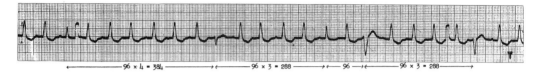

Figure 9-10. Ventricular parasystole. The basic sinus rhythm is interrupted by APCs and a ventricular parasystole. The features of the parasystole include varying coupling to the preceding sinus impulse, a constant interectopic interval of 960 ms, with the longer intervals a multiple of the basic interval, and fusion complexes (i.e., the third, the tenth, and the third from the end).

ID: 001088581

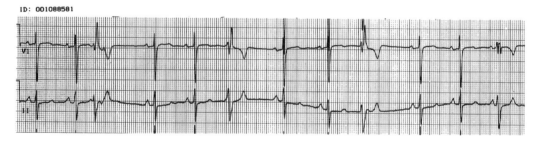

Figure 9-11. Ventricular parasystole. The basic rhythm is sinus with an R-R of approximately 800 ms. The parasystolic complexes with RBB configuration exhibit varying coupling to the preceding QRS complex, a fixed interectopic interval of 2600 ms, and a fusion manifest by the last QRS complex.

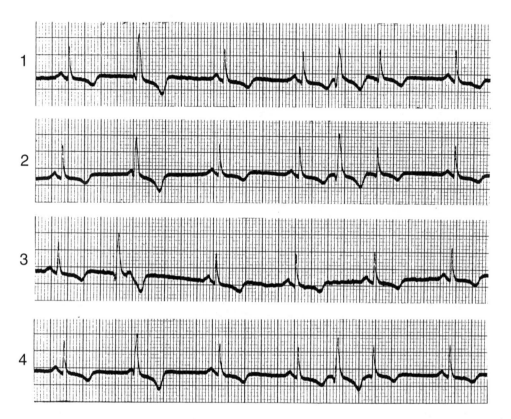

Figure 9-12. Ventricular parasystole with ventricular reentry. The basic rhythm is sinus with a ventricular parasystole. Some of the parasystolic impulses are followed by ventricular reentry. The parasystolic interectopic interval is 2470 ms. The ventricular reentry is indicated by: 1) a normal QRS complex following a parasystolic QRS complex by an interval too short to be sinus in origin, and 2) failure of reentry when a sinus P wave conceals into the AV junction blocking the reentry. The first parasystolic QRS complex in each row maintains a close temporal relationship with the sinus P wave, which reaches the junction, blocks retrograde conduction, and prevents reentry. The second parasystolic impulse in rows one, two, and four are followed by a retrograde P and ventricular reentry. The close temporal relation of the sinus P wave and the parasystolic QRS complex suggests that interruption of reentry by the nonconducted sinus impulse is the most likely mechanism of failure of reentry.

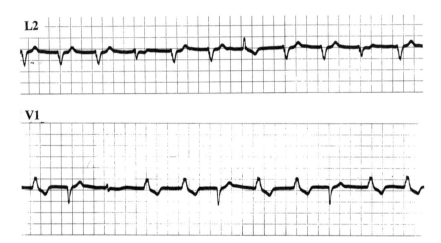

Figure 9-13. Parasystolic VT. The narrow QRS complexes are supraventricular in origin. The complexes with RBBB and left axis deviation are parasystolic in origin. The interectopic interval is 680 ms or a multiple thereof. The fifth and the 11th complexes in L2 and the third in lead V_1 are fusions. The rhythmicity of the VT is not interrupted. Although a parasystole is most likely, it is also possible that the protection is the result of a rapidly discharging ventricular focus with an area of refractoriness and, thus, a dissociation rather than a true protected parasystolic focus.

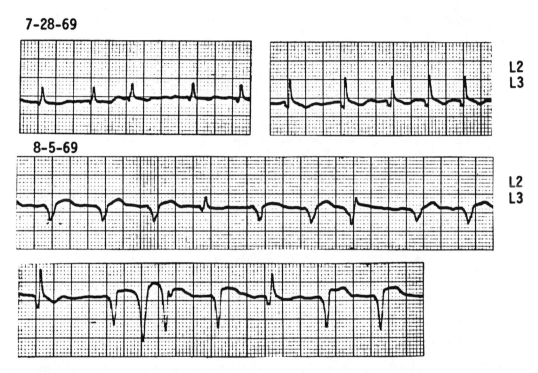

Figure 9-14. Parasystolic VT. The basic rhythm is atrial fibrillation with supraventricular QRS complexes recorded in the top panel. The bottom panel shows atrial fibrillation and VT with a basic RR interval of 600 ms. The longer intervals of 1200 and 1800 encompassing a supraventricular QRS complex or VPC or both are a multiple of the basic VT interval of 600 ms. In the bottom tracing, the first QRS complex is supraventricular. The second and fourth are ventricular complexes and encompass a VPC. The VPC does not disturb the rhythmicity of the parasystolic tachycardia. Failure of the supraventricular impulse or the VPC or both to disturb the rhythmicity of the VT indicate a protected VT. Because of the rapid rate of the ectopic focus, the protection may be caused by physiological interference rather than true parasystole (see Figure 9-13). From Fisch C. Digitalis induced tachycardia. In Surawicz B, Reddy CP, Prystowsky EN (eds): *Tachycardias.* Boston: Martinus Nijhoff Publishers; 1984:399.

References

1. Kaufmann R, Rothberger CJ. Beitrag zur Kenntnis der Entsehungsweise extrasystolischer Allorhythmien. *Z Ges Exp Med* 1920;11:40.
2. Lewis T. *The Mechanism and Graphic Registration of the Heart Beat.* 3rd ed. London: Shaw and Sons; 1925:393.
3. Mobitz WL. Ueber die verschiedene Eststehungsweise extrasystolischer Allorhythmien beim menschen, ein Beitrag zur Frage der Interferenz mehrerer Rhythmen. *Z Ges Exp Med* 1923;34:491.
4. Rothberger CJ. Normale und Pathologische Physiologie der Rhythmik and Koordination des Herzens. *Ergebn Physiol* 1931;32:472.
5. Wenckebach KF, Winterberg H. *Die Unregelmaessige Herztaetigkeit.* Leipzig: W Engelemann; 1927:313.
6. Scherf D. Experimental parasystole. *Am Heart J* 1951;42:212.
7. El-Sherif N, Samet P. Multiform ventricular ectopic rhythm—evidence for multiple parasystolic activity. *Circulation* 1975;51:492.
8. Pick A. Parasystole. *Circulation* 1953;8:243.
9. Hiejima K, Poh TD. Double ventricular parasystole—supernormal phase of conduction as a mechanism of intermittent parasystole. Report of a case. *Circulation* 1976;53:572.
10. Nau GJ, Aldariz AE, Acunzo RA, et al. Modulation of parasystolic activity by non-parasystolic beats. *Circulation* 1982;66:462.
11. Jalife J, Moe GK. Effect of electronic potentials on pacemaker activity of canine Purkinje fibers in relation to parasystole. *Circ Res* 1976;39:801.
12. Jalife J, Michaels DC, Langendorf R. Modulated parasystole originating in the sinoatrial node. *Circulation* 1986;74:945.
13. Moe GK, Jalife J, Mueller WJ, Moe B. A mathematical model of parasystole and its application to clinical arrhythmias. *Circulation* 1977;56:968.
14. Cohen H, Langendorf R, Pick A. Intermittent parasystole—mechanism of protection. *Circulation* 1973;68:761.
15. Steffens TG. Intermittent ventricular parasystole due to entrance block failure. *Circulation* 1971;64:442.
16. Langendorf R, Pick A. Parasystole with fixed coupling. *Circulation* 1967;35:304.
17. Scherf D, Yildiz M, DeArmas D. Atrial parasystole. *Am Heart J* 1959;57:507.
18. Schamroth L. Sinus parasystole. *Am J Cardiol* 1967;20:434.
19. Friedberg HD, Schamroth L. Atrial parasystole. *Br Heart J* 1970;32:172.
20. Lesser M, Plotkin P, Levin B. Atrial parasystole with interpolation observations on prolonged sinoatrial conduction. *Am Heart J* 1962;63:649.
21. Tenczer J, Littman L. Double irregular ventricular parasystole: Rate dependent entrance block and "supernormal" exit conduction. *Circulation* 1978;53:723.

10

Reentry

The conditions necessary for reentry include dual pathways, slowing or asynchrony of conduction, unidirectional block, and recovery of excitability in order for a tissue to be reexcited.

Historical Perspective

"I shall now describe a type of rhythm which I have observed occasionally in the course of experiments where two chambers of the heart were used and where rhythmic stimulation at a fairly high pace had been applied. The phenomenon to which I refer may be called reciprocating rhythm. I have seen it in three experiments on the auricle-ventricle preparation of the heart of the electric ray, and in one experiment on the ventricle-bulbus preparation from the frog. The preparations were, before stimulation, either quiescent or giving infrequent spontaneous beats.

"After the application of rhythmic stimuli at some particular rate, the cessation of the stimuli was followed by a quick reciprocating movement of auricle and ventricle or of ventricle and bulbus. The appearance of the heart gave the impression that the beats of the ventricle were caused by those of the auricle or bulbus, while these in turn were caused by the ventricle. This was confirmed by observation of the effect of sending in a single shock, either to the auricle or to the ventricle. This, if timed properly, instantly arrested both chambers . . .

"A slight difference in the rate of recovery of two divisions of the AV connexion might determine that an extra systole of the ventricle, provoked by a stimulus applied to the ventricle shortly after activity of the AV connexion, should spread up to the auricle by that part of the AV connexion having the quicker recovery process and not by the other part. In such a case, when the auricle became excited by this impulse, the other portion of the AV connexion would be ready to take up the transmission again back to the ventricle. Provided the transmission in each direction was slow, the chamber at either end would be ready to respond (its refractory phase being short) and thus the condition once established would tend to continue, unless upset by the interpolation of a premature systole. The experiments I have been able to make have given results in accord with this conclusion."[1]

So wrote Mines in 1913, describing the concept of and the conditions necessary for reentry. His experimental preparation was an electric ray and a frog, and the recording equipment was a smoked drum. That the "impulse travels over different pathways on entering and reentering the depressed region" was confirmed by Schmitt and Erlanger in 1928.[2]

The first electrocardiographic record of reentry was published by White[3] in 1915. The reentry was manifest by a normal QRS complex, a retrograde negative P wave, and a second, reentrant normal QRS complex.

As indicated, conditions necessary for reentry include: 1) dual pathways; 2) slowing or asynchrony of conduction; 3) unidirectional block; and 4) recovery of excitability.[4]

Electrocardiographic Characteristics

Although the initial description of reentrant rhythm was that of the ventricle, of the AV node,[5,6] and of the atrium, reentry has since been documented for the SAN,[7] the His-Purkinje fibers,[6,8] the bundle of His, and the myocardium.[2,7]

If the origin of reentry is in the AV node, the first QRS complex is normal, providing there is no BBB or aberration (Figures 10-1 and 10-2) followed by a negative

P wave and a normal QRS complex. If the impulse originates in the ventricle, as is often the case, the first QRS complex is abnormal and is followed by a retrograde P and, most often, a normal QRS complex (Figures 10-3 and 10-4).[9] Reentry originating in the atrium inscribes a normal P wave followed by a normal QRS complex and this, in turn, by a retrograde P wave (Figure 10-5).[10]

In addition to the classic ECG manifestations of reentry described above, reentry can be seen with VT (Figures 10-6, 10-7, and 10-8) and artificial electronic pacemakers, among other conditions. Reentry can occur within the AV node without involving the ventricle (Figures 10-9, 10-10, 10-11, and 10-12). In such cases, the ECG would inscribe a sequence of a normal and a retrograde P wave. Reentry without involvement of the atrium will be manifest by two consecutive normal QRS complexes.

In cases of reentrant tachycardia, the reentry can take place in the AV node (AVNRT) or may include an accessory pathway as one of the limbs of the reentrant loop (AVRT).

Although retrograde conduction is common during VT, ventricular reentry[11,12] is rare. Because of the rapid ventricular rate, either the return pathway does not recover in time or the ventricle is still refractory. However, if reentry does take place, the ECG includes a sequence of a QRS complex of the VT, a retrograde P wave followed by a normal QRS complex, or a ventricular fusion (Figures 10-6 and 10-7).[13]

While a normal QRS complex that follows an interpolated VPC may be sinus in origin, often the normal QRS complex represents a ventricular reentry. This is true in the presence or absence of a recognizable retrograde P wave. The P wave may not be recognizable when superimposed on the T wave, or the reentry may be intranodal without involvement of the atrium. Reentry time does not vary by more than 60 ms in any given tracing.[14] This is in keeping with intranodal reentry even in the absence of retrograde P waves. A diagnosis of intranodal reentry based on accurate coupling is possible in atrial fibrillation or complete A-V block or in other conditions in which retrograde conduction is not possible (Figure 10-13).

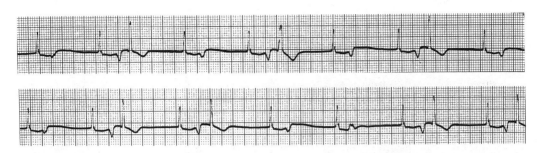

Figure 10-1. L2. Ventricular reentry, atrial fusion. The junctional R-R intervals of 160 ms are followed by retrograde, negative P waves at an R-P interval of 360 ms and a P-R interval of 220 to 240 ms. Ventricular reentry is inscribed following junctional QRS complexes 2, 4, and 6 in the top and 2, 3, 6, and 7 in the bottom tracing, respectively. P waves 1, 3, 5, and 7 and 1, 4, and 5 in the top and bottom tracings, respectively, are atrial fusions. The ventricular reentry fails in the presence of atrial fusion. An atrial fusion implies that the junctional impulse reached the atrium. Therefore, failure to reciprocate cannot be due to failure of the retrograde impulse to reach the atrium. It is more likely that the sinus impulse conceals into the return limb of the dual pathway and blocks reentry. This mechanism is supported by the fact that reentry fails only after an atrial fusion. The R-R interval from reentrant QRS complex to the next junctional impulse measures 1040 ms, or 120 ms less than the dominant junctional R-R interval of 1160 ms. The shorter R-R interval indicates that the reentry or the "turnaround" discharges and resets the junctional pacemaker before the QRS complex is inscribed. The true intrajunctional interval is still 1160 ms, even though the manifest junctional R-R interval is only 1040 ms.

L-3

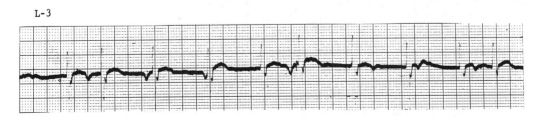

Figure 10-2. Ventricular reentry. The basic rhythm is junctional with an R-R interval of 800 ms. Each QRS complex is accompanied by a negative inverted P wave. The relationship of the P wave to the preceding QRS complex varies. The first, the fourth, and seventh junctional impulses are followed by a negative P wave and a ventricular reentry. The reentry is manifest by a normal junctional QRS complex followed by a retrograde P wave and reentry to the ventricle inscribing a normal QRS complex.

LII

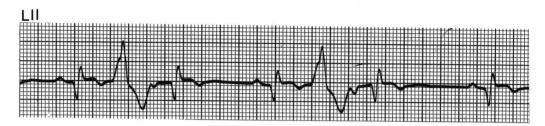

Figure 10-3. Ventricular reentry. Each of the two VPCs are followed by a retrograde, negative P wave and a ventricular reentry. The reentrant QRS complex suggests an inferior myocardial infarction.

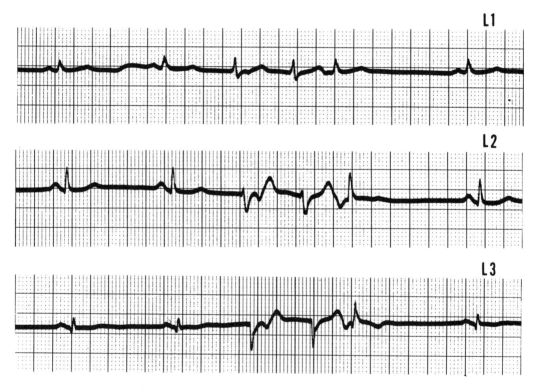

Figure 10-4. Retrograde Wenckebach conduction and ventricular reentry. The basic sinus rhythm with a P-P interval of 1120 ms is interrupted by ventricular premature couplets. The ventricular premature of the couplet conducts retrogradely with an R-P interval of 200 and 430 ms, respectively. The second retrograde P wave is followed by ventricular reentry. The minimal aberration of the reentrant QRS complex is due to a shorter R-R interval.

L2

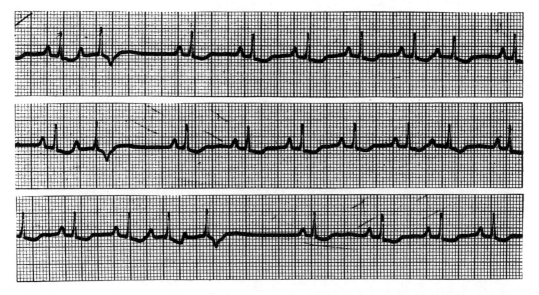

Figure 10-5. Atrial reentry. The basic rhythm is sinus with APCs. The P-R intervals of the APCs vary from 200 to 280 ms. The APCs with a P-R interval of 240 and 280 ms reenter the atrium inscribing a negative P wave. The prolonged P-R interval reflects conduction along the slowly conducting limb of a dual pathway, allowing sufficient time for the atrium to recover and for reentry to occur.

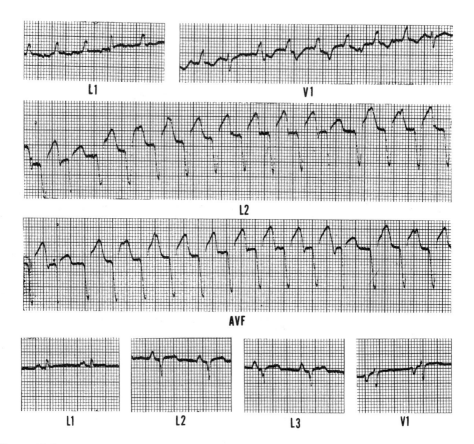

Figure 10-6. VT with retrograde Wenckebach conduction and ventricular reentry. The dominant rhythm is VT with an R-R of 400 ms. The successively longer R-P intervals and the gradually more distinct inverted P waves are best seen in the middle of lead AVF. Following the longest R-P interval, a ventricular reentry inscribes a normal QRS complex. The R-R interval of the reentrant complex is 40 ms shorter than the R-R interval of the VT. The ventricular reentry with a normal QRS complex is diagnostic of VT by excluding preexisting BBB or rate-dependent aberration.

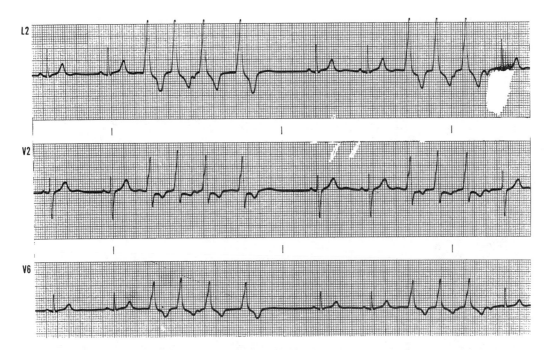

Figure 10-7. Ventricular reentry. The basic rhythm is sinus with a P-P of 1040 ms interrupted by runs of VT. Retrograde conduction is indicated by the inverted P waves. The second run of VT is followed by a retrograde P wave with an R-P interval of 400 ms and a ventricular reentry with a P-R interval of 280 ms.

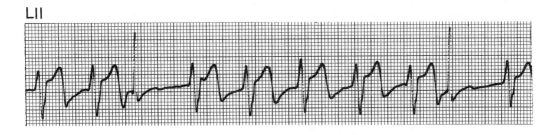

Figure 10-8. VT with ventricular reentry. The basic rhythm is VT with an R-R of 640 ms. Retrograde conduction, indicated by deeply inverted P waves, follows ventricular ectopy and a normal QRS complex.

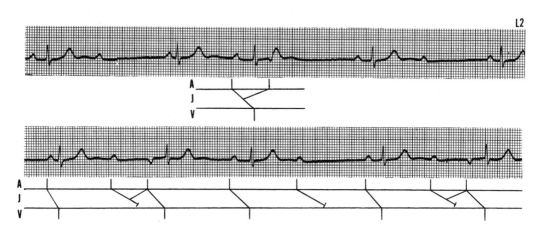

Figure 10-9. Type I Wenckebach A-V block with concealed intranodal reentry. In the middle of the top tracing, Wenckebach periodicity is interrupted by an atrial reentry manifest by a retrograde, negative P wave. In the lower tracing, the first P wave conducts with the P-R interval of 200 ms, and the second, fourth, and the sixth sinus P waves are blocked. The second and the sixth P waves are followed by a retrograde, reentrant P wave. The atrial reentry is, in turn, followed by a ventricular reentry with a P-R interval of 300 ms. The appearance of retrograde P waves only after the longest P-R interval, or after a blocked sinus P wave, supports reentry as the mechanism of the negative P wave. Were the negative P waves APCs rather than reentrant P waves, a random relationship of the negative P to the preceding P-R interval would be expected with some APCs following the shorter P-R intervals. Sinus P waves followed by retrograde P waves, without an intervening QRS complex, indicate concealed intranodal reentry.

L II

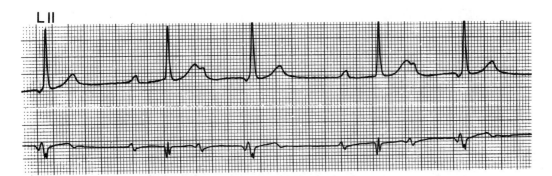

Figure 10-10. Type I Wenckebach A-V block with concealed intranodal reentry. The basic rhythm is sinus with a P-P of 920 ms. A negative P wave with a P-P of 560 ms follows the blocked P of the Wenckebach sequence. This P wave reflects an atrial reentry with the "turnaround" within the AV node, an example of concealed intranodal reentry (see Figure 10-9).

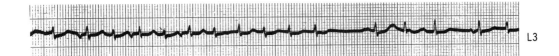

L3

Figure 10-11. Reciprocating AVNRT. The AVNRT is associated with a 2:1 retrograde conduction with failure of retrograde conduction preceding cessation of the tachycardia. The mechanism of the tachycardia is unclear. Alternating retrograde conduction and ultimately failure of retrograde conduction rules out the "incessant" form of reentrant tachycardia, AVRT, and atrial tachycardia. The R-P longer than the P-R rules out the usual form of AVNRT, since a retrograde P of AVNRT is usually inscribed within or at the end of the QRS complex. The most likely mechanism is an uncommon form of AVNRT with fast anterograde and slow retrograde conduction. The junctional tachycardia continues at the same rate but without intervening QRS complex, indicating concealed intranodal reentry.

V1

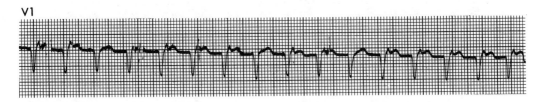

Figure 10-12. AVNRT with concealed reentry. The basic rhythm is AVNRT with retrograde P waves inscribed as a pseudo r^1. The R-R measures 440 ms. Following the third, eighth, and 11th QRS complexes, there is no evidence of retrograde conduction. The rhythmicity, however, is undisturbed. The AVNRT is uninterrupted without evidence of atrial involvement, suggesting that the atrium may not be a necessary component of the reentrant loop.

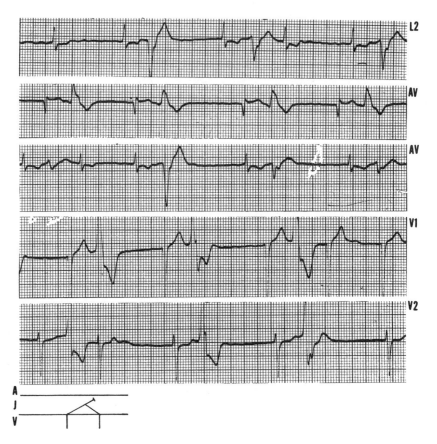

Figure 10-13. Atrial fibrillation with concealed ventricular reentry. The basic rhythm is atrial fibrillation with an AV nodal rhythm at an R-R of 1000 ms. The VPCs are accurately coupled and have a relatively uniform configuration, indicating a unifocal origin. Some of the VPCs are followed by a junctional impulse with a shorter fixed junctional to junctional R-R of 900 ms. Early normal QRS complexes with a constant coupling to the VPC indicates reentry within the AV node, a manifestation of concealed intranodal reentry.

References

1. Mines GR. On dynamic equilibrium in the heart. *J Physiol* 1913;46:349.
2. Schmitt FO, Erlanger J. Directional differences in the conduction of the impulse through heart muscle and then possible relation to extrasystolic and fibrillating contractions. *Am J Physiol* 1928–29;87:326.
3. White PD. A study of atrioventricular rhythm following auricular flutter. *Arch Intern Med* 1915;16:517.
4. Moe GK, Preston JB, Burlington H. Physiologic evidence for a dual A-V transmission system. *Circ Res* 1956;4:357.
5. Goldreyer BN, Bigger JT Jr. The site of reentry in paroxysmal supraventricular tachycardia. *Circulation* 1971;43:15.
6. Akhtar M, Damato AN, Batsford WP, Ruskin JN, Ogunkelu JB, Varga G. Demonstration of reentry within the His-Purkinje system in man. *Circulation* 1974;50:1150.
7. Paulay KL, Varghese PJ, Damato AN. Atrial rhythms in response to an early atrial premature depolarization in man. *Am Heart J* 1973;85:323.
8. Cranefield PF, Klein HO, Hoffman BE. Conduction of cardiac impulse delay, block and one-way block in depressed Purkinje fibers. *Circ Res* 1971;28:199.
9. Kistin AD. Multiple pathways of conduction and reciprocal rhythm with interpolated ventricular premature systoles. *Am Heart J* 1963;65:162.
10. Kistin AD. Atrial reciprocal rhythm. *Circulation* 1965;32:687.
11. Grau S, Gouaux JL. Paroxysmal ventricular tachycardia with second degree V-A block and reciprocal rhythm. *Circulation* 1950;2:422.
12. Katz LN, Pick A. *Clinical Electrocardiography. I. The Arrhythmias.* Philadelphia: Lea and Febiger; 1956:144.
13. Vermeulen A, Wellens HJJ. Paroxysmal ventricular tachycardia showing fusion with reciprocal ventricular beats. *Br Heart J* 1971;33:320.
14. Pick A, Langendorf R. A case of reciprocal beating with evidence of repetitive and blocked reentry of the cardiac impulse. *Am Heart J* 1950;40:13.

11

Supernormal Conduction
and Excitability

Supernormal excitability can be recorded during a brief period of recovery of the TAP, in which excitation is possible in response to an otherwise subthreshold stimulus (Figure 11-1). A stimulus of the same strength fails to elicit a response either earlier or later in the cardiac cycle. An impulse that arrives during the supernormal period of recovery will conduct better than expected or will conduct when block had been expected (Figures 11-2 and 11-3). Supernormal conduction depends on supernormal excitability. When supernormal excitability is eliminated, supernormal conduction is no longer possible.[1] In the ECG, the supernormal period of excitability occurs during a brief period at the end of the T wave or at the beginning of isoelectric diastole (Figures 11-3, 11-4, 11-5).

Historical Perspective

In 1925, Lewis wrote,

> *"There is a case recently reported from my laboratory, in which an auricular rhythm and a much slower ventricular rhythm interplay and produce almost accurate coupling . . . In the whole series of curves, response of the ventricle is invariably coupled to any auricular systole which falls between the summit of T and its endpoint. There is no response to an auricular systole falling in any other part of the ventricular cycle . . . In other words, over this phase there has been an overswing in the recovery curve of responsiveness, reminiscent of or identical with the 'supernormal' phase of recovery described by Adrian and Lucas."[2]*

The above appears to be the earliest report of "supernormal" conduction in the human—in this instance, in the presence of a complete heart block.

At about the same time, Mackenzie published tracings that were recorded in 1913 in a patient with RBBB and paroxysmal A-V block. Resumption of sinus rhythm was possible due to "supernormal" conduction induced by retrograde conduction of an escape impulse.

The supernormal phase of excitability was first observed by Adrian and Lucas[3] in nerve tissue, and by Adrian[4] in the frog ventricle. It has been recorded in a compressed turtle atrium,[5] in dog myocardium, and in the intact dog.[6] With the advent of cellular electrophysiology, the supernormal period was demonstrated in the Purkinje fiber[7] and in the specialized atrial tissue.[8] The supernormal period is recorded earlier with shortening of the transmembrane potential; however, its duration, configuration, and minimal stimulus strength required to elicit a response remain unchanged.

The Clinical Picture

In the clinical setting, "supernormality" of conduction is manifested by better than expected conduction, but not by conduction that is more rapid than normal. Thus, the term relative "supernormality" is more appropriate when applied to the ECG. In humans, supernormal conduction is recorded only in abnormally functioning cardiac tissue. It has been demonstrated in the His-Purkinje fibers but not in the AV node, the His bundle, or atrial or ventricular myocardium. In fact, its existence in tissue other than the His-Purkinje fibers is denied by most investigators. The paradox of unexpected improved A-V conduction ascribed to supernormal A-V nodal conduction can be explained by a number of different mechanisms such as, for example, the "GAP," "peeling," or dual A-V nodal conduction.

In humans, the most common manifestation of supernormal conduction is an unexpected normalization of bundle branch conduction at an R-R interval shorter than the R-R with bundle branch aberration (Figures 11-6, 11-7, 11-8, and 11-9).[9] The diagnosis of supernormal conduction is strengthened by a P-R interval that is constant or actually shortened. This rules out equal prolongation of conduction in the two bundles as a mechanism of unexpected normalization of the QRS complex (Figures 11-10 and 11-11). Supernormal conduction has been recorded with A-V block (Figure 11-12).

With BBB, the "supernormal" period is shifted to the right because of delayed activation of the bundle by concealed transseptal conduction from the contralateral bundle branch.[10]

Supernormal excitability is most often noted in the presence of a malfunctioning electronic pacemaker and is manifested by an unexpected response to an otherwise subthreshold stimulus (Figures 11-5 and 11-13).

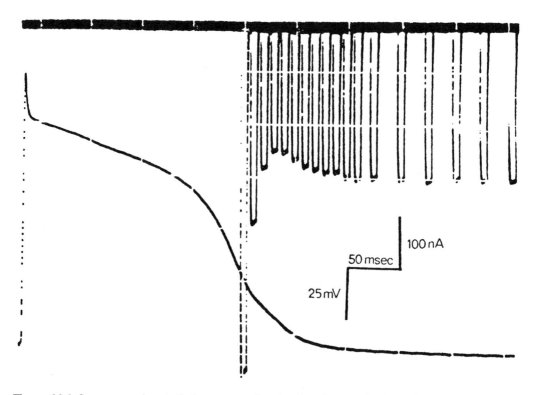

Figure 11-1. Supernormal period of recovery of excitation of canine Purkinje fiber. The TAP of the Purkinje fiber is scanned with a stimulus (vertical bars). The strength necessary to excite the cell is indicated by the length of the bar. During a brief period at the end of phase 3 (T wave of the ECG), a stimulus of lesser strength elicits a response. This is the supernormal period of excitability. Courtesy of Dr. John C. Bailey.

426445
1/27/60

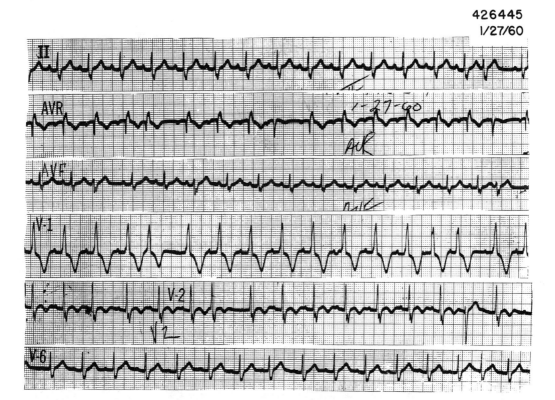

Figure 11-2. Supernormal conduction of the RBB. The basic rhythm is sinus with RBBB and a P-P interval of 640 ms interrupted by APCs. The APCs conduct normally or with RBBB. The APCs with a normal QRS complex are coupled with an R-P interval of 400 to 420 ms. The APC with a shorter coupling, an R-P interval of 250 to 320 ms, conduct with RBBB as do sinus impulses with an R-P interval of 480 or longer. The first APC in lead V_1 is followed by an accelerated junctional escape. RBBB is present at an R-R interval of 380 to 480 ms, a normal QRS complex is present at an R-R interval of 500 to 520 ms, and RBBB is present at an R-R interval of 580 ms or longer. The normal QRS complex at a coupling of 400 to 420 ms and RBBB with either shorter or longer coupling indicates that the normal QRS complex conducts during the supernormal phase of the RBB (see Figure 11-3). From Mihalick MH, Fisch C. Supernormal conduction of the right bundle branch. *Chest* 1970;57:395.

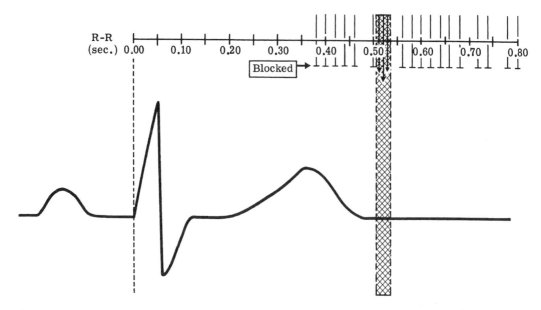

Figure 11-3. Supernormal period of the RBB. The diagram is based on data from Figure 11-2. The crossbar identifies the supernormal period during which the P waves conduct with a normal QRS complex. At an R-R interval shorter or longer than that identified by the crossbar, conduction of the RBB is blocked. From Mihalick MH, Fisch C. Supernormal conduction of the right bundle branch. *Chest* 1970;57:395.

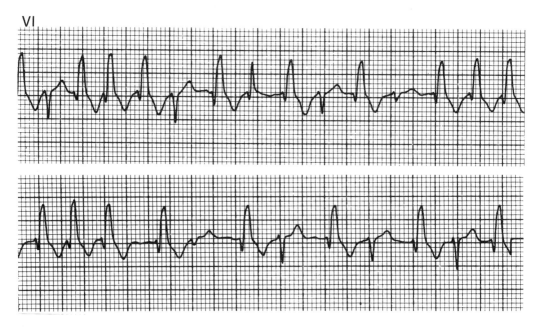

Figure 11-4. Supernormal conduction of the RBB. The basic rhythm is atrial fibrillation with R-R intervals varying from 260 to 520 ms. At an R-R of 320 to 360 ms, the QRS complex is normal, inscribed during the supernormal period of recovery of the RBB.

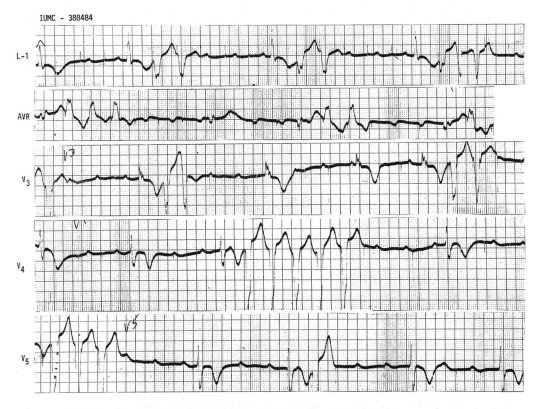

Figure 11-5. Supernormal excitability of the myocardium. The basic rhythm is sinus with a P-P interval of 600 ms and complete A-V block with an idioventricular rate of approximately 35 per minute. There is a malfunctioning fixed-rate electronic pacemaker with a pacing cycle of 520 ms. Only stimuli falling at the end of the T wave of the idioventricular complex, the supernormal period of recovery of excitability, elicit a propagated response. Intermittently, one to four additional consecutive stimuli fall during the supernormal period of the preceding pacemaker-induced complex, resulting in a run of two to five consecutive QRS complexes, all the result of supernormal excitability. From Davis RH, Knoebel SB, Fisch C. Pacemaker-induced arrhythmias. *Cardiovasc Clin* 1970:2:163.

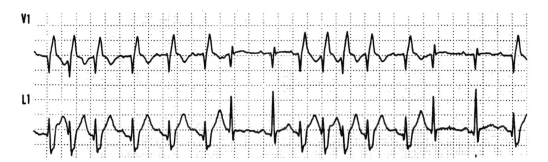

Figure 11-6. Acceleration-dependent RBB with supernormal conduction. The basic rhythm is si-nus with APCs, some in runs. Following a prolonged compensatory pause due to an APC, the QRS conduction is normal, indicating that the RBBB represents acceleration-dependent aberration. Similarly, APCs closely coupled to the previous QRS complex conduct normally. This paradoxical normalization of intraventricular conduction at a shorter R-R interval is due to conduction during the supernormal period of recovery of the RBB.

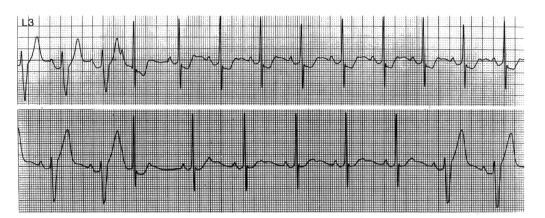

Figure 11-7. Supernormal conduction of the LBB. The basic rhythm is sinus with an R-R interval of approximately 900 ms interrupted by an APC. In the top tracing, the first three QRS complexes con-duct with LBBB due to acceleration-dependent aberration. The APC conducts with a normal QRS complex. This is followed by a compensatory pause that is longer than the R-R of the aberrant QRS complex, and a normal QRS complex. In the bottom strip, the first two complexes are aberrant due to acceleration-dependent aberration. These are followed by an APC, which conducts with a nor-mal QRS complex. Because the compensatory pause following the APC is longer than the R-R of the aberrant complexes, the QRS complexes following the pause are normal. The normalization of the QRS complex following a longer R-R interval indicates acceleration-dependent aberration. At the shorter R-R, the APC conducts paradoxically with a normal QRS complex because it conducts during the supernormal period of recovery of the LBB.

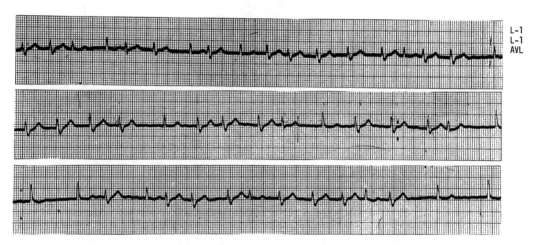

L-1
L-1
AVL

Figure 11-8. Supernormal conduction of the RBB. The basic rhythm is atrial fibrillation with R-R intervals varying from 360 to 920 ms. The normalization of the QRS complex at long R-R cycles indicates acceleration-dependent aberration. Normal QRS complexes are also recorded at R-R intervals shorter than those with aberrant QRS conduction. In the top row, the first two QRS complexes, at an R-R interval of 520 ms, are aberrant. The third and fourth QRS complexes are normal at an R-R interval of 400 and 640 ms, respectively. The fourth complex from the end is also normal at an R-R interval of 400 ms. Similarly and unexpectedly, normal QRS complexes at short R-R intervals are recorded in the middle and bottom rows. Normalization of the QRS complexes at long cycles indicates acceleration-dependent aberration while normalization at paradoxically short intervals indicates conduction during the supernormal phase of bundle branch recovery.

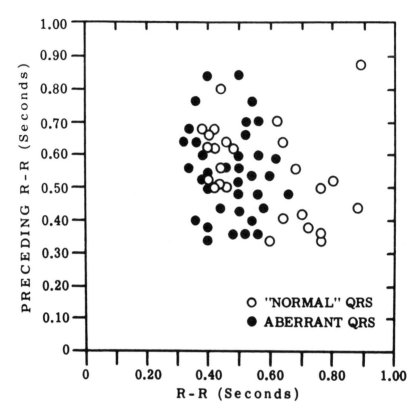

Figure 11-9. Supernormal conduction of the RBB. This figure illustrates the relationship of the normal and aberrant QRS complexes (abscissa) to the preceding cycle lengths (ordinate), based on Figure 11-8. The normal QRS complexes are identified by the open circles and the aberrant QRS complexes are identified by the solid circles. At cycle lengths shorter than 0.40 s, the conduction is aberrant, while in a range of 0.40 to 0.50 s, the QRS complex is normal, and at cycle lengths of 0.50 to approximately 0.64 s, the QRS is aberrant. It is of interest to note that the normal QRS complexes at a cycle range of 0.40 to 0.50 s follow the longer preceding cycles, the opposite of the expected Ashman phenomenon. Therefore, the paradox is not only one of a short R-R interval with a normal QRS complex but also of a normal QRS complex following a prolonged preceding R-R interval. Both support "supernormal" His-Purkinje conduction as the mechanism of the unexpectedly normal QRS complexes at short R-R intervals. Lack of directional relationship of the R-R interval of the paradoxically normal QRS complexes and the duration of the preceding cycle suggests that the location of the supernormal period responsible for normalization of conduction shifts only slightly. The supernormal period is expected to shift to the right as the preceding cycle and the duration of the TAP lengthens. It is likely that more accurate measurement than that possible on the surface ECG would disclose a shift of the supernormal period in parallel with the duration of the TAP and of the preceding cycle.

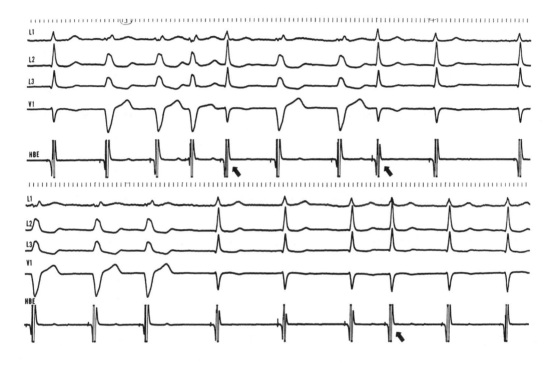

Figure 11-10. Acceleration-dependent LBBB and supernormal conduction. The basic rhythm is atrial fibrillation with LBBB at cycle lengths of 700 ms or less and normal QRS complexes at cycles of 650 ms and longer. Normalization of the QRS complexes at cycles of 650 ms or longer indicates that the LBBB is acceleration-dependent. The unexpected normalization of the QRS complexes following at short R-R intervals (arrow) may be due to either supernormal conduction or equal delay of conduction in the two bundle branches. However, the constant H-V interval with both the normal QRS complexes and LBBB indicates that the paradoxical normalization of the QRS complex is because of supernormal conduction. Equal prolongation of His-Purkinje conduction would prolong the H-V interval. The unexpected LBBB after the first relatively long R-R cycle in the bottom row is due to concealed transseptal activation of the LBB. The concealed conduction shortens the LBB-to-LBB interval, resulting in LBBB.

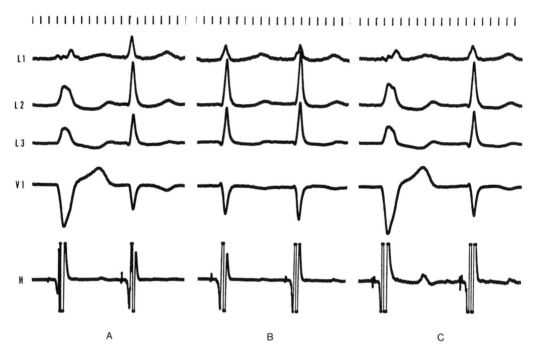

Figure 11-11. Supernormal conduction of the LBB. Panels A, B and C illustrate normal QRS complexes following short R-R intervals. The H-V interval is constant at 45 ms regardless of the QRS pattern. The fixed H-V interval rules out equal prolongation of the His-Purkinje conduction as the mechanism of the unexpected normalization of the QRS complexes at short R-R intervals, leaving supernormal conduction as the mechanism of the paradoxical QRS normalization.

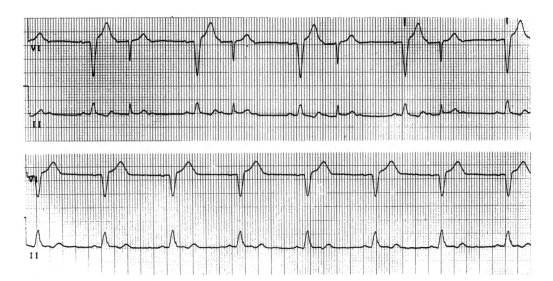

Figure 11-12. Supernormal conduction. In the top panel, the basic rhythm is sinus with Wencke-bach Type 1 3:2 A-V block. The first QRS complex with LBBB is preceded by a P-R interval of 160 ms. The next QRS complex, with an R-R of 600 ms and a P-R interval of 240 ms, is normal. The next P wave is blocked. In the bottom tracing, the rhythm is a sinus bradycardia at a rate of approximately 60 per minute and LBBB. The unexpected normalization of the QRS complexes in the top panel is most likely due to conduction during the supernormal phase. It is, however, possible that the LBBB represents deceleration-dependent aberration. The latter is supported by the sinus bradycardia with LBBB recorded in the bottom panel.

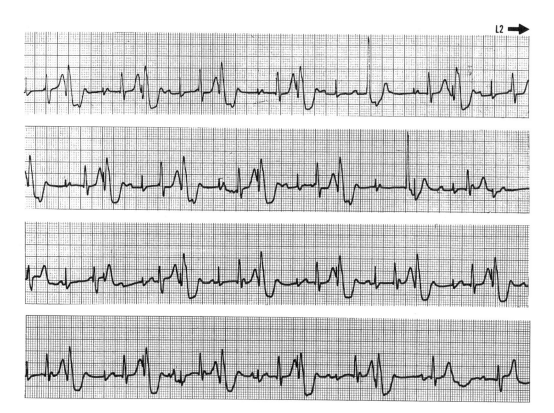

Figure 11-13. Supernormal period of ventricular excitability. The basic rhythm is sinus with complete A-V block and a malfunctioning fixed-rate electronic pacemaker with a cycle length of 680 ms. The interectopic idioventricular intervals, based on the first two cycles in the third row and the last cycle in the bottom row, vary from 1160 to 1120 ms. The pacemaker stimuli, with the coupling to the idioventricular QRS complexes of 380 to 450 ms, falling on the down slope of the T wave, elicit a propagated ventricular response. Pacemaker stimuli falling later in the cardiac cycle fail to elicit a response. The interval between 380 and 450 ms, measured from the spontaneous ventricular QRS complex to the pacemaker-induced QRS complex, defines the supernormal period of recovery. The exceptions are two escapes, one each in the top and second-to-top rows. All idioventricular impulses follow the pacemaker-induced QRS complex by an interval of approximately 1080 ms. This interrelationship of the idioventricular QRS complex to the artificial stimulus forces a bigeminal pattern, a form of escape (idioventricular) capture (pacemaker) bigeminy. The return cycle of 1080 ms following the artificial stimulus is shorter than the spontaneous idioventricular cycle of 1160 to 1200 ms. This may be because of electrotonic modulation of phase 4 of the TAP of the idioventricular impulse by the pacemaker-induced QRS complex, the latter making the slope of phase 4 much steeper.

References

1. Moore NE, Spear JF, Fisch C. Supernormal conduction and excitability. *J Cardiovasc Electrophysiol* 1993;4:330.
2. Lewis T, Master AM. Supernormal recovery phase, illustrated by two clinical cases of heart block. *Heart* 1925;11:371.
3. Adrian ED, Lucas K. On the summation of propagated disturbances in the nerve and muscle. *J Physiol* 1912;44:69.
4. Adrian ED. The recovery process of excitable tissue. *J Physiol* 1920;54:1.
5. Ashman R. Conductivity in compressed cardiac muscle: Supernormal phase in conductivity in compressed auricular muscle of turtle heart. *Am J Physiol* 1925;74:140.
6. Arbel E, Sasyniuk BI, Moe GK. Supernormal ventricular conduction in the dog heart. *Fed Proc* 1971;30:553.
7. Spear JF, Moore EN. Supernormal excitability and conduction in the His-Purkinje system of the dog. *Circ Res* 1974;35:782.
8. Agha AS, Castillo CA, Myerburg RS, Castellanos A. Supernormality in the human atria. *Circulation* 1970;42:67.
9. Fisch C, Knoebel SB. Vagaries of acceleration dependent aberration. *Br Heart J* 1992;67:1.
10. Levi RJ, Salerno JA, Nau GJ, Elizari MV, Rosenbaum MB. A reappraisal of supernormal conduction. In Rosenbaum MB, Elizara MV (eds): *Frontiers of Cardiac Electrophysiology.* Boston: Martinus Nijhoff Publishers; 1983:437.

12

Vulnerability

The vulnerable period is a brief period during recovery of excitability when the heart is vulnerable to ventricular fibrillation or VT.

Historical Perspective

"The fiber during the interval may be expected to reach varying levels of repolarization; and, therefore, the applied stimuli may elicit action potentials with different amplitudes, durations, and velocities of depolarization. This may produce sufficient amounts of asynchrony to generate fibrillation."[1]

General Background

The vulnerable period in humans has been recorded with fixed-rate artificial pacemakers (Figures 12-1 and 12-2) and with VPCs interrupting the T wave (Figures 12-3, 12-4, 12-5, 12-6, and 12-7).[2-6] In the intact heart, the vulnerable period occurs during the mid portion of the T wave—more precisely, during a 30-ms period at the apex of the T wave (Figure 12-8).[7,8,10]

Asynchrony of conduction and refractoriness is the fundamental disorder responsible for the manifestations of vulnerability, namely ventricular fibrillation or VT.[7-9] Factors that enhance asynchrony of conduction and refractoriness and increase the vulnerability for ventricular fibrillation or VT include prolongation of the QT interval, congenital (Figure 12-9) or acquired (Figure 12-10), increased heart rate, mass of the myocardium exhibiting asynchrony, ischemia (Figure 12-4),[10] hypocalcemia, hyperkalemia (Figure 12-5), a variety of other pathological states, and severity of aberration of the first ectopic QRS complex.[4,5,10,11]

The vulnerable period of the atria is manifest by atrial fibrillation initiated by an APC during the vulnerable period of atrial recovery (Figure 12-11).[12]

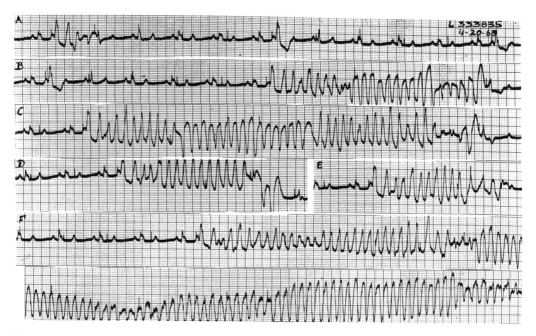

Figure 12-1. Ventricular vulnerability with torsades de pointes. The basic rhythm is sinus with 2:1 A-V block and a malfunctioning fixed-rate electronic pacemaker. The pacemaker stimulus scans the entire cardiac cycle. At a coupling interval of pacemaker stimulus to the preceding QRS complex of 0 to 320 ms, no response is elicited. At a coupling interval of approximately 320 ms, the stimulus followed by a latent period varying from 80 to 100 ms induces either an isolated QRS complex or nonsustained VT. The QRS vector of the VT rotates 180°, characteristic of torsades de pointes. In this instance, however, the QT interval is normal rather than prolonged as in the case with ordinary torsades de pointes. The period during which the stimulus induces the ventricular arrhythmia is the vulnerable period. The latent period occurs during ventricular repolarization and electrotonic spread of the stimulus. From Tavel ME, Fisch C. Repetitive ventricular arrhythmia resulting from artificial internal pacemakers. *Circulation* 1964;30:493. By permission of the American Heart Association, Inc.

V5

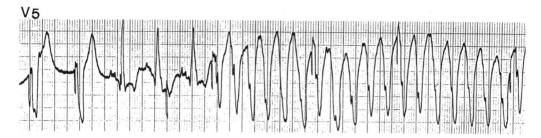

Figure 12-2. Vulnerable period of the ventricle. The basic rhythm is sinus tachycardia with a fixed-rate electronic pacemaker. The electronic stimulus falling on the nadir of the T wave, the vulnerable period, elicits VT.

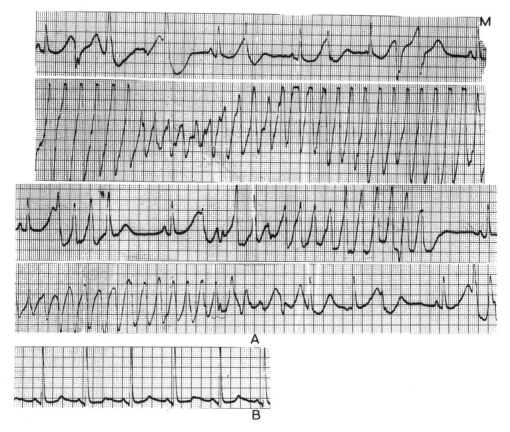

Figure 12-3. Ventricular vulnerability manifest by torsades de pointes. In panel A, the VPC falling on the peak of the T wave, the vulnerable period of ventricular recovery, induces non-sustained polymorphic (torsades de pointes) VT. The prolongation of the QT interval is caused by phenothiazine. Panel B, which was recorded after the drug was discontinued, is a normal ECG recording.

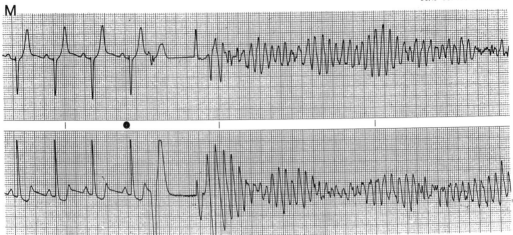

Figure 12-4. Ventricular vulnerability manifest by torsades de pointes. The sinus rhythm is interrupted by a VPC and a junctional escape. A closely coupled VPC (R on T) initiates a torsades de pointes VT.

PLASMA K⁺ 1.7 MEQ/L

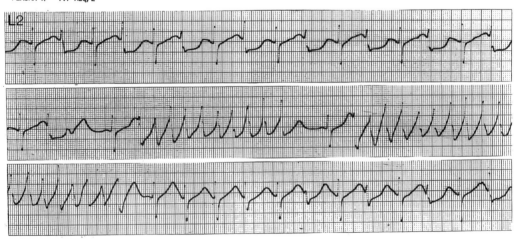

Figure 12-5. Nonsustained VT due to hypokalemia. The top row illustrates a prolonged QT interval and a ventricular bigeminy. The middle row illustrates the R on T phenomenon. The VPC falling during the vulnerable period elicits a nonsustained VT. In the bottom row, the VT is terminated with a run of NPJT and ventricular bigeminy.

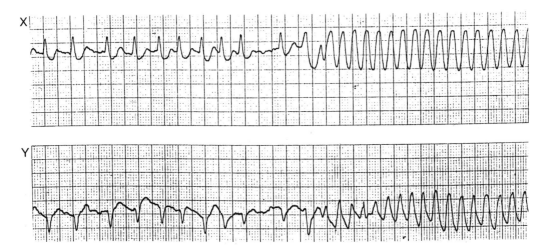

Figure 12-6. Ventricular vulnerability. The basic rhythm is atrial fibrillation. Following the prolonged R-R, a VPC falling during the vulnerable period initiates VT. Following the prolonged R-R the TAP is also prolonged, thereby shifting the vulnerable period to the right. Now the VPC falls during the vulnerable period of the ventricle initiating the VT.

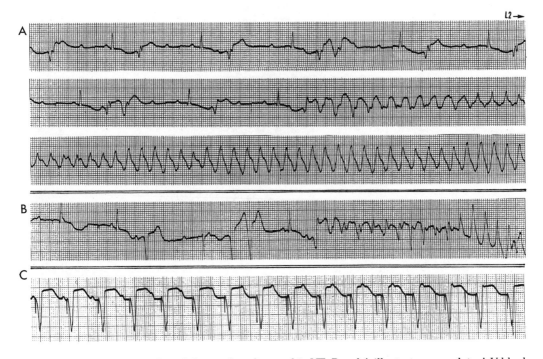

Figure 12-7. Ventricular vulnerability with polymorphic VT. Panel A illustrates complete A-V block with ventricular bigeminy and a malfunctioning electronic pacemaker. The QT interval measures approximately 640 ms. In the middle of the second tracing, a VPC initiates a nonsustained polymorphic VT which ceases spontaneously (not shown). The arrhythmia recurs in panel B. In panel C, pacing the heart at a rate of approximately 100 per minute controls the ventricular arrhythmia. The prolonged QT interval is probably due to bradycardia, which contributes to asynchrony of recovery. A stimulus during the QT, the vulnerable period, initiates the nonsustained polymorphic VT.

IUMC 388471-887

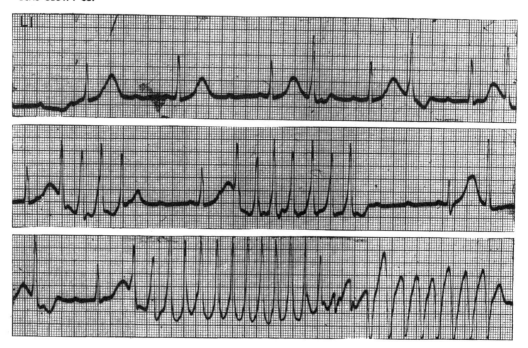

Figure 12-8. Ventricular vulnerability with torsades de pointes. The basic rhythm is sinus with a P-P interval of 520 ms and a high degree of A-V block. The coupling of the VPC shortens gradually and, at a coupling of 560 ms, is followed by nonsustained VT. Further shortening of the coupling interval to 560 ms, the vulnerable period, initiates a VT. In the bottom row, the VPC, coupled at an interval of 560 ms, is followed by VT with torsades de pointes configuration. From Fisch C, McHenry PL, Knoebel SB. Cardiac arrhythmias. In *Tice's Practice of Medicine.* Philadelphia: Harper and Row; 1970:1–29.

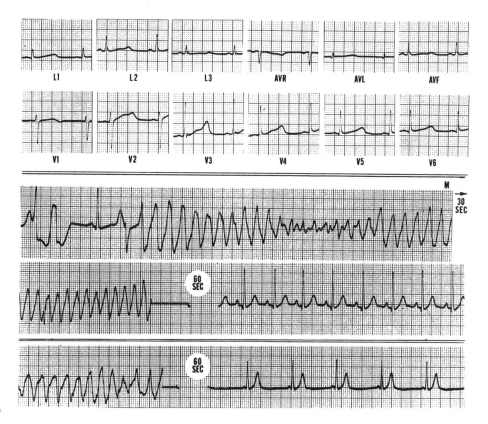

Figure 12-9. Ventricular vulnerability with polymorphic VT. In the top panel, the control tracing, the QT interval is prolonged, measuring approximately 540 ms with a notched T wave. The lead in the bottom panel is a monitor lead. In the top row of the bottom panel, a VPC falling during the T wave (the vulnerable period) initiates nonsustained polymorphic VT. A 30-second section is deleted for mounting purposes. In the middle of the row, the arrhythmia is followed by normal sinus rhythm. The bottom row records termination of the VT, sinus rhythm with a short P-R interval, and a "tented" T wave. The normalization of the QT interval coupled with a significant shortening of the P-R interval and the tented T wave strongly suggests that these changes are a result of the release of catecholamines or potassium or both, in response to the VT and flutter. From Fisch C. Electrocardiography and vectrocardiography. In Braunwald E (ed): *Heart Disease.* 3rd ed. Philadelphia: W.B. Saunders; 1988:180.

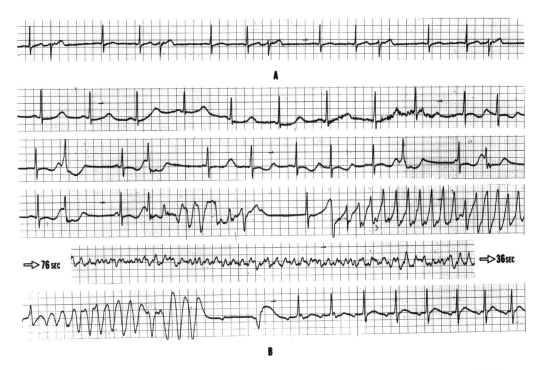

Figure 12-10. Ventricular vulnerability manifest by torsades de pointes and ventricular fibrillation. In panel A, the control tracing, the rhythm is sinus with ventricular trigeminy. The QT interval measures approximately 360 ms with a coupling interval of the VPC of approximately 480 ms. In panel B, which was recorded after administration of quinidine, the QT interval is prolonged to 700 ms. There are APCs, VPCs, and an occasional junctional escape. The bottom three rows are continuous, with 76- and 36-second sections omitted for mounting purposes. The third VPC in row three initiates a 122-second run of ventricular arrhythmia including VT, flutter, and perhaps fibrillation. These cease spontaneously. The run is followed by three nonconducting negative P waves and a VPC. The remainder represents an ectopic atrial tachycardia. In panel B, because of the prolonged QT interval, the VPC falls during the vulnerable period and induces the ventricular arrhythmias. This occurs despite the fact that the coupling of the VPC in panel B is considerably longer than that in panel A.

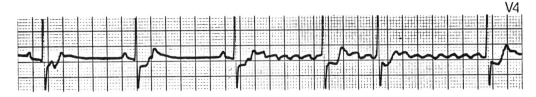

Figure 12-11. Atrial vulnerability manifest by atrial fibrillation. The basic rhythm is sinus with non-conducted APCs in a bigeminal pattern. The APC with the shortest coupling interval falls during the vulnerable period of atrial recovery and initiates atrial fibrillation.

References

1. Wiggers CJ, Wegria R. Ventricular fibrillation due to single localized induction and condenser shocks applied during the vulnerable phase of ventricular systole. *Am J Physiol* 1940;128:500.
2. Surawicz B, Steffens T. Cardiac vulnerability. In Fisch C (ed): *Complex Electrocardiography*. Philadelphia: FA Davis; 1977:159.
3. Smirk FH. R waves interrupting T waves. *Br Heart J* 1949;11:23.
4. Smirk FH, Palmer DG. A myocardial syndrome. With particular reference to the occurrence of sudden death and of premature systoles interrupting antecedent T waves. *Am J Cardiol* 1960;6:620.
5. Tavel ME, Fisch C. Repetitive ventricular arrhythmia resulting from artificial internal pacemaker. *Circulation* 1964;15:493.
6. Garrey WE. The nature of fibrillatory contractions of the heart—its relation to tissue mass and form. *Am J Physiol* 1914;33:397.
7. Lewis T, Feil HS, Stroud WD. Observations upon flutter and fibrillation. *Heart* 1918–1920;7:247.
8. Moe GK, Harris AS. Repetitive focal discharges and conduction changes related to induction of ventricular fibrillation. *Am J Physiol* 1941;133:390.
9. Moe GK, Harris AS, Wiggers CJ. Analysis of the initiation of fibrillation by electrographic studies. *Am J Physiol* 1941;134:473.
10. Wegria R, Moe GK, Wiggers CJ. Comparison of the vulnerable period and fibrillation thresholds of normal and idioventricular beats. *Am J Physiol* 1941;133:651.
11. Palmer DG. Interruption of T waves by premature QRS complexes and the relationship of this phenomenon to ventricular fibrillation. *Am Heart J* 1962;63:367.
12. Killip T, Gault JH. Mode of onset of atrial fibrillation in man. *Am Heart J* 1965;70:172.

13

Exit and Entrance Blocks

Exit Block

The concept of exit block was invoked to explain the failure of a parasystolic impulse to elicit a ventricular response at a time when the heart is no longer refractory.

Historical Perspective

Since the early observations of Kaufmann and Rothberger, in 1920,[1] of exit block during ventricular parasystole (see Figure 9-4), exit block has been described with nearly all spontaneous and artificially induced rhythms, including those of the SAN, the atrium (Figures 13-1, 13-2, and 13-3), the node (Figures 13-4, 13-5, and 13-6), the bundle of His, the Purkinje system (Figures 13-7, 13-8, and 13-9), and the ventricular myocardium.[2] Laboratory studies and occasional ECGs suggest that exit block is a function of altered conduction in the surrounding tissue, rather than of abnormal impulse formation.[3]

Electrocardiography of Exit Block

Exit block from a parasystolic atrial or ventricular focus should be suspected whenever "group beating," a repetitive sequential pattern of P or R waves, is present. Exit block may exhibit the classic Wenckebach periodicity of the P-P or R-R intervals, with a gradual shortening of the respective cycles and ultimate failure of a P or R wave to manifest (Figure 13-6). Type I exit block can be recognized only in the presence of normal sinus rhythm; otherwise, it may be impossible to differentiate it from sinus arrhythmia. When the long cycle is a multiple of the basic interectopic interval, the exit block is Type II (Figure 13-6).[4] The long pause in Type II exit block may be slightly shorter than expected because the conduction following the long pause is accelerated due to the longer period of recovery.

ECG records of exit block from an ectopic atrial focus are relatively rare,[5-7] while exit block from the junctional and ventricular ectopic pacemakers are common.

Wenckebach exit block from a reentrant pathway has been proposed. It is manifest by progressive prolongation of VPC coupling with ultimate failure of the VPC to manifest.[8] There also is evidence to suggest that in some instances the block is a result of delay of conduction once the impulse exits from the reentrant pathway rather than a result of an abnormal conduction within the reentrant pathway (Figure 13-10).

For additional discussion of Wenckebach periodicity and Wenckebach exit block, see Chapter 16.

Entrance Block Electrocardiography

Entrance block denotes failure of an impulse to reach, enter, suppress, reset, or discharge a dominant pacemaker.

Although entrance block is characteristic of parasystole, it has been noted with nearly all pacemakers, either primary or secondary (Figures 13-11, 13-12, 13-13, and 13-14). Entrance block may be a normal event or a manifestation of an altered electrophysiological state. An early impulse may encounter physiological refractoriness surrounding a pacemaker and thus fail to reach the pacemaker. In the strict sense of the word, however, this is not an entrance block but rather manifestation of physiological interference. True entrance block occurs after the surrounding tissue has recovered (Figure 13-13). In such a case, the entrance block is an abnormal finding and a result of an abnormally prolonged refractory period or local impairment of conduction.

An interpolated impulse may delay the exit of the subsequent impulse from its pacemaker site. The delayed exit is recognized by the fact that the cycle encompassing the interpolated impulse is longer than the basic cycle length (Figure 13-11). Occasionally, the interpolated impulse may prevent the exit of the subsequent impulse. In such cases, the interval encompassing the entrance-blocked (interpolated) impulse is a multiple of the basic cycle length.

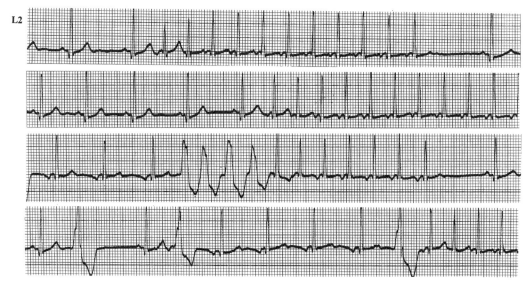

Figure 13-1. Junctional tachycardia with a 2:1 exit block. The basic rhythm is sinus interrupted by a junctional tachycardia manifest by inverted P waves, a P-R interval of approximately 80 ms, and an R-R of 360 ms. In the third row from the top, the junctional rhythm at an R-R interval of 720 ms is twice as long as the basic 360 ms, indicating a 2:1 exit block from the tachycardia focus. The run of the bizarre complexes may represent VT but, since the rate equals the junctional tachycardia, it is more likely a junctional tachycardia with aberration. In the bottom row, the junctional rhythm at an R-R of 720 ms is twice as long as that of the more rapid tachycardia at an R-R of 360 ms, reflecting a 2:1 exit block from the ectopic focus.

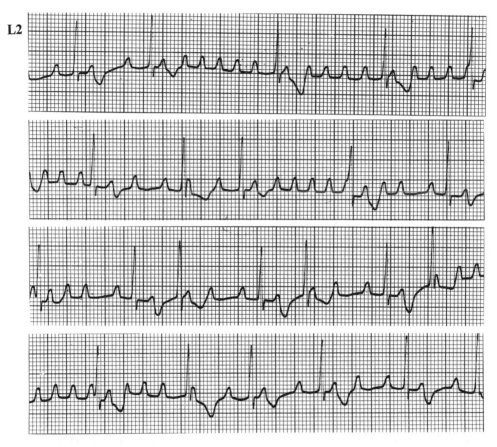

Figure 13-2. Atrial flutter with 2:1 and 3:2 Type I exit block. The basic rhythm is atrial flutter with an FL-FL interval of approximately 180 ms. Episodes twice the length of the basic FL-FL cycle are recorded in the top, second from bottom, and bottom rows. In addition, there are sequences of short–long cycles. The short cycle is longer than the basic FL-FL interval while the longer cycle is shorter than the sum of two basic FL-FL intervals. The sum of the short–long cycles equals three basic FL-FL cycles. This is the pattern of a 3:2 Type I exit block from the flutter focus.

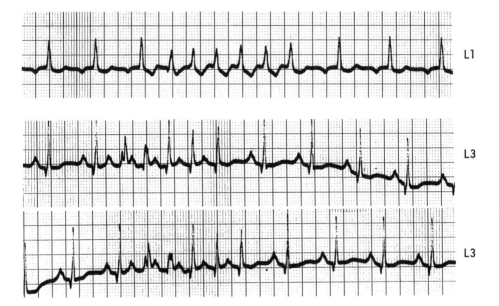

Figure 13-3. Ectopic atrial tachycardia with a 2:1 exit block. The negative P waves in lead L1 indicate an ectopic rhythm. Doubling of the P-P interval from 340 to 680 ms indicates a 2:1 Type II exit block from the ectopic atrial focus. The QRS aberration is either rate-dependent or an Ashman phenomenon. The normalization of the QRS complex following the first two aberrant QRS complexes in lead L3 is due to time-dependent shortening of the refractory period.

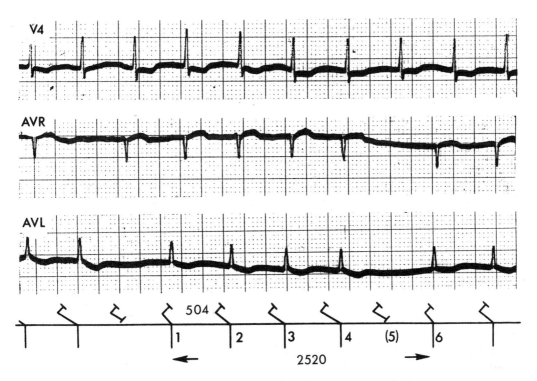

Figure 13-4. NPJT with Wenckebach Type I exit block. NPJT with a regular R-R interval of 528 ms is recorded in lead V_4. In AVR and AVL, repetitive "group beating" is present with a gradual shortening of the R-R interval followed by a long cycle. The latter is shorter than two preceding cycles. This grouping reflects a Wenckebach sequence. The rate of the junctional pacemaker is estimated by adding the cycles of the Wenckebach sequence, in this instance five. The sum is 2520 ms. This sum is divided by the five junctional cycles, giving an interectopic interval of 504 ms.

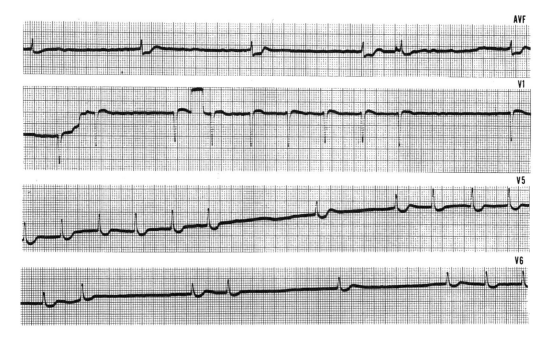

Figure 13-5. Junctional rhythm with Wenckebach Type I exit block. The basic rhythm is atrial fibrillation with a junctional rhythm. The junctional rhythm exhibits a repetitive "group beating." The R-R interval shortens gradually with the long pauses less than the sum of two preceding cycles. This pattern indicates a Wenckebach Type I exit block.

Figure 13-6. NPJT with Mobitz Type II exit block. The basic rhythm is atrial fibrillation with NPJT. The basic R-R of the NPJT is 680 ms. The long cycles are a multiple of this basic cycle, reflecting either a 2:1 or 3:1 exit block. Since the long R-R is an exact multiple of the basic R-R, the exit block is Mobitz Type II.

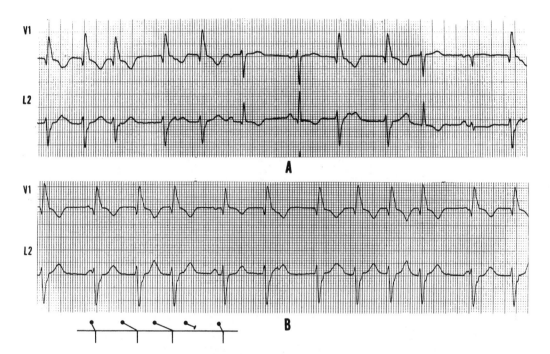

Figure 13-7. VT with Wenckebach Type I exit block. The basic rhythm is VT with repetitive "group beating." In panel A, the next to the last QRS complex and in panel B, the fifth QRS complex are fusions, confirming the ventricular origin of the arrhythmia. In panel B, as indicated by the Lewis diagram, there is a gradual shortening of the R-R interval, with the long pauses less than the sum of two preceding cycles. This is the Wenckebach structure with Wenckebach Type I exit block from the ventricular pacemaker.

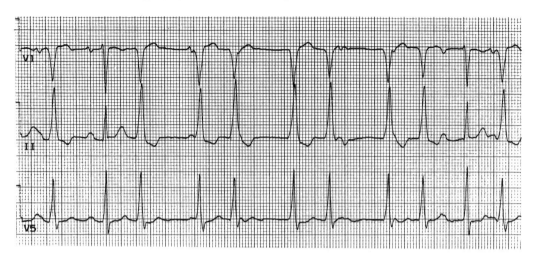

Figure 13-8. VT with a 3:2 exit block. The ventricular rate is 143 per minute with an R-R of 423 ms, derived from a sum of short and long cycles divided by three, the number of ectopic cycles. The captures, second and tenth QRS complexes, confirm the ventricular origin of the arrhythmia. The short R-R intervals are constant and the long cycle is less than twice that of the short cycle, indicating the 3:2 Wenckebach Type I exit block.

IUMC 512798-1379

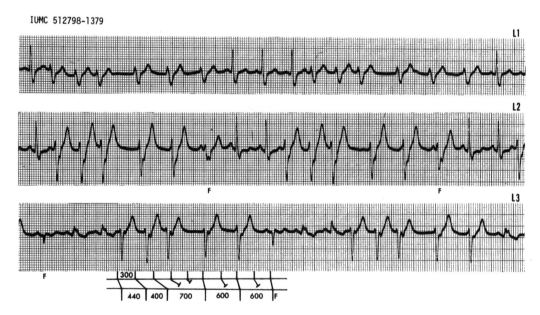

Figure 13-9. VT with Type I exit block. The basic rhythm is sinus with a P-P interval of 520 ms, a P-R interval of 120 ms, and RBBB. There are six runs of VT, each beginning with an accurately coupled VPC and each exhibiting an almost identical repetitive R-R sequence consisting of R-R cycles of 440, 400, 700, 600, and 600 ms, respectively. Fusion complexes (F) are present in lead L2 and lead L3, confirming the diagnosis of VT. Although the VT appears to be grossly irregular, the nearly identical repetitive "group beating" R-R cycles suggest a common denominator, i.e., a common basic interectopic interval. The first three cycles of each sequence measure 440, 400, and 700 ms, respectively, the sum of the three cycles being 1540 ms. These three manifest R-R cycles encompass five basic interectopic intervals. Therefore, the basic interectopic cycle length is 1540 divided by 5 or 306 ms. This estimate is supported by the two cycles that follow, each measuring 600 ms, or twice the estimated basic interectopic interval.

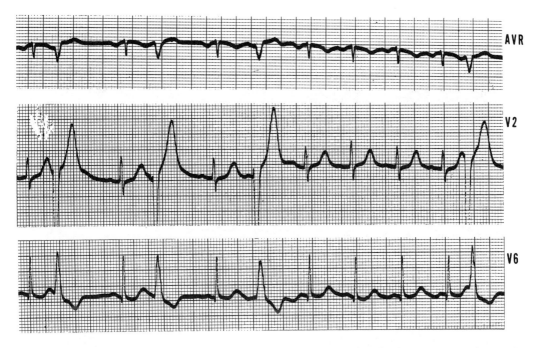

Figure 13-10. Wenckebach exit from a reentrant pathway. The basic rhythm is sinus with ventricular bigeminy. There is progressive prolongation of the coupling interval suggesting Wenckebach-like delay of the conduction in the reentrant pathway or during exit.

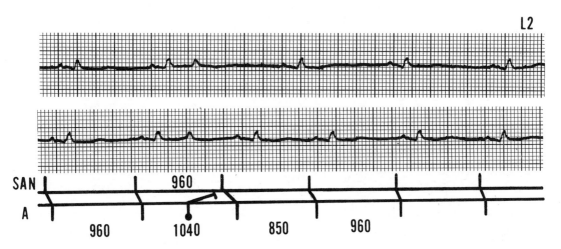

Figure 13-11. APCs with SA nodal entrance block and exit delay. The basic rhythm is a sinus bradycardia with a P-P interval of 950 ms. In the top tracing, the nonconducted APC discharges the SAN. In the bottom tracing, the APC is interpolated. The sinus interval encompassing the interpolated APC measures 1040 ms. The subsequent P-P intervals measure 850, 960, and 920 ms, respectively. The Lewis diagram indicates that exit time from the SAN to the atrium (A) is regular, with a cycle length of 950 ms, while the manifest P-P intervals vary from 920 to 960 ms. The interpolated APC, while failing to discharge the SAN, postpones the next P wave by 80 ms (1040 minus 960 equals 80). The next P-P interval measures 850 ms, with a normal exit time of the SAN to the atrium. Although the interpolated APC fails to discharge the SAN, it delays the SAN exit, displacing the manifest P wave to the right and shortening the P-P interval to 850 ms.

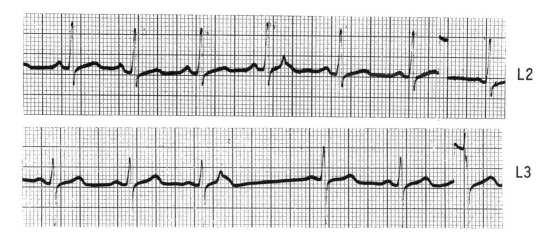

Figure 13-12. APCs with SAN entrance block. The basic rhythm is sinus, with a P-P interval of 680 ms, interrupted by two APCs. The APC in lead L2 is interpolated, with a sinus cycle encompassing the premature of 760 ms. The APC in lead L3 is followed by a compensatory pause and a return cycle of 960 ms, 200 ms longer than the basic P to P interval. The failure of the interpolated APC to alter the sinus rhythm indicates an entrance block. In lead L3, the APC with a somewhat longer coupling interval reaches the SAN after the perinodal tissue recovers and discharges the sinus node. A compensatory pause follows. The return cycle longer than the basic sinus cycle may be due to suppression of the sinus node, conduction of the APC to the SAN, and conduction from the SAN to the atrium. Assuming that there is no suppression of the SAN and that the conduction time of APC to sinus node and from sinus node to the atrium are equal, the exit time can be calculated by dividing 200 ms, prolongation of the return cycle, by a factor of 2. The SAN exit time is approximately 100 ms.

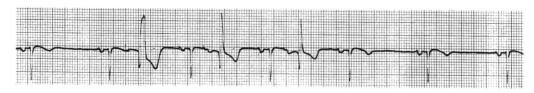

Figure 13-13. APCs with SAN entrance block. The sinus cycle length is 1280 ms. The APCs do not disturb the sinus node rhythmicity. The fact that the APCs, with aberration, do not disturb the sinus node rhythmicity indicates an APC to SAN entrance block.

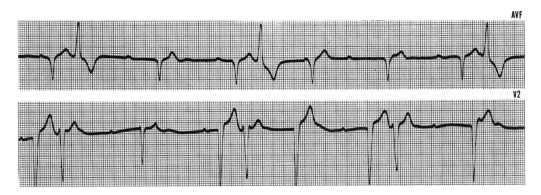

Figure 13-14. Idioventricular rhythm with VPCs and entrance block. The basic rhythm is sinus with a P-P interval of 840 ms, complete A-V block, and idioventricular rhythm with an interectopic interval of 1440 ms. The idioventricular rhythm is interrupted by a VPC with fixed coupling. Two of the VPCs (AVF, V_2) are interpolated and do not disturb the idioventricular rhythm, indicating an entrance block. The interectopic interval encompassing the blocked VPC equals the basic cycle of 1440 ms. The remaining VPCs discharge the idioventricular pacemaker and are followed by a return cycle of approximately 1560 ms.

References

1. Kaufmann R, Rothberger CJ. Beitrage der Entstehungsweise extrasystolischer Allorhythmien. Vierte Mitteilung. Uber Parasystolie, eine besondere Art extrasystolischer Rhythmusstorungen. *Z Gesamte Exp Med* 1920;11:40.
2. Greenspan K, Anderson GJ, Fisch C. Electrophysiological correlate of exit block. *Am J Cardiol* 1971;28:197.
3. Fisch C, Greenspan K, Anderson GJ. Exit block. *Am J Cardiol* 1971;28:402.
4. Katz LN, Pick A. *Clinical Electrocardiography. I. The Arrhythmias.* Philadelphia: Lea and Febiger; 1957:531.
5. Rosen KM, Rahimtoola SH, Gunnar RM. Pseudo A-V block secondary to premature nonpropagated His bundle depolarization—documentation by His bundle electrocardiography. *Circulation* 1970;42:367.
6. Calvino JM, Azan L, Castellanos A. Paroxysmal atrial tachycardia with exit block. *Am Heart J* 1957;54:444.
7. Phibbs B. Paroxysmal atrial tachycardia with block around the ectopic pacemaker. *Circulation* 1963;28:949.
8. Mirvis DM, Bandura JP, Brody DA. Wenckebach type exit block from an ectopic focus as a cause of variable coupling. *J Electrocardiol* 1976;9:365.

14

Electrical Alternans

Table 14-1

Anatomic Structures Involved in Conduction Alternans

Atria
AV junction
Bundle branches
  Single
  Both
  Fascicles
Distal Purkinje fibers
Ventricular myocardium
Accessory AV pathways
  Confined to the accessory pathway
  Fusion of impulses conducted via AV node and accessory pathway
Various combinations of the above

Modified from Surawicz B, Fisch C. Cardiac alternans: Diverse mechanisms and clinical manifestations. *J Am Coll Cardiol* 1992;20:483–499.

"In occasional electrocardiograms from man and animal, alternate complexes are conspicuously different, not only in height but in form,"[1] thus defining electrical alternans. Electrical alternans is a property of all cardiac tissue and of all phases of electrical activity including depolarization, repolarization, impulse formation, and conduction (Table 14-1).[2]

Historical Perspective

Alternation of amplitude and direction of the QRS complex, and alternation of A-V conduction in the presence of depressed A-V conduction as well as with rapid atrial stimulation, were recorded in 1910 by Lewis and Mathison[1] and in 1918 by Lewis, Feil, and Stroud.[2] This was followed by recognition of S-T segment,[3,4] T,[5,6] and U[7] wave alternans. P wave alternans is common in the experimental setting but rare in humans (Figure 14-1). When present, it is usually accompanied by QRS, ST, and T alternans, so-called total alternans.

    In the clinical setting, except for some cases of AV alternans, electrical alternans in most instances is a manifestation of severe myocardial disorder often caused by ischemia or by metabolic and electrolyte disturbances. In the absence of pericardial effusion, the mechanism of electrical alternans is obscure.[8] It has been suggested that the alternans is the result of a nonuniform refractoriness caused by a nonuniform duration of the excited state of the myocardium or of the conduction system. However, alternans of TAP of a single cell has been recorded, suggesting that the alternans is caused primarily by altered ionic fluxes.[9] Electrical alternans has been observed with normal heart rates, during tachycardia, and as a transient postextrasystolic phenomenon.

Alternans of Atrioventricular and Intraventricular Conduction

Although all components of the ECG are subject to electrical alternans, the discussion that follows deals primarily with alternans of A-V and intraventricular conduction. In addition, alternans secondary to recognizable mechanisms such as exit delay and block, Ashman phenomenon, concealed conduction (Figure 14-2), supernormal conduction, dual A-V transmission, and WPW is discussed in the respective chapters in greater detail.

Alternation of A-V conduction, either anterograde (Figure 14-3) or retrograde (Figure 14-4), has been observed with normal as well as rapid heart rates.[10] It can be accompanied by QRS and cycle length alternans. Proposed explanations include: 1) conduction during the supernormal phase of recovery[11,12]; 2) concealed A-V conduction of APCs with lengthening of the subsequent P-R interval; 3) concealed His bundle discharge; and 4) dual AV nodal pathways.

Alternation of either RBBB or LBBB with normal QRS complexes (Figure 14-5), referred to as 2:1 BBB, may be tachycardia- or bradycardia-dependent. Although the mechanism is not always clear, it has been suggested that every second impulse conducts during the supernormal period of recovery of excitability. Others have proposed that alternating cycle length results from transseptal retrograde penetration of the affected bundle branch.

Alternation of complete RBBB and LBBB (Figure 14-5) during normal sinus rhythm is rare. Even rarer is alternation of complete with incomplete BBB (Figure 14-5) or a combination of P-R alternans with simultaneous BBB alternans. Alternating conduction along the LAF and the LPF (Figure 14-6) is most often accompanied by an incomplete or complete RBBB, and represents bidirectional VT. His bundle studies have shown that, in most cases, bidirectional tachycardia originates in the LBB with conduction alternating between anterior and posterior fascicles, and is thus a form of VT.

Subtle changes in QRS duration or amplitude or both without changes in the QRS axis have been observed in the presence of ectopic SVTs with normal QRS durations (Figure 14-7). In patients with spontaneous or induced SVT with a narrow QRS complex, QRS alternans has been observed with AVRT with retrograde conduction along an accessory pathway (Figure 14-7). While additional studies tend to support these findings, others have suggested that during rapid pacing, alternans is primarily a function of the heart rate. It has also been suggested that alternans during narrow QRS tachycardia and VT (Figures 14-8 and 14-9) are most likely due to changing refractoriness of the peripheral Purkinje system or of ventricular myocardium.

Alternation of conduction has been recorded between accessory and AV nodal pathways (Figures 14-10 and 14-11) and between two separate accessory pathways (Figure 14-12).

In acute ischemia, the risk of ventricular fibrillation increases with increasing magnitude of ST alternans (Figures 14-12 and 14-13), particularly when the ST segment alternans is discordant (that is, the ST changes in the adjacent leads are out of phase). Arrhythmias also have been aggravated by changes in the configuration of ST alternans induced by ventricular premature impulses.

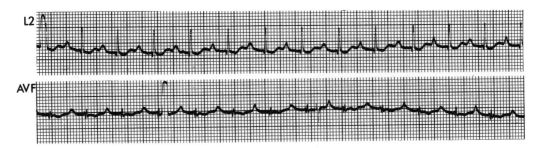

Figure 14-1. Alternans of the P wave. The basic rhythm is sinus with a P-P interval of 460 ms. The configuration of the P wave changes from one with a rounded summit to one with a summit that is pointed. The P-R interval measures 220 ms and is constant.

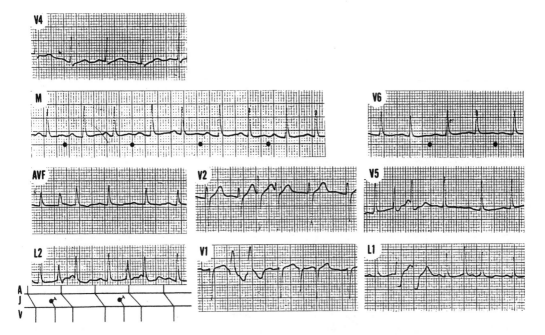

Figure 14-2. AV alternans caused by concealed His discharge. Sinus rhythm with a normal P-R interval is recorded in lead V_4, the control lead. AV and R-R alternans are recorded in leads M (monitor) and V_6. The P-R interval alternates between 160 and 220 ms. In lead AVF, an interpolated JPC is followed by AV alternans. The R-R interval encompassing the interpolated JPC is the same as the longer R-R intervals in leads M and V_6. The shorter R-R intervals encompass a P-R interval of 160 ms and the longer R-R intervals encompass a P-R interval of 220 ms. The prolongation of the P-R interval is due to concealed junctional discharge indicated by the solid circles. The same sequence of events is recorded in leads V_2 and V_5. Manifest junctional trigeminy, with or without aberration, is recorded in leads L2, V_1, and L1 in the bottom row. The analysis is aided by the Lewis diagram. The R-R intervals encompassing the manifest junctional complexes, being equal to the R-R cycles encompassing the prolonged P-R interval but without manifest junctional impulses, support concealed junctional discharge as the mechanism of the AV alternans. The prolonged P-R intervals, whether or not preceded by a manifest interpolated junctional complex, are the same in duration, lending further support to concealed discharge as the mechanism of the P-R alternans. From Fisch C. Concealed conduction. In Zipes D (ed): *Cardiology Clinics. Symposium on Arrhythmias I.* Philadelphia: W.B. Saunders; 1983:63.

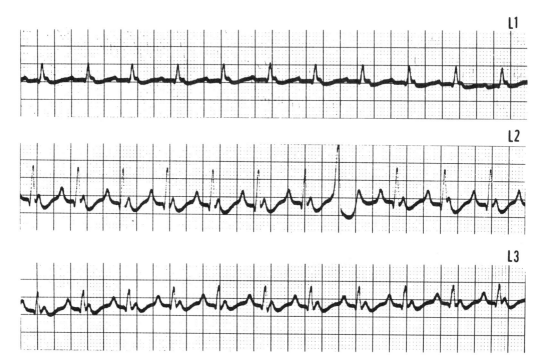

Figure 14-3. Alternans of the P-P interval. The basic rhythm is an atrial tachycardia with a 2:1 A-V block. The P-P intervals alternate from approximately 250–260 to 280–300 ms, with the shorter P-P interval encompassing the QRS complex. The mechanism of alternation is unclear. The assumption of an automatic pacemaker and alternating exit time is possible. Similarly, alternation of the rate of rise of phase 4 would explain the P-P intervals. Both could be influenced by the QRS complex in a manner similar to ventriculophasic arrhythmia. The vagal effect is usually manifest approximately 600 ms after ventricular contraction and may depress phase 4 of the TAP of the pacemaker, thus resulting in alternation of the P-P interval. If reentry is the mechanism of the tachycardia, two alternate pathways could create the short–long P-P sequence. It is also possible that the mechanism is reentry with alternation of the exit time.

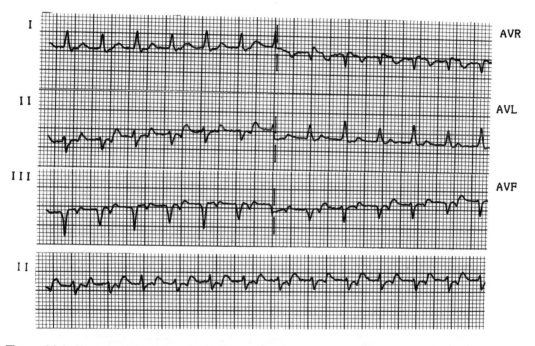

Figure 14-4. Alternans of retrograde (V-A) conduction. The basic rhythm is an NPJT with an R-R interval of 400 ms. The R-P interval varies from 160 to 180 ms. Since the R-R is constant, the most likely mechanism of alternans of the retrograde conduction is the presence of dual AV nodal pathways. From Surawicz B, Fisch C. Cardiac alternans: Diverse mechanisms and clinical manifestations. *J Am Coll Cardiol* 1992;20:483–499.

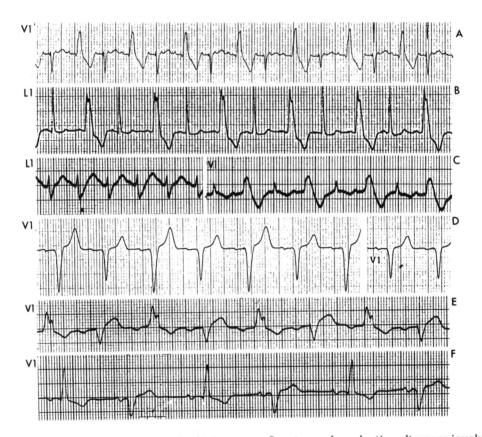

Figure 14-5. Alternans of the His-Purkinje system. Spectrum of conduction alternans involving the His-Purkinje system. A. RBBB and normal QRS complex; B. LBBB and normal QRS complex; C. complete and incomplete RBBB; D. complete and incomplete LBBB; E. RBBB and LBBB; F. RBBB, LBBB, and P-R interval (see Chapter 18). From Surawicz B, Fisch C. Cardiac alternans: Diverse mechanisms and clinical manifestations. *J Am Coll Cardiol* 1992;20: 483–499.

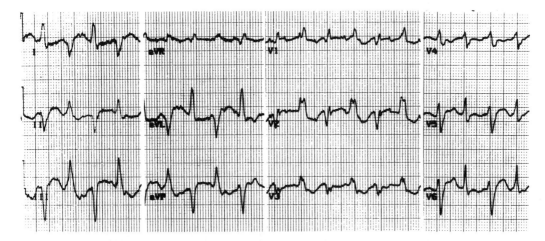

Figure 14-6. Bidirectional VT. The basic rhythm is atrial flutter at a rate of 300 per minute with RBBB. The ventricular rate is approximately 150 per minute. The constant R-R interval indicates a unifocal origin of the VT with conduction along the LAF alternating with conduction along the LPF. This arrhythmia was once thought to represent an NPJT, with RBBB aberration and alternation of conduction along the LAF and LPF responsible from the changing frontal axis. However, His bundle studies indicate that the arrhythmia is VT, most likely originating within the LBB with alternate conduction along the LAF and the LPF. From Surawicz B, Fisch C. Cardiac alternans: Diverse mechanisms and clinical manifestations. *J Am Coll Cardiol* 1992;20:483–499.

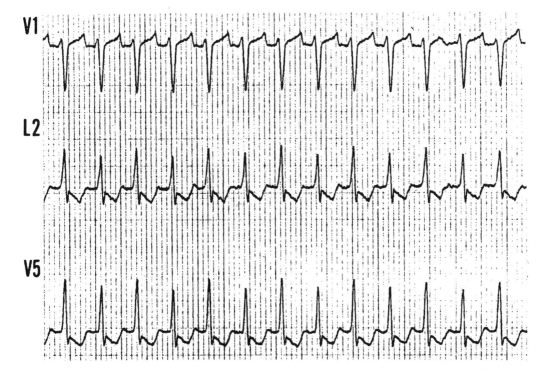

Figure 14-7. Alternans of QRS amplitude. The R-P interval of 160 ms and a negative P wave suggest AVRT with QRS alternans. While supporting AVRT, the alternans may also be a function of the tachycardia.

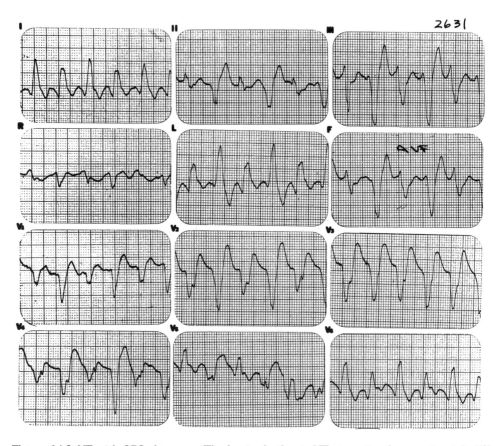

Figure 14-8. VT with QRS alternans. The basic rhythm is VT at a rate of approximately 150 per minute with alternans of QRS duration and amplitude. The alternans is probably due to changing refractoriness of the peripheral Purkinje system or of the ventricular myocardium. Supporting this hypothesis is the laboratory observation of alternating QRS axis during ventricular pacing from a single site.

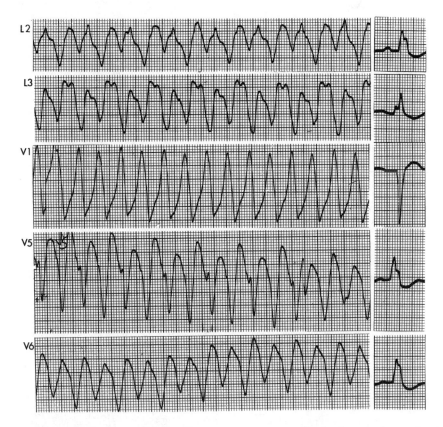

Figure 14-9. VT with QRS alternans. The alternans is most likely due to alternating intraventricular conduction time or alternating pathways of ventricular excitation due to alternating refractoriness of the Purkinje fibers or of the myocardium (see Figure 7-11). From Surawicz B, Fisch C. Cardiac alternans: Diverse mechanisms and clinical manifestations. *J Am Coll Cardiol* 1992;20:483–499.

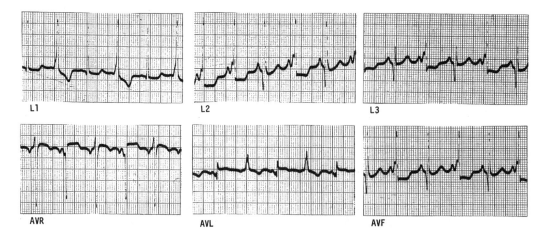

Figure 14-10. WPW with alternans of conduction along the AV node and the accessory pathway. WPW is manifest by a short P-R interval and a delta wave. Conduction along the AV node is indicated by a normal P-R interval and an initial Q wave in leads L2 and L3 and AVF. The conduction alternates between the AV node and the accessory pathway.

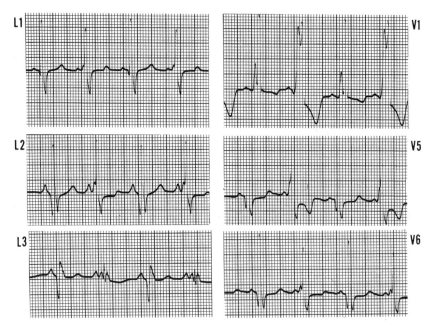

Figure 14-11. WPW with alternans. The basic rhythm is sinus with a P-P interval of 640 ms and RBBB. The conduction proceeds alternately along the AV junction and the accessory pathway. In lead V_1, the first and the third QRS complexes are due to conduction along the AV node while the second and the fourth QRS complexes result from the conduction along the accessory pathway and manifest by a short P-R interval and a delta wave. AVRT with an R-R interval of 280 ms and RBBB is recorded in the bottom tracing. The impulse conducts anterogradely through the AV node and retrogradely through the bypass. It is also possible, but unlikely, that the tachycardia is an AVNRT.

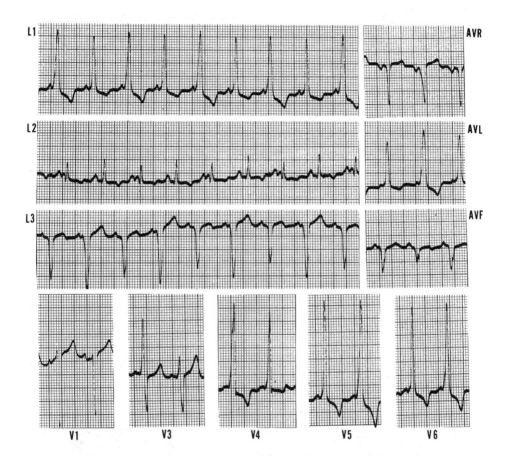

Figure 14-12. WPW with alternans of conduction along accessory pathways. The basic rhythm is sinus with a regular P-P interval of 530 ms and WPW. The P-J interval in lead L2 alternates between 210 and 220 ms. A possible explanation for the alternation is a change of speed of conduction along the accessory pathway. Another mechanism, although less likely, is the presence of two distinct accessory pathways with conduction alternating between the two. The alternation of conduction through the accessory pathway alters the ventricular mass activated and this, in turn, results in alternation of the delta wave, the QRS complex, and the ST-T segment.

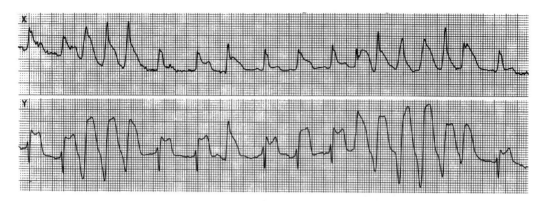

Figure 14-13. Alternans of the ST segment and T wave. The record was obtained from a patient with vasospastic angina pectoris associated with brief episodes of VT. Brief episodes of polymorphic VTs are interrupted by sinus tachycardia with alternans of the ST segment and T wave.

References

1. Lewis T, Mathison GC. Auriculo-ventricular heart block as a result of asphyxia. *Heart* 1910;2:47.
2. Lewis T, Feil H, Stroud WD. Some effects of rhythmic stimulation of the auricle. *Heart* 1918–20;7:247.
3. Hellerstein HK, Liebow IM. Electrical alternation in experimental coronary artery occlusion. *Am J Physiol* 1950;160:366.
4. Kleinfeld MJ, Rozanski JJ. Alternans of the S-T segment in Prinzmetal's angina. *Circulation* 1977;55:574.
5. Kimura E, Yoshida K. A case showing electrical alternans of the T wave without change in the QRS complex. *Am Heart J* 1963;65:391.
6. Fisch C, Edmands RE, Greenspan K. T wave alternans: An association with abrupt rate change. *Am Heart J* 1971;81:817.
7. Bashour T, Rios JC. U wave alternans and increased ventricular irritability. *Chest* 1972;64:377.
8. Feigenbaum H, Zaky A, Grabhorn L. Cardiac motion in patients with pericardial effusion. A study using reflected ultrasound. *Circulation* 1966;34:611.
9. Kleinfeld M, Magin J, Stein E. Electrical alternans in single ventricular fibers of the frog heart. *Am J Physiol* 1956;187:139.
10. Moe GK, Childers RW, Merideth J. An appraisal of "supernormal" A-V conduction. *Circulation* 1968;38:5.
11. Levi RJ, Salerno JA, Nau GJ, Elizari MV, Rosenbaum MB. A reappraisal of supernormal conduction. In Rosenbaum MB, Elizari MV (eds): *Frontiers of Cardiac Electrophysiology.* Boston: Martinus Nijhoff; 1983:427.
12. Moe GK, Preston JB, Burlington H. Physiologic evidence for a dual A-V transmission system. *Circ Res* 1956;4:357.

15

Wolff-Parkinson-White Syndrome

In 1913, Cohn and Fraser[1] published an ECG with a short P-R interval, a prolonged QRS complex, and an intermittent SVT (Figure 15-1). In 1930, this ECG constellation was recognized as a specific ECG syndrome, the WPW syndrome.[2] Shortly thereafter, ventricular preexcitation was proposed as the mechanism, and this concept has stood the test of time.[3]

Typically, WPW, or preexcitation, is an ECG pattern characterized by a short P-R interval ($\geq$0.12 s), a prolonged QRS complex ($\geq$ 0.12 s), a slur on the upstroke of the QRS complex (delta wave), and, as a rule, a normal P-J interval and secondary ST segment and T wave changes.[2] SVT is recorded in approximately 50% of patients with WPW (Figure 15-2).

Accessory A-V connections are responsible for the WPW pattern.[4,5] In addition to the most common accessory connection, the bundle of Kent, other accessory connections have been described, including atriofascicular pathways (James fibers) that insert in the bundle of His,[6] and Mahaim connections that may exit from the AV node (nodoventricular) from the bundle of His or from the bundle branches (fasciculoventricular) (Figure 15-3).[7–9]

Accessory pathways may conduct anterogradely and retrogradely or only retrogradely (concealed retrograde pathway) (Figure 15-4). The latter is responsible for approximately 30% of the reciprocating SVTs in WPW. Concealed retrograde conduction is suspected because of extremely rapid rates, but can be diagnosed only with electrophysiological studies.[9]

The diagnosis of WPW can be confirmed with intracardiac studies.[10] With a progressively shorter coupling of an electronic stimulus to the basic drive impulse, conduction through the AV node is gradually prolonged while conduction through the accessory pathway remains unchanged. Consequently, the H-V interval becomes progressively shorter and the H may be superimposed on the V or may be recorded after the V complex. The earliest inscription of the QRS complex in any of the surface leads indicates the V wave.

In WPW, the QRS complex is a fusion between the impulse traversing the accessory pathway and the AV junction. The magnitude of the delta wave varies depending on the mass of ventricular myocardium activated through the bypass. In the presence of A-V conduction delay, all of the ventricle may be preexcited, and the entire QRS complex represents a delta wave (Figure 15-5).

Traditionally, WPW has been classified into type A and type B. Type A is characterized by a prominent positive initial QRS deflection in leads V_1 and V_2, and type B is characterized by a predominantly negative deflection in leads V_1 and V_2. In type A, the initial inscription of the QRS complex—the delta wave—reflects early activation of the posterior left ventricle, and in type B, the delta wave reflects early activation of the anterior superior right ventricle. A type C WPW, characterized by a negative delta wave in the left lateral leads, has also been described. However, a number of other preexcitation sites have been identified during studies using surface potential mapping, through epicardial mapping during surgery, and during intracardiac electrophysiological studies.[10–12] The exact location of the bypass is of concern to individuals performing ablation of the accessory pathway.

The pattern of WPW varies depending not only on the anatomical location, but on the site of origin and insertion of the accessory pathway. The delta wave may be insignificant or absent with a left lateral pathway because ventricular activation may be largely through the AV node. Similarly, in the presence of an atriofascicular bypass, the delta is absent. The P-R interval is normal in the presence of a fasciculoventricular bypass and may vary when associated with a nodoventricular bypass, depending on the point of origin of the accessory pathway. Presence of more than one wide QRS pattern, usually with atrial fibrillation, suggests the possibility of multiple bypass tracts.

The conduction and duration of the refractory period of the bypass can be estimated with atrial pacing with progressively shorter pacing intervals.

Wolff-Parkinson-White Syndrome and Atrial Fibrillation

Atrial fibrillation with conduction along the accessory pathway inscribes a bizarre QRS complex (Figure 15-6). Such a QRS complex indicates total ventricular activation along the accessory pathway. Since the refractory period of the bypass may be as short as 200 ms or less, the ventricular rate may be as rapid as 300 (Figures 15-7, 15-8, and 15-9). The rhythm at such extreme rates may be perfectly regular and due to ventricular activation immediately at the end of the refractory period or may indicate atrial flutter with 1:1 conduction across the accessory pathway (Figure 15-7). Repetitive concealed conduction into the bypass may result in pauses sufficiently long to allow AV recovery and, thus, intermittent normal A-V conduction with normal QRS complexes (Figures 15-7 and 15-9).

Supraventricular Tachycardia with Wolff-Parkinson-White Syndrome

SVT is common in WPW because of the presence of two pathways with differing conduction times and refractoriness, a milieu for unidirectional block. The conduction is sufficiently slow in one pathway to allow for recovery of the alternate pathway of the reentrant loop. Most often, the reentrant loop includes anterograde conduction through the AV node, with a normal QRS complex in the absence of BBB or aberration, and retrograde conduction through the bypass (Figures 15-2 and 15-10). In the presence of such an orthodromic (anterograde along the AV node) reentrant tachycardia, a diagnosis of WPW is difficult. WPW is suggested by a shortening of the R-R cycle of the tachycardia when an ipsilateral BBB disappears,[9,13,14] by a negative P in lead I with an R-P interval of 100 ms or longer, and, perhaps, by alternans of the QRS amplitude (Figures 15-11 and 15-12).

During tachycardia, the QRS complex may be aberrant if the anterograde conduction is through the accessory pathway and the retrograde conduction is through the AV node (Figure 15-13). More often, however, the wide QRS complex recorded during reciprocating tachycardia is because of an acceleration-dependent RBBB or LBBB (Figures 15-14 and 15-15) with anterograde conduction through the AV node (Figures 15-11, 15-12, and 15-13). Supernormal[15] and concealed conduction in the bypass may alter the classic WPW pattern (Figure 15-16). Similarly, first, second, and third degree A-V block[16,17] and RBBB and LBBB have been reported in association with WPW.[18,19]

Incessant Supraventricular Tachycardia

A recurrent reentrant tachycardia that may last for hours or days and one that uses a bypass tract has been described and is referred to as "incessant SVT" or paroxysmal junctional reentrant tachycardia.[20–22] The P waves in leads II, III, and AVF are negative and the R-P interval is longer than the P-R interval. The prolonged retrograde conduction is due to AV nodal-like characteristics of the accessory pathway (Figure 15-17).

Lown-Ganong-Levine Syndrome (see also Chapter 2)

Sinus rhythm with a short P-R interval and a normal QRS complex with frequent SVTs is known as Lown-Ganong-Levine syndrome and is considered to be a variant of WPW. The most likely mechanism is an accessory pathway (James fibers) bypassing the AV node with insertion into the bundle of His that results in a short P-R interval and normal QRS complex (see Figures 2-30 and 2-31).

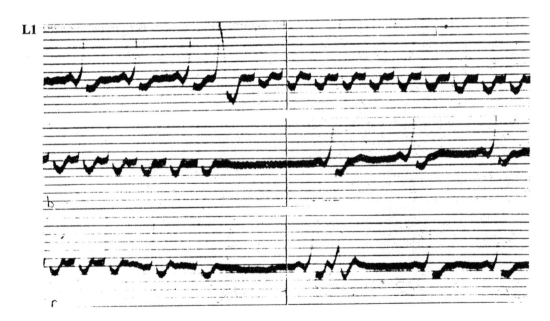

Figure 15-1. WPW with intermittent AVRT. This tracing, published in 1913 by Cohn, illustrates a short P-R interval, a prolonged QRS complex, and an intermittent SVT. In 1930, this ECG constellation was recognized as a specific ECG syndrome, WPW. The first three complexes in the top row are WPW followed by a VPC and an SVT, AVRT. The arrhythmia ceases spontaneously and is followed by a WPW pattern and, again, by an SVT. A sinus complex with WPW conduction and an APC follow. The last two complexes are sinus with WPW.

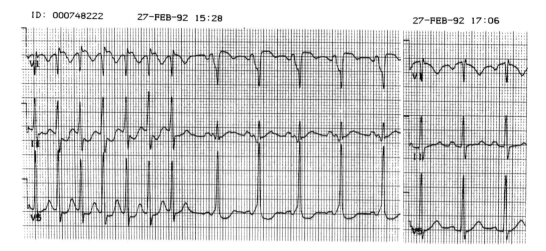

Figure 15-2. WPW with AVRT. The initial part of the tracing is an SVT, an AVRT, with an R-P interval in lead L2 of approximately 160 ms. WPW with an R-R interval of 600 ms follows. The right panel, a control tracing, illustrates normal sinus rhythm.

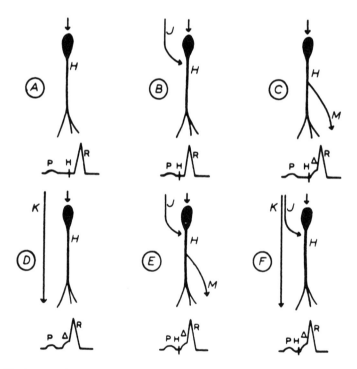

Figure 15-3. Various pathways of preexcitation. This now historical figure illustrates various pathways of preexcitation. A. Normal conduction; B. James fibers bypassing the AV node and inserting into the bundle of His, manifest by a short P-R interval and normal QRS complex; C. Mahaim fibers originating in the bundle of His manifest by a normal P-R interval and aberrant QRS complex with a delta wave; D. bundle of Kent with a short P-R interval and a delta wave; E. James and Mahaim fibers manifest by a short P-R interval and a delta wave. Not shown is the nodoventricular connection. From Coumel P, et al. Syndrome de pre-excitation ventricular associant PR court et ende delta, sans elargissement de QRS. *Arch Mal Coeur Vaiss* 1971;64:1234.

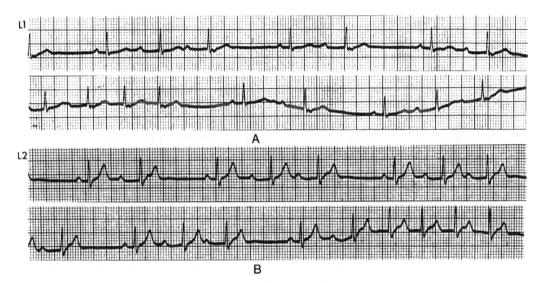

Figure 15-4. Wenckebach Type I A-V block with atrial reentry. The basic rhythm is sinus with a P-P of approximately 740 ms. Wenckebach Type I A-V block is present in panels A and B. Each Wenckebach sequence is terminated by an atrial reentry manifest by a negative P wave. A short run of AVRT is present in panel A, row 2 and in panel B, bottom row. The exact mechanism of the A-V block in the presence of WPW is unclear. It may be that conduction along the accessory pathway is blocked, forcing the impulse down the AV node with preexisting Type I block.

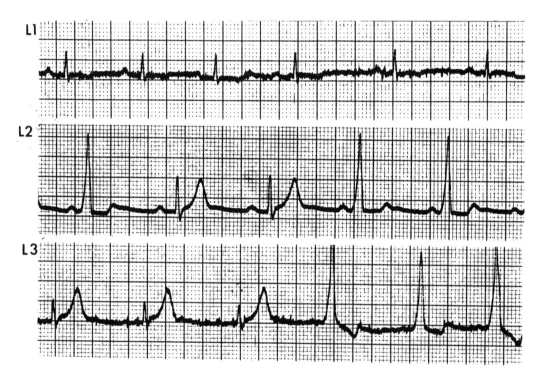

Figure 15-5. WPW and A-V block. This figure was recorded from the same patient as in Figure 15-4. The basic rhythm is sinus with a P-P interval of approximately 1000 ms and a P-R interval of 220 ms. Intermittent WPW with a short P-R interval and a delta wave is present in lead L2 and lead L3.

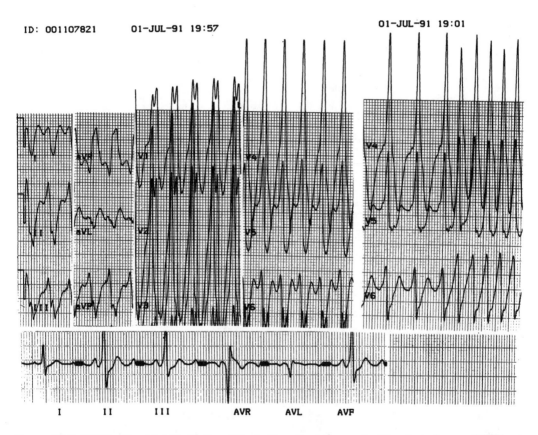

Figure 15-6. WPW with atrial fibrillation. The bottom row, the control tracing, shows a WPW pattern. Atrial fibrillation is recorded in the top panel, with runs of perfectly regular rhythm at a rate of approximately 300 to 150 per minute. For additional comments, see Figures 15-7 and 15-8.

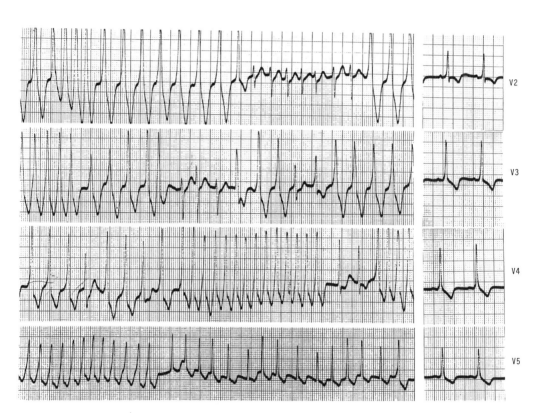

Figure 15-7. WPW with atrial fibrillation. Sinus rhythm with WPW is recorded in the right panel, the control tracing. In the left panel, the basic rhythm is atrial fibrillation with WPW and total activation via the accessory pathway at an RR interval of 200 or 400 ms. Normal QRS complexes and fusions interrupt the WPW complexes. Because the refractory period of the bypass is approximately 200 ms or shorter, a ventricular rate of 300 per minute is possible. The perfectly regular ventricular response suggests that the bypass was traversed at the exact moment the refractory period ended. The regular R-R intervals at 400 ms suggest a 2:1 block in the bypass with prompt conduction at the end of the refractory period induced by the blocked impulse. Repetitive concealment of the fibrillatory waves with block of conduction within the accessory pathway allows the AV junction to recover and to conduct with normal QRS complexes. From Heger JJ, Fisch C. Cardiac arrhythmias. In Spittell JA Jr. (ed): *Clinical Medicine.* Philadelphia: Harper and Row; 1982.

IUMC - 429411
L-2

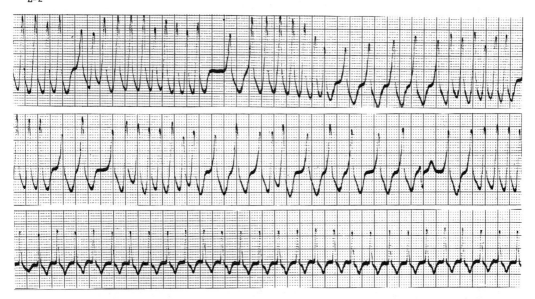

Figure 15-8. WPW with atrial fibrillation. Atrial fibrillation with conduction along the accessory pathway at rates of 300 or 150 per minute are shown in the upper two rows, with runs of regular rhythm. In the bottom row, AVRT with an R-P interval of approximately 160 ms is present. The regular rate of 300 may be due to a 1:1 flutter across the accessory pathway or conduction immediately at the end of each refractory period. The refractory period of the bypass may be as short as 200 ms or less, thus allowing for a rate as rapid as 300 per minute. The rate of 150 per minute may be due to atrial flutter with a 2:1 block in the bypass.

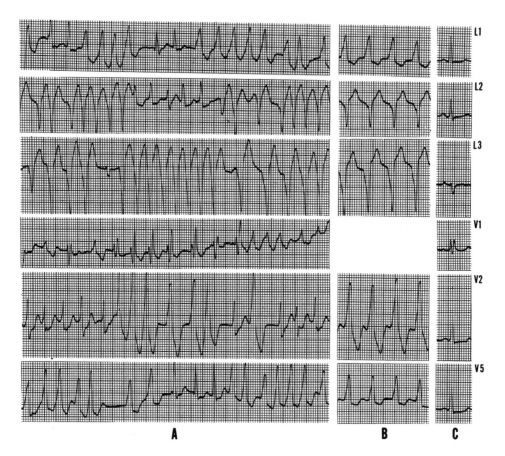

Figure 15-9. WPW and atrial fibrillation. Panel C, the control tracings, shows sinus rhythm with WPW and incomplete RBBB. In Panel B, the entire ventricle is activated along the accessory pathway with regular R-R intervals at 400 ms. Panel A shows atrial fibrillation with WPW with total activation of the ventricle along the accessory pathway with the R-R varying from 240 to 440 ms. The WPW is interrupted by QRS complexes with incomplete RBBB with conduction along the AV node. The refractory period of the bypass, being approximately 200 ms or less, allows for conduction at an R-R of 240 ms. In panel B, the regular R-R at 400 ms suggests a 2:1 block in the bypass. For additional comments, see Figures 15-6 through 15-9.

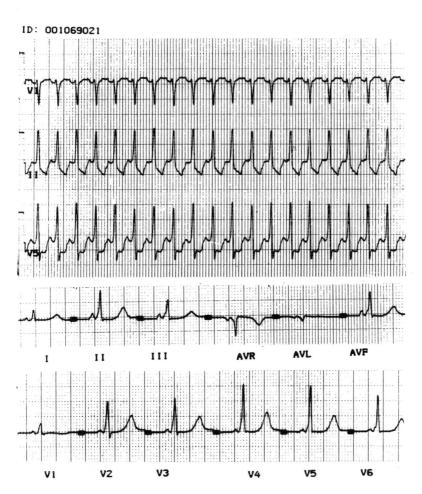

Figure 15-10. WPW with AVRT. The top panel illustrates WPW and AVRT with an R-P interval of approximately 140 ms. The nonspecific ST-T changes are most likely related to the WPW or to the rate or to both. The control WPW is recorded in the bottom panel.

NL QRS   BBB

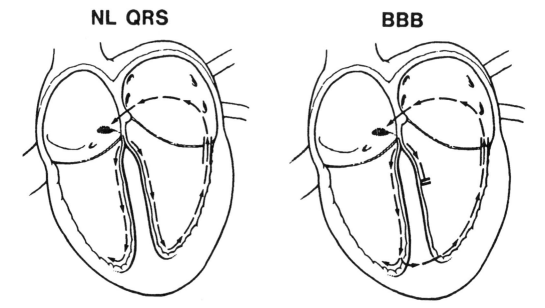

Figure 15-11. LBBB and AV nodal reciprocating tachycardia. In the left panel, the impulse responsible for the AV reciprocating tachycardia conducts anterogradely along the AV node, the LBB, the left lateral accessory pathway, and the atrium. In the right panel with LBBB, the reciprocating pathway conducts anterogradely along the AV node, the RBB, the left lateral accessory pathway, and the atrium. The pathway is longer; therefore the cycle length is longer and the rate of the tachycardia is slower.

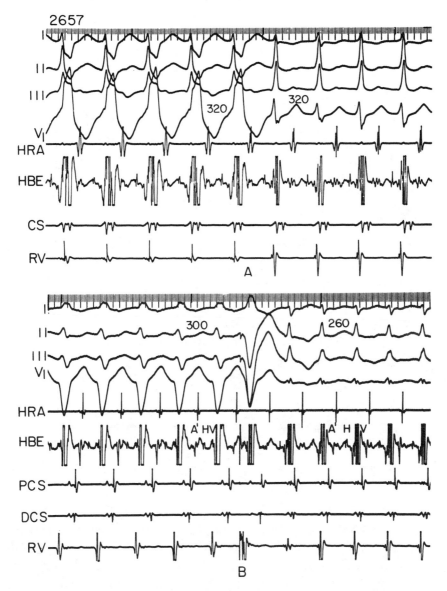

Figure 15-12. BBB and the cycle length of an AV nodal reciprocating tachycardia. The tracings include leads I, L2, L3, V_1, and electrograms recorded from the high right atrium (HRA), His bundle (HBE), proximal coronary sinus (PCS), distal coronary sinus (DCS), and right ventricle (RV). In panel A, the reciprocating tachycardia is accompanied by RBBB and the R-R interval is 320 ms. With normalization of the QRS complex, the tachycardia continues with the R-R interval unchanged at 320 ms. Since the bypass was on the left side and the impulse conducted anterogradely through the AV node and LBB, and retrogradely through the accessory pathway, the RBB did not affect the cycle length or the duration of conduction through the reciprocating pathway. In panel B, the reciprocating tachycardia with LBBB conducts anterogradely through the AV node and the RBB, and retrogradely through a left-sided accessory pathway. With normalization of the QRS complex induced by a premature stimulus, the reciprocating pathway is shortened from 300 to 260 ms because the impulse conducts anterogradely along the AV node and both the LBB and the RBB reach the accessory pathway and the atrium earlier.

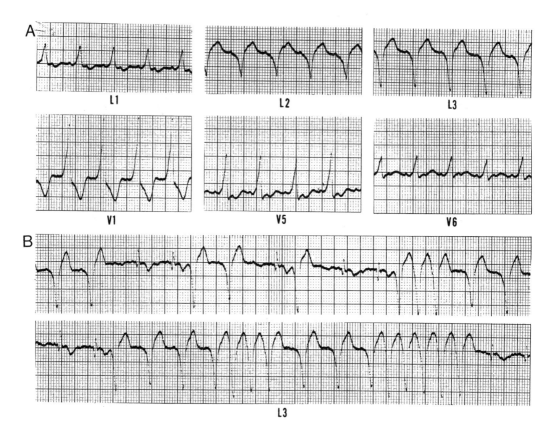

Figure 15-13. WPW with atrial tachycardia and A-V block. Panel A illustrates an atrial tachycardia with a P-P interval of 270 ms and 2:1 A-V block. In the top row of panel B, the first two WPW complexes with a 2:1 A-V block are followed by a 3:1 and 2:1 A-V block with normal QRS complexes. This sequence is repeated in the bottom row. 1:1 conduction is recorded in the right-hand side of the bottom row, with a P-P of 270 ms—exactly one half of that recorded in panel A with a 2:1 block. The A-V block excludes reentry as a mechanism of the tachycardia. The mechanism of changing block within the accessory pathway is unclear. Ventricular refractoriness is an unlikely cause in view of the fact that the ventricle is capable of responding to cycles of 270 ms. It is possible that the atrial impulses reach the accessory pathway near the end of each refractory period. If for some reason the impulse arrives earlier, 2:1 block results; however, if the impulse arrives slightly later, 1:1 conduction through the accessory pathway is possible. Similarly, a slight variation in the duration of the refractory period of the bypass in the presence of a constant atrial rate may be responsible for the changing A-V conduction. In essence, simultaneous failure of conduction through the AV junction and the accessory pathway is difficult to explain on the basis of the ECG alone.

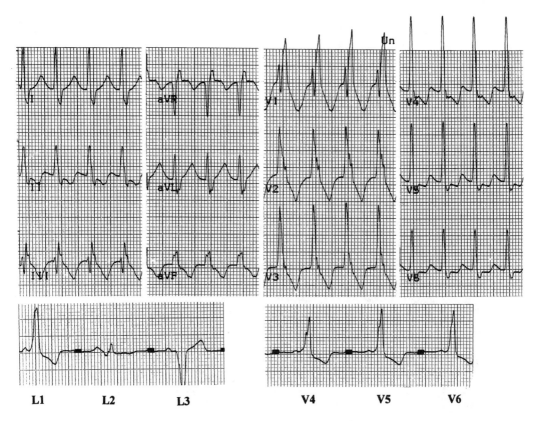

Figure 15-14. WPW, AVRT with RBBB aberration. The bottom row, the control tracing, shows a WPW pattern. The top panel reflects an AVRT with an R-P interval of approximately 160 ms. The conduction is retrograde through the accessory pathway and anterograde through the AV node (orthodromic) with RBBB aberration.

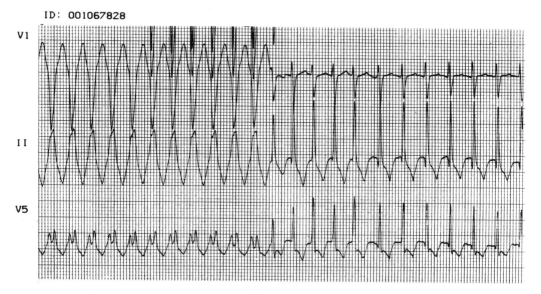

Figure 15-15. WPW, AVRT with aberration. The basic rhythm is an orthodromic AVRT with an R-P interval of approximately 160 ms. The first part of the tracing reflects rate-related LBB aberration with conversion to normal QRS. The normalization of LBB conduction is most likely due to shortening of its refractory period in response to the rate.

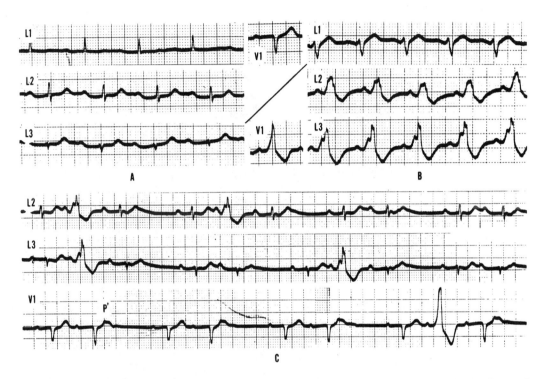

Figure 15-16. WPW with A-V block and supernormal conduction of the accessory pathway. In panel A, the control tracing, the basic rhythm is sinus with P-P and P-R intervals of 830 and 320 ms, respectively. WPW with a P-R interval of 140 ms is recorded in panel B. In panel C, Wenckebach periodicity is interrupted by a retrograde P (P'). The QRS complexes are either normal or WPW. P waves with an R-P interval of approximately 370 ms conduct to the ventricle through the bypass. P waves with the longer R-P interval conduct through the AV junction. A possible mechanism of the unexpectedly rapid A-V conduction via the bypass at an R-P interval of 370 ms is supernormal conduction of the accessory pathway. The supernormal conduction is the result of concealed retrograde conduction. In support of this mechanism and, more specifically, of concealed retrograde conduction in the accessory pathway, are the fully conducted retrograde P waves (P'). The fact that the P' is recorded only after the longer of the two P-R intervals indicates that the P' is due to reentry rather than an APC. From McHenry PL, Knoebel SB, Fisch C. The WPW syndrome with supernormal conduction through the anomalous bypass. *Circulation* 1966;34:734. By permission of the American Heart Association, Inc.

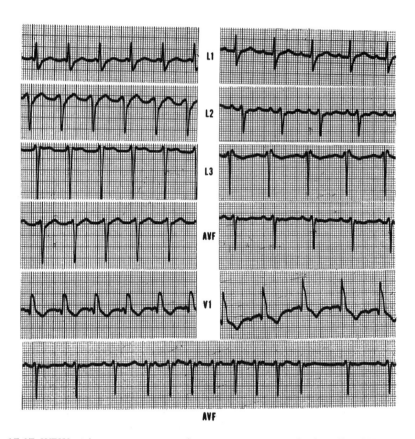

Figure 15-17. WPW with an accessory pathway inserting into the bundle of His. In the right panel, the control tracing, the dominant rhythm is sinus with a P-R interval of 220 ms and RBBB with LAFB. On the left, the P-R interval is shortened to approximately 100 ms without any significant change in the QRS configuration. The bottom tracing illustrates AVRT with an R-R interval of approximately 360 ms and retrograde P waves inscribed in the ST segment. The combination of tachycardia and a short P-R interval, without significant change in the QRS from control, suggests a James bundle inserting into the bundle of His above its bifurcation. The short P-R interval, normal QRS complex, and tachycardia are referred to as the Lown-Ganong-Levine syndrome (see Figures 2-32 and 2-33).

References

1. Cohn AE, Fraser FR. Paroxysmal tachycardia and the effect of stimulation of the vagus nerves by pressure. *Heart* 1913;5:93.
2. Wolff L, Parkinson J, White PD. Bundle branch block with short P-R interval in healthy young people prone to paroxysmal tachycardia. *Am Heart J* 1930;5:685.
3. Holzmann N, Scherf D. Ueber Elektrokardiogramme mit verkuerzter Vorhof-Kammer-Distanz and positiven P-Zacken. *Z Klin Med* 1932;121:404.
4. Kent AFS. Research on the structure and function of the mammalian heart. *J Physiol* 1893;14:222.
5. Wood FC, Wolferth CC, Geckeler GD. Histologic demonstration of accessory muscular connections between auricle and ventricle in a case of short P-R interval and prolonged QRS complex. *Am Heart J* 1943;25:454.
6. Lev M, Leffler WB, Langendorf R, Pick A. Anatomic findings in a case of ventricular pre-excitation (WPW) terminating in complete atrioventricular block. *Circulation* 1966;34:718.
7. Mahaim I, Winston MR. Recherches D-anatomie comparee et de pathologie experimentale sur les connexions hautes du faisceau de His-Tawara. *Cardiologia* 1941;5:189.
8. Mahaim I. Kent's fibers and the AV paraspecific conduction through the upper connections of the bundle of His-Tawara. *Am Heart J* 1947;33:651.
9. Coumel P, Attuel P. Reciprocating tachycardia in overt and latent preexcitation. Influence of bundle branch block on the rate of the tachycardia. *Eur J Cardiol* 1974;1:423.
10. Gallagher JJ, Pritchett ELC, Sealy WC, Kasell J, Wallace AG. The preexcitation syndromes. *Prog Cardiovasc Dis* 1978;20:285.
11. Giorgi C, Ackaoui A, Nadeau R, Savard P, Primeau R, Page P. Wolff-Parkinson-White VCG patterns that mimic other cardiac pathologies: A correlative study with the preexcitation pathway localization. *Am Heart J* 1986;111:891.
12. Benson DW, Sterba R, Gallagher JJ, Waltson A II, Spach MS. Localization of the site of ventricular preexcitation with body surface maps in patients with WPW syndrome. *Circulation* 1982;65:1259.
13. Kerr CR, Gallagher JJ, German LD. Changes in ventriculoatrial intervals with bundle branch block aberration during reciprocating tachycardia in patients with accessory atrioventricular pathways. *Circulation* 1982;66:196.
14. Pritchett ELC, Tonkin AM, Dugan FA, Wallace AG, Gallagher JJ. Ventriculo-atrial conduction time during reciprocating tachycardia with intermittent bundle branch block in the Wolff-Parkinson-White syndrome. *Br Heart J* 1976;38:1058.
15. McHenry PL, Knoebel SB, Fisch C. The Wolff-Parkinson-White (WPW) syndrome with supernormal conduction through the anomalous bypass. *Circulation* 1966;34:734.
16. Probst P, Pachinger O, Steinbach K, Kaindl F. Preexcitation of the ventricle associated with total intra His Bundle block. *Am Heart J* 1977;94:96.
17. Seipel L, Both A, Briethardt G, Loogen F. His bundle recordings in a case of complete atrioventricular block combined with preexcitation syndrome. *Am Heart J* 1976;92:623.
18. Krikler D, Coumel P, Curry P, Oakley C. Wolff-Parkinson-White syndrome type A obscured by left bundle branch block. *Eur J Cardiol* 1977;5:49.
19. Pick A, Fisch C. Ventricular preexcitation (WPW) in the presence of bundle branch block. *Am Heart J* 1958;55:504.
20. Coumel PH, Attuel P, Slama R, Curry P, Krikler D. "Incessant" tachycardias in Wolff-Parkinson-White syndrome. II: Role of atypical cycle length dependency and nodal-His escape beats in initiating reciprocating tachycardias. *Br Heart J* 1976;38:897.
21. Coumel P. Junctional reciprocating tachycardias. The permanent and paroxysmal forms of AV nodal reciprocating tachycardias. *J Electrocardiol* 1975;8:79.
22. Krikler D, Curry P, Attuel P, Coumel PH. "Incessant" tachycardias in Wolff-Parkinson-White syndrome. I. Initiation without antecedent extrasystoles or P-R lengthening, with reference to reciprocation after shortening of cycle length. *Br Heart J* 1976;38:885.

Atrioventricular and Ventriculoatrial Conduction and Blocks, GAP, and Overdrive Suppression

Historical Perspective

In 1925, Lewis and Master[1] studied the conduction and refractoriness of the A-V system of the dog heart. They defined the absolute (effective), the relative, and the functional refractory periods. The effective refractory period, 250 to 300 ms in duration, is the shortest P-P interval that conducts to the ventricle; the relative refractory period is the shortest interval between a first conducted APC of a series of APCs and the first normally conducted APC. The functional refractory period is the shortest QRS to QRS interval in response to any P-P interval, and indicates the most rapid ventricular rate possible (Figure 16-1).

Lewis and Master also noted that the P-R and R-P intervals manifest an inverse relationship in that the shorter the R-P, the longer the P-R and the longer the R-P, the shorter the P-R (Figures 16-2 and 16-3).[1] The prolonged P-R interval is due to conduction during the relative refractory period while failure of conduction is due to attempted conduction during the absolute refractory period (Figure 16-4). The occasional sudden prolongation of the P-R interval ("jump") may be due to conduction along the slow limb of a dual pathway (see Chapter 17).

If the relative refractory period is brief, the difference between the R-P interval of conducted and blocked P waves may be extremely short and is referred to as the "critical" conduction period (Figure 16-5).

Atrioventricular Block: General Classification

A-V blocks are classified as first, second, and third degree (see Chapter 5).

First Degree Block

First degree A-V block is present when the P-R interval exceeds 0.20 s or 0.22 s. Although most often caused by delay within the AV node (Figure 16-6), it may rarely result from delay within the atrium, the His bundle, the Purkinje system, or a combination of the above (Figure 16-7).

Second Degree Block

Based on the relationship of the jugular a-c waves, Wenckebach[2] described A-V block characterized by a gradual prolongation of the a-c interval and an ultimate failure of conduction manifest by the absence of the c wave followed by a pause.

In 1906, Wenckebach[3] and Hay[4] independently described two types of second degree A-V block. In 1924, Mobitz[5] classified the two forms as Type I or Wenckebach and Type II or Mobitz II A-V block. Presently, the two forms of A-V block are referred to simply as Type I and Type II A-V block. Type I A-V block is characterized by a gradual prolongation of the P-R interval prior to block of conduction (Figures 16-8 and 16-9). In Type II A-V block, the P-R interval preceding the block remains constant. In either type, the first P-R interval of the sequence may be normal or prolonged.[6,7]

Occasionally Type I, but more often Type II, A-V block is associated with block of two or more consecutive P waves. This type of block (block of two or more consecutive P waves), initially considered by Mobitz[5] and Wenckebach and Winterberg[8] to be Type II block, was found by Langendorf to be an occasional manifestation of Type I block. On the basis of P-R interval variations, block of two or more consecutive P waves can be classified as a variant of either Type I or Type II. It is, however, commonly referred to as advanced second degree A-V block. Advanced A-V block may be interrupted by isolated junctional or ventricular escapes or by intermittent AV dissociation with ventricular captures (Figure 16-10) (see below).

In Type I second degree A-V block with a normal QRS complex, the block is nearly always at the level of the AV node. Type II block is nearly always at the level of the His-Purkinje system and, as a rule, is caused by bilateral BBB with an abnormal QRS. Type I block within the His-Purkinje system is rare,[9] and when present may be impossible to differentiate from Type I block at the level of the AV node.[6-8] Type II A-V block with a normal QRS has been ascribed to block within the bundle of His.[6]

Third Degree Block

Third degree or complete A-V block is characterized by failure of any of the P waves to conduct. The rate of the subsidiary pacemaker is slow—approximately 40 to 50 per minute with a junctional pacemaker and approximately 30 per minute with a ventricular pacemaker. A-V block should not be confused with AV dissociation caused by physiological interference (Figure 16-10).

Electrocardiography of Specific Types of Block

Wenckebach Type I Second Degree Block

Type I second degree A-V block (Wenckebach) can be typical or atypical. The typical form of Wenckebach periodicity is characterized by a progressive prolongation of the P-R interval, with the largest increment following the second conducted P wave. The gradual prolongation of the P-R interval but with decreasing increments results in a progressively shorter R-R interval. The pause that follows the blocked P wave that ends the sequence is less than the sum of two preceding sinus cycles.

In *atypical Type I A-V block*, the P-R and R-R intervals terminating the Wenckebach sequence are longer than expected and may be the longest of the sequence (Figure 16-11). Other atypical manifestations include a number of P-R intervals of the same duration, an unexpected decrease of a P-R interval, or failure of the second P-R interval to show the maximal increase in duration. The prevalence of atypical Type I A-V block exceeds 50%, with the incidence of the atypical form increasing with the length of a Wenckebach sequence. At a ratio of 6:5, all Type I A-V blocks are atypical.

Occasionally, the P-R interval exceeds the P-P interval and one or more P waves are "skipped" by the P-R interval. The skipped P wave can be seen with typical or atypical Type I block (Figure 16-12).

Wenckebach Type I block may be a manifestation of any ectopic pacemaker and is recognized by the Wenckebach periodicity of P or QRS waves. Pacemaker impulses exiting in the Wenckebach mode may originate in the SAN,[10,11] the atrium,[12] the AV node,[13] the Purkinje fibers, and possibly the ventricular myocardium (Figures 16-13 and 16-14).[14] Exit delay and block have also been observed with electronic pacemakers (see Chapter 15).

In the presence of Type I exit block from the SAN, the AV junction, or a ventricular pacemaker, the rate of the ectopic pacemaker can be estimated by measuring the interval from the first complex of the Wenckebach sequence to the complex that terminates the long pause. This interval is divided by the number of manifest P-P or R-R cycles, adding one for the cycle "lost" because of block of conduction. Having identified and plotted the interectopic intervals and the manifest P wave or QRS complex, the conduction time from the ectopic focus to the manifest P or QRS can be estimated. This method is valid only if the ectopic rhythm is regular and the exit delay follows the classic Wenckebach pattern. The method of estimating the interectopic interval and conduction time from the ectopic focus to the surrounding tissue is illustrated in Figure 13-4.

Alternating Wenckebach Block

Alternating Wenckebach block is manifest by a progressive prolongation of the P-R interval of the every other conducting P wave of a 2:1 A-V block.[15-17] The pause following the block encompasses two and sometimes three nonconducted P waves. This arrhythmia is usually associated with an accelerated sinus rate, and the A-V block is usually at the level of the His-Purkinje system. It has been suggested that some atypical forms of atrial flutter and atrial tachycardias are examples of alternating Wenckebach with two levels of block[16-18] in the AV node (Figure 16-15).

Atrioventricular Block Due to Concealed Conduction

Anterograde concealed conduction of ectopic P waves may block two or more consecutive sinus P waves, resulting in a 3:1 or greater ratio of A-V block. Localized concealed discharges of the His bundle may simulate either Type I (Figure 16-16) or Type II (Figure 16-17) block. On occasion, the longest P-R interval of a Wenckebach sequence is followed by an atrial reentry interrupting the Wenckebach sequence (Figure 16-18). Similarly, concealed V-A conduction may block P wave conduction, suggesting that concealed reentry may be one of the mechanisms of Wenckebach block.[19,20]

2:1 Atrioventricular Block

2:1 A-V block may be Type I or Type II, and the differential diagnosis may be difficult or impossible. While the P-R interval is not helpful, a normal QRS complex supports the diagnosis of Type I block and a prolonged QRS complex favors Type II block.

AV dissociation with captures interrupting second degree A-V block may aid in the differentiation of Type I and Type II blocks. If the QRS complex is normal,

Type I block is likely. If the QRS is prolonged, Type II should be considered. Similarly, if the P-R interval of all of the capture complexes is constant despite a varying R-P interval, Type II A-V block is present. Conversely, if the P-R interval varies inversely with the R-P interval, Type I A-V block is the more likely diagnosis.[21]

With Type II A-V block, conduction may be unexpectedly altered by conduction during the supernormal period of recovery of the His-Purkinje system. The supernormal conduction may be induced by an anterograde or attempted (concealed) retrograde conduction of an extraneous impulse. Given an appropriate sinus rate, the 2:1 Type II A-V block may be interrupted by 1:1 A-V conduction,[21] with each impulse conducting during the supernormal period. The supernormal conduction is that of the His-Purkinje tissue. Supernormal conduction of AV node has yet to be demonstrated.[17]

Paroxysmal Atrioventricular Block

Paroxysmal A-V block is manifest by abrupt and persistent A-V block in the presence of an otherwise normal A-V conduction.[22] The block may be initiated by a conducted or blocked APC or VPC, or simply by acceleration or slowing of the sinus rate (Figures 16-19 and 16-20). Once a sinus P wave is blocked, the A-V block usually persists until it is terminated by an escape impulse with a predictable temporal relationship to the sinus P wave. Occasionally, however, conduction may resume without the presence of an escape complex. The configuration of the escape QRS is frequently similar to that of the dominant QRS complex. Paroxysmal A-V block is most likely subnodal and is probably caused by BBB.

The electrophysiological mechanism of paroxysmal A-V block is unclear. Repetitive concealed conduction has been proposed as one possible mechanism. Resumption of normal A-V conduction has been variously ascribed to conduction during the supernormal period of recovery following the idioventricular impulse, summation of anterograde and retrograde impulses, and Wedensky facilitation, in which a properly timed retrograde impulse makes it possible for an otherwise nonthreshold anterograde impulse to conduct and "peel" back the refractory period.

Ventriculoatrial Conduction

Retrograde V-A conduction may coexist with normal or abnormal anterograde A-V conduction. The retrograde conduction can be initiated by idioventricular impulse, VPCs, VT, or electronic pacing.

The first clinical case of V-A conduction was reported in a patient with a VT by Sir Thomas Lewis[23] in 1909. In subsequent studies, Lewis found V-A conduction in the dog to be a frequent phenomenon.[24] V-A conduction may be difficult to recognize in the ECG because of superimposition of the retrograde P wave on the ST segment or the T wave (Figure 16-21). V-A conduction depends to a large extent on the relation of the VPC to the sinus-induced junctional refractoriness and, therefore, to the prematurity of the VPC. The more premature the VPC, the less likely is V-A conduction. The potential for V-A conduction of properly timed VPCs may approach 100% (Figures 16-22 and 16-23).[25] Retrograde activation of the His bundle proceeds most often along the LBB, less frequently along both bundles, and least often along the RBB.[26] The retrograde conduction may manifest a 1:1 or a varying ratio of QRS complex to P wave (Figure 16-24). The V-A interval may be constant or may exhibit retrograde Wenckebach periodicity. Ventricular reentry is present in approximately 30% of patients with V-A conduction.[25]

V-A conduction in the presence of A-V block was reported in 1914,[27] and the subject was critically reviewed in 1944.[28] The retrograde conduction can be manifest or concealed.[29] In contrast to the high prevalence of V-A conduction during normal A-V conduction, V-A conduction in the presence of delayed or complete anterograde block of conduction is much less common (Figures 16-25, 16-26, and 16-27). Only isolated cases of V-A conduction have been reported in the presence of complete anterograde block. The reason for the differences in anterograde and retrograde conduction in the presence of A-V block is unclear (Figure 16-26). Although V-A conduction may occur along an accessory pathway, the long R-P interval, the increment in R-P with stimulation, and the retrograde Wenckebach periodicity—all features of junctional physiology—indicate that the V-A conduction proceeds along the AV nodal pathway.[30]

Overdrive Suppression of Atrioventricular Conduction

Depression of a preexisting A-V conduction abnormality by ventricular pacing was reported by Langendorf and Pick.[31] The duration of the depression is related directionally to the duration and the rate of the pacing (Figures 16-28 and 16-29). A likely mechanism of the depression of conduction is overdrive "fatigue" of the His-Purkinje tissue. The lesion is in the distal conduction system with prolongation of the H-V interval or Type II block. It has been suggested that when the QRS complex is normal, the block is most likely within the His bundle. In the presence of a bifascicular block, the pacing-induced complete A-V block is caused by block of conduction in the remaining fascicle.[32]

Atrial pacing also may exaggerate a preexisting AV junction conduction abnormality. The effect, however, is less pronounced than when the pacing is ventricular.

The GAP Phenomenon

An APC conducts to the ventricle and, with shortening of the R-P interval, conduction is blocked. With further shortening of the R-P interval, conduction is resumed. This sequence is a manifestation of the GAP phenomenon (Figures 16-30 and 16-31).[33–35]

The paradox of the resumption of conduction at a shorter R-P interval is possible because the early APC is delayed proximally in the AV node, allowing for recovery of tissue distal to the area of the block. When the proximal delay is at the level of the AV node with A-H prolongation, Type I GAP is present. When the delay is at the upper His-Purkinje level with H-V prolongation, Type II GAP is present.[35,36] Despite the paradox of resumption of conduction at a shorter R-P interval, the QRS to QRS interval in the ECG or the H1–H2 or V_1–V_2 intervals in the His bundle ECG are prolonged. This is because of the proximal delay with prolongation of the H1–H2 (Type I GAP) and H2–V_2 (Type II GAP) intervals. With resumption of conduction, the QRS may be normal or aberrant. With a shorter proximal delay, the QRS may be aberrant and with a longer delay, the QRS may be normal.

The two types of GAP are easily differentiated with an His bundle electrogram.[36] In Type I GAP, the H1–H2 interval that allows for recovery and conduction is prolonged. In Type II GAP, the H2–V_2 interval is prolonged.

Surface ECG differentiation of the two types of GAP is difficult if not impossible. If the resumption of conduction is associated with a normal QRS, Type I GAP is likely. If the QRS is aberrant, either Type I or Type II GAP may be present.

A Type III GAP has been suggested. It differs from Type I and Type II GAP in that resumption of A-V conduction occurs without prolongation of either the H1–H2 interval or the H2–V_2 interval. The mechanism of this type of GAP is obscure, and supernormality or dual conduction have been offered as possible explanations.[37]

Because in humans the effective refractory period of the His-Purkinje system rarely exceeds the functional refractory period of the AV node, and since the APCs are usually blocked at the AV nodal level, the GAP phenomenon is infrequent.[35]

The GAP phenomenon has been recorded with V-A conduction with the site of block either proximal or distal to the His bundle. The former is Type I, and the latter Type II, GAP.[38]

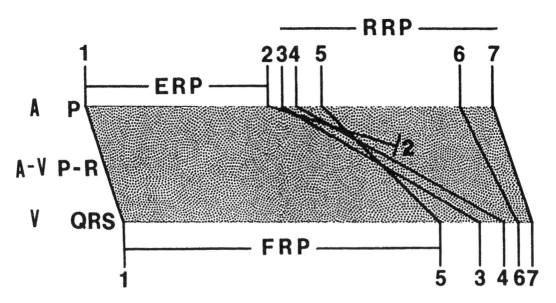

Figure 16-1. Refractory period of the AV node, derived from the surface ECG and HBE. The A, A-H, and V of the HBE and the respective ECG components, namely the P wave, P-R interval, and QRS complex, are indicated on the left. The effective refractory period (ERP) is the longest P1–P2 (A1–A2) interval at which P2 (H2) is blocked. The functional refractory period (FRP) is the shortest QRS 1–QRS 2 (H1–H2) interval possible, in this instance QRS 1–QRS 5. The relative refractory period (RRP) is the shortest interval between the first conducted P wave (A) and the final normally conducted P wave (A). In this figure, the interval between P3 and P7 (A3 to A7) defines the RRP.

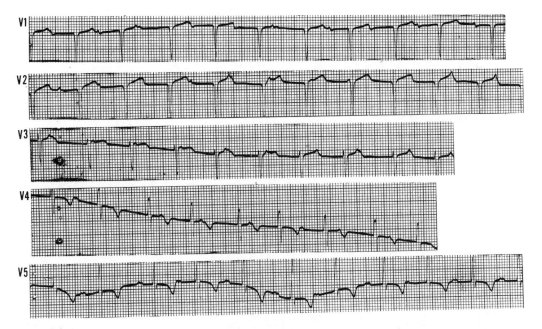

Figure 16-2. R-P and P-R intervals. The rhythm is sinus with APCs, some in the form of bigeminy. The R-P intervals vary from 240 to 600 ms, with the respective P-R intervals of 570 and 200 ms. The relationship between the R-P and P-R intervals is plotted in Figure 16-3.

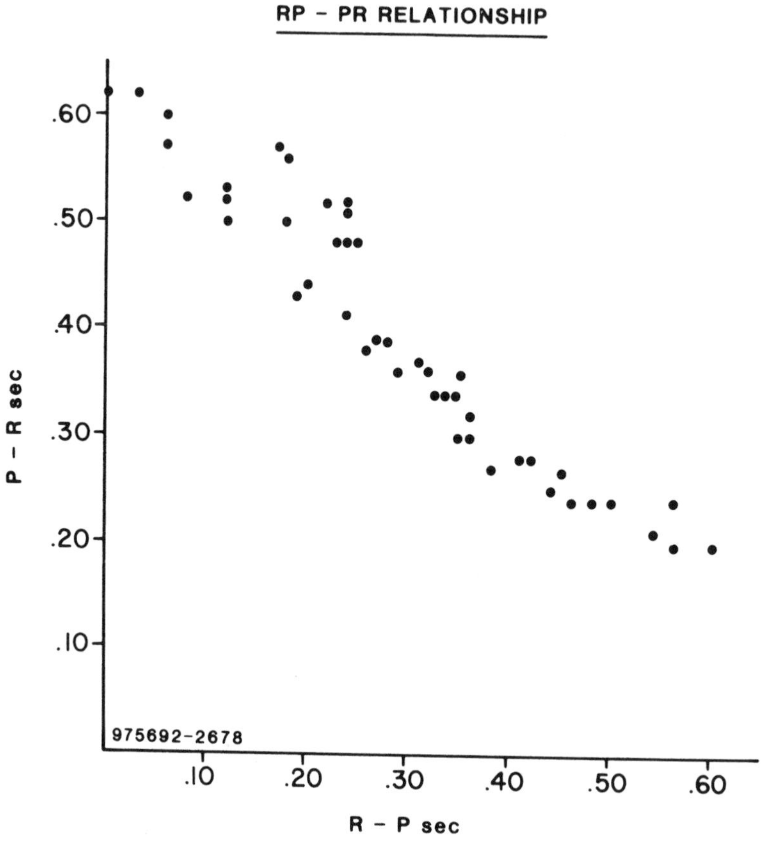

RP – PR RELATIONSHIP

Figure 16-3. R-P to P-R relationship. The data from Figure 16-2 illustrate the inverse relationship between the R-P, shown on the abscissa, and the P-R shown on the ordinate. In this instance, the relationship is nearly linear.

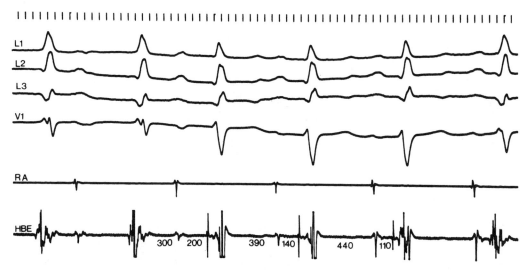

Figure 16-4. R-P to P-R relationship. The tracing includes leads I, L2, L3, V₁, right atrial (RA), and His bundle electrogram (HBE). The first two and the last QRS complexes are ventricular in origin, as indicated by the absence of a His potential preceding the QRS complex. A normal H-V interval precedes the three sinus QRS complexes. The R-P intervals measure 300, 390, and 440 ms, and the respective A-H (P-R) intervals measure 200, 140, and 110 ms, illustrating the inverse relationship of the R-P interval to the P-R interval. The longer the R-P interval, the more time for recovery of the AV node and, thus, the shorter the A-H (P-R) interval. Similarly, the shorter the R-P interval, the less time allowed for recovery of the AV node, the longer the A-H (P-R) interval.

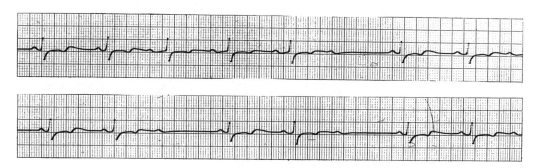

Figure 16-5. A-V block and the "critical" R-P interval. The basic rhythm is sinus, with a P-P interval of 1040 ms. In the top tracing, the first APC conducts with a P-R interval of 320 ms while the second APC is blocked. In the bottom tracing, both APCs are blocked. The R-P intervals of the four APCs are 680, 630, 680, and 640 ms, respectively. The longest R-P in which A-V conduction is blocked is 680 ms and the shortest R-P at which a P wave conducts is also 680 ms. The range during which the P wave conducts or blocks is narrow, with conduction or failure of conduction depending on a small "critical" R-P interval change, a change not easily recognizable on the surface ECG. Block of conduction at an R-P interval of 680 ms indicates an abnormally prolonged absolute (effective) refractory period of the AV junction.

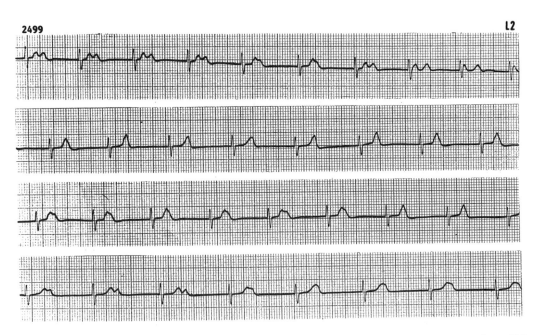

Figure 16-6. First degree A-V block. The basic rhythm is sinus with a P-P interval varying from 860 (first two P waves in the top row) to 1100 ms (first two P-P intervals in the bottom row). The fact that the P-R interval is constant at approximately 720 ms, while the duration of the P-P and R-R intervals change in parallel, indicates that the P waves conducted to the ventricle with 1:1 ratio.

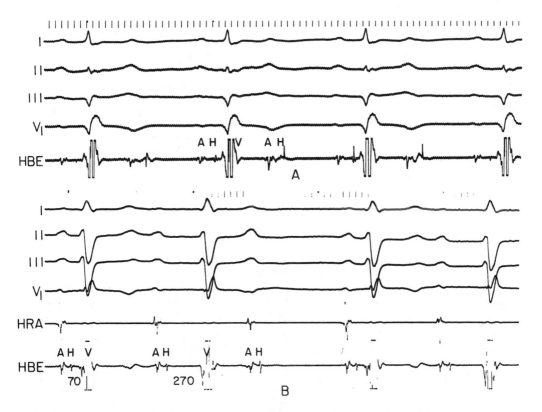

Figure 16-7. Type I (Wenckebach) and Type II (Mobitz II) A-V block below the bundle of His. The tracings include leads I, II, III, V_1, and a His bundle electrogram (HBE) in panel A and a high right atrial (HRA) and HBE electrograms in panel B. In panel A, the rhythm is sinus with a 2:1 A-V block and RBBB. A-V conduction fails below the bundle of His, as indicated by the His potential recorded after the blocked A (P) wave. In panel B, there is a 3:2 Type I A-V block. The configuration of the QRS complex is that of RBBB with LAFB with a gradual prolongation of the P-R interval and block of the third P wave. Although the level of block cannot be determined from the ECG, the HBE indicates that the prolongation of the P-R interval occurs below the His bundle at the H-V level. The H-V interval prolongs from 70 to 270 ms with block of the third A(P) below the bundle of His. The tracing in panel B indicates that despite the presence of RBBB with LAFB, Type I A-V block may occur below the bundle of His, an extremely rare finding.

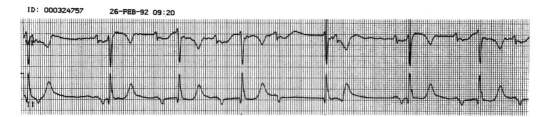

Figure 16-8. Ectopic atrial rhythm with a Type I A-V block. The ectopic rhythm is indicated by an inverted P wave in lead II and a prominent P wave in V_1. The P-P is regular. There is a gradual prolongation of the P-R interval, with the fifth P wave blocked. The long pause is terminated by a junctional escape. The next P wave is blocked because it falls during absolute refractory period induced by the junctional escape. The next P wave is conducted, with a P-R interval of 180 ms, and initiates a Wenckebach sequence.

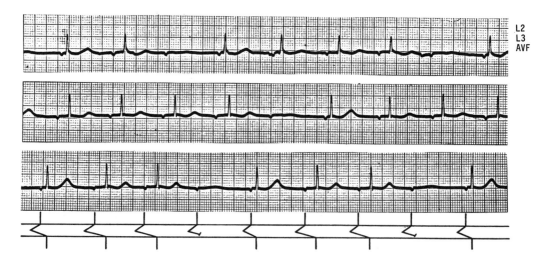

Figure 16-9. AV junctional rhythm with anterograde Type I A-V block and a 1:1 constant retrograde conduction. The interpretation is aided with the Lewis diagram. Negative P waves with a P-R interval of less than 120 ms in leads II, III, and AVF indicate a junctional origin of the P wave. The nearly regular P-P intervals indicate uniform retrograde conduction with a gradual delay of anterograde conduction. The gradual shortening of the R-R interval and the fact that the long pause is shorter than the sum of the two preceding R-R cycles, indicate an anterograde Type I A-V block. When an ECG fails to record a complete Wenckebach sequence, comparison of the last R-R cycle before the pause with the cycle immediately after the pause, the latter being longer, indicate Wenckebach periodicity.

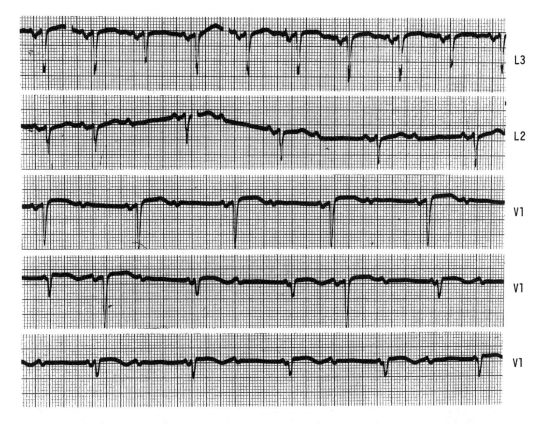

Figure 16-10. Advanced A-V block. Lead III, the control tracing, illustrates sinus rhythm at a rate of 83 per minute and a normal P-R interval. Lead II and V_1 illustrate 2:1 A-V block. In the middle V_1 tracing, sinus conducted impulses are interrupted by junctional escape complexes at an interval of 1280 seconds. The bottom tracing illustrates complete AV dissociation with an R-R interval of 1360 seconds.

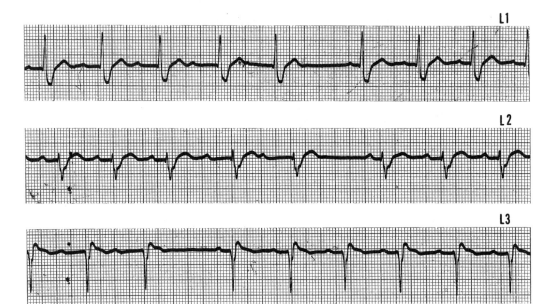

Figure 16-11. Atypical Type I A-V block. The basic rhythm is sinus with a P-P interval of 750 ms, RBBB, and LAFB. The P-R interval increases gradually from 240 to 380 ms with a sinus pause, most likely due to 2:1 SA block, although sinus arrest cannot be ruled out. The Wenckebach periodicity is atypical, with the last P-R interval being the longest of the sequence. The site of A-V conduction delay, whether above (A-H) or below (H-V) the bundle of His, cannot be determined from the ECG. In light of the RBBB and LAFB, it is possible that the Wenckebach block is at the His-Purkinje level (see Figure 16-7).

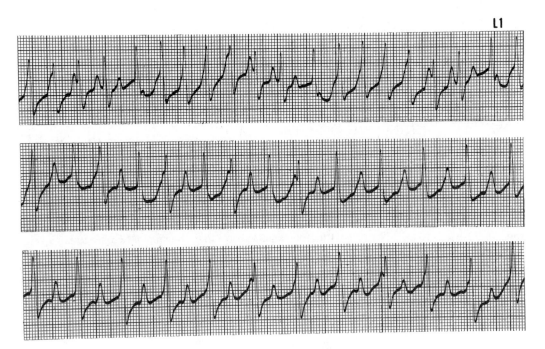

Figure 16-12. Wenckebach A-V block with "skipped" P waves. The basic rhythm is an atrial tachycardia with a rate of 200 per minute. The "skipped" P waves are best seen in the top row. Beginning with the fifth P wave and a P-R interval of 300 ms, the next P wave conducts to the ventricle, thus "skipping" the next P wave. This sequence continues until the P wave is blocked (middle of the tracing). The next P wave conducts with a P-R of 280 ms and the cycle is repeated. In keeping with the Wenckebach sequence the P-R interval lengthens from 280 to 440 ms before block of the P wave. In the middle row, a 3:2 Wenckebach block gives way to 2:1 conduction, which continues in the bottom row. The "skipped" P wave is the result of the P-R interval being longer than the R-R interval. The P-R interval is measured from the P wave to the next QRS complex.

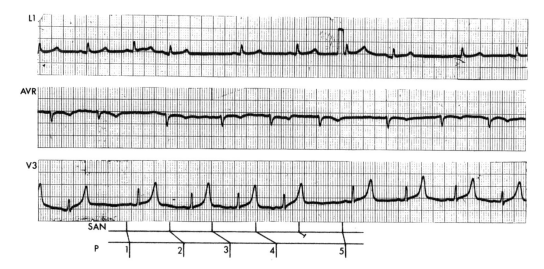

Figure 16-13. SA Type I block. The exit from the sinus node is gradually prolonged until the fifth sinus impulse fails to exit. The pause that follows is shorter than the sum of two preceding cycles, indicating a Type I exit block. The diagnosis is supported by repetitive group beating with the respective P-P intervals of each sequence being equal, and with a gradual shortening of the P-P interval.

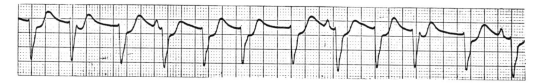

Figure 16-14. VT with Wenckebach exit block. The VT exhibits a repetitive pattern ("group beating") of R-R intervals. The longest R-R intervals measure 727 and 740 ms, respectively, and the R-R cycles that follow measure 640, 600, and 600 ms, respectively. The long cycle is less than the sum of two of the shorter cycles. The duration of the true interectopic cycle is calculated by dividing the sum of the five cycles, R3–R7 (2520 ms) by 5 for an interectopic interval of 504 ms. The maximal delay of conduction from the Purkinje is calculated by subtracting from the sum of three manifest cycles R1–R4 (1800 ms) the sum of three 504-ms interectopic intervals (504 × 3 = 1512 ms). The maximal delay calculates to be 288 divided by 3, or 96 ms. From Fisch C, Greenspan K, Anderson GJ. Exit block. *Am J Cardiol* 1971;28:402.

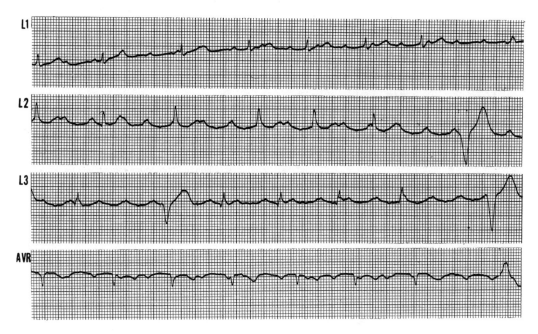

Figure 16-15. Atrial tachycardia with alternating Wenckebach periodicity. The dominant rhythm is atrial tachycardia with a 2:1 A-V block. The 2:1 block is associated with a gradual prolongation of the P-R interval of the conducting P wave, terminating with a block of the P wave. Such a sequence is illustrated in L2 beginning with the seventh P wave. The Wenckebach pause is terminated by a ventricular escape. The alternating Wenckebach is most likely due to two levels of A-V block, 2:1 high level and a 3:1 or 4:3 Type I low level block (see figures of atrial flutter).

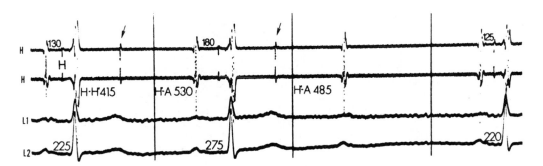

Figure 16-16. Concealed His bundle impulses (H′) with pseudo Type I A-V block. The A-H interval prolongs from 130 to 180 ms with block of the next A wave by the H′ (arrow). In the ECG, this is manifest by prolongation of the P-R interval from 225 to 275 ms, and block of the third P wave. The P-R interval following the pause is 220 ms. This sequence of events is consistent with Type I A-V block. In this instance, however, the block is due to concealed His discharge and, thus, a pseudo Type I A-V block. The temporal relationship of H′ to the subsequent A wave determines whether the conduction is delayed or blocked. As the H′-A interval shortens from 530 to 485 ms, the third A wave finds the AV junction refractory and is blocked.

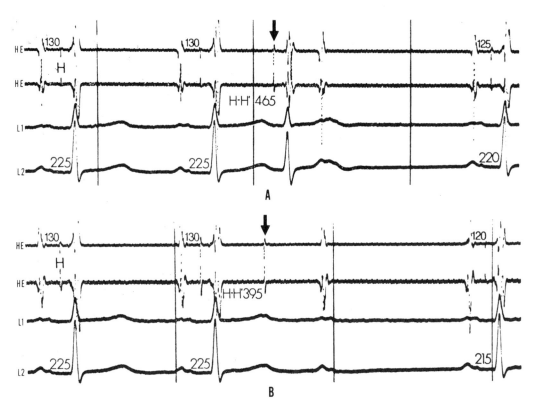

Figure 16-17. Concealed, premature His discharge with pseudo Type II A-V block. In panel A the H′ preceded by an H-H′ interval of 465 ms conducts to the ventricle (V, QRS). The A (P) wave that follows is blocked and is followed by a compensatory pause. In panel B, the H′ following a shorter H-H′ interval of 395 ms fails to reach the ventricle. However, this nonconducted impulse induces local refractoriness and blocks the subsequent sinus P (A) wave. The P (A) wave blocks without any antecedent prolongation of the P-R (A-H) interval, and suggests Type II A-V block. In reality, however, the block is caused by a concealed His bundle discharge (H′), and is therefore a pseudo Type II A-V block. From Fisch C, Zipes DP, McHenry PL. Electrocardiographic manifestations of concealed junctional ectopic impulses. *Circulation* 1976;53:217. By permission of the American Heart Association, Inc.

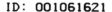

ID: 001061621

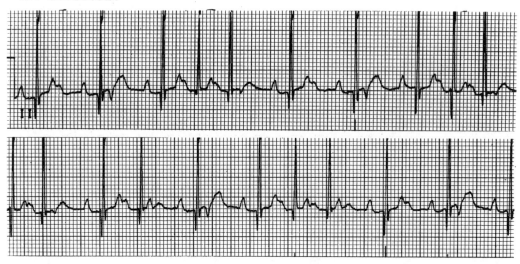

Figure 16-18. Type I A-V block with atrial reentry. The basic rhythm is a sinus tachycardia with Wenckebach A-V block. The Wenckebach sequence ends with block of a sinus P wave or a retrograde P wave, an atrial reentry. The eighth P wave in the top tracing and the second P wave in the bottom tracing are fusions between the sinus and reentrant P waves.

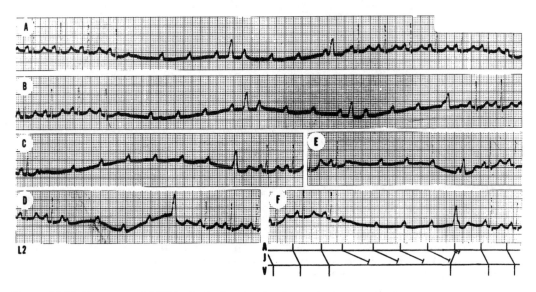

Figure 16-19. Paroxysmal A-V block. Each episode of ventricular standstill is initiated by a blocked APC and is terminated by a sinus impulse. Each follows the preceding idioventricular impulse by nearly the same interval. This suggests that the conduction was possible because of conduction during the supernormal period of recovery following the idioventricular impulse. The Lewis diagram suggests repetitive concealment as the cause of the A-V block. However, other mechanisms may be operative (see Figure 16-20).

LI

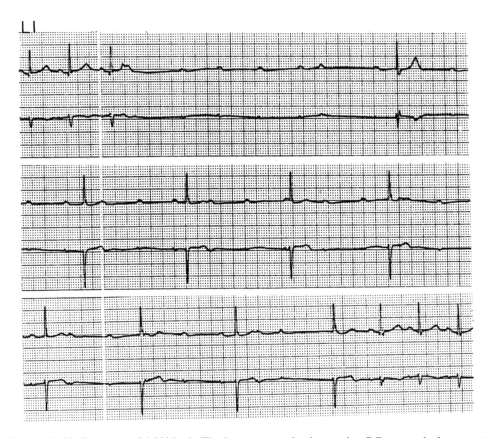

Figure 16-20. Paroxysmal A-V block. The basic sinus rhythm with a P-P interval of approximately 700 ms is interrupted by an APC with a sinus return cycle of approximately 1000 ms. The ventricular standstill and the gradually accelerating sinus rate are interrupted by an occasional APC and an escape. The site of origin of the escape impulse is most likely the junction. The mechanism responsible for initiation and perpetuation of A-V block is unclear. Concealed conduction of the APC followed by repetitive AV nodal concealment of the nonconducted P waves may be one mechanism. It has also been suggested that the prolonged P-P interval following the APC associated with deceleration-dependent (phase 4) depolarization of the lower part of the junction and resultant A-V block. Resumption of normal conduction has been variously ascribed to conduction during the supernormal period of recovery following the idioventricular escape impulse, summation of anterograde and retrograde impulses, or Wedensky facilitation, in which a properly timed retrograde impulse makes it possible for an otherwise nonthreshold anterograde impulse to conduct and, finally, "peeling" back of the refractory period.

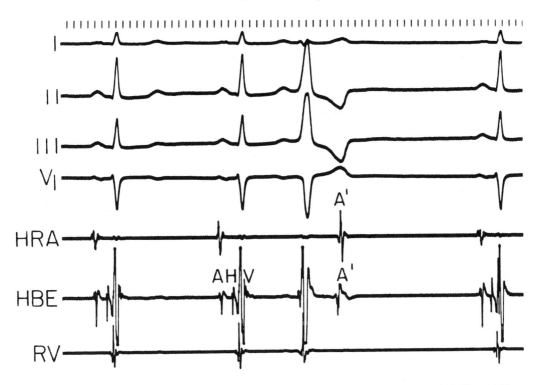

Figure 16-21. VPCs with retrograde V-A conduction. The tracing includes leads I, II, III, and V_1 as well as high right atrial (HRA), His bundle (HBE), and right ventricular (RV) electrograms. The basic rhythm is sinus with VPCs with retrograde conduction to the atria, the latter indicated by A′.

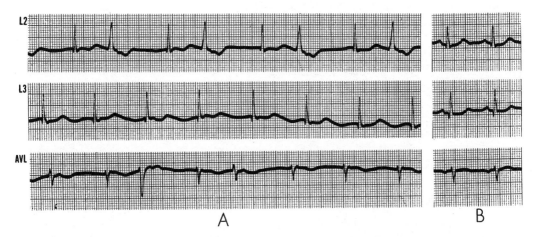

Figure 16-22. Retrograde (V-A) conduction. The basic sinus rhythm with a P-R of 160 ms and a normal QRS is shown in panel B. In panel A, the basic rhythm is junctional with retrograde P waves recorded at the end of the QRS complex. In L2, there is ventricular bigeminy, with V-A conduction of the VPC. Junctional rhythm with V-A conduction is illustrated in L3. In AVL, the junctional impulses and the VPC conduct retrogradely.

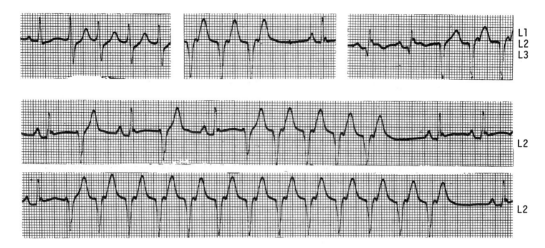

Figure 16-23. VT with retrograde conduction. This figure illustrates nonsustained monomorphic VT complicating acute inferior infarction conducting retrogradely with a 1:1 ratio of the QRS complex to the retrograde P wave.

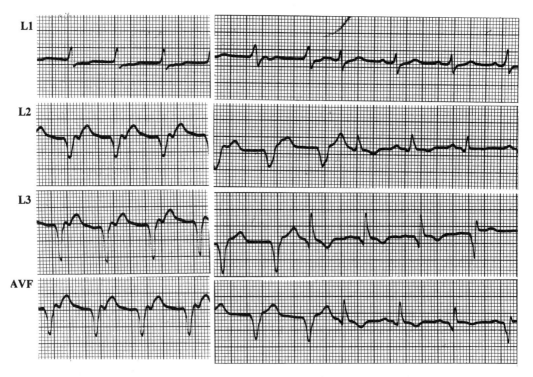

Figure 16-24. VT with retrograde conduction. VT with 1:1 V-A conduction is recorded in the left panel. In the right panel, VT is terminated with resumption of normal sinus rhythm. There is an underlying inferior myocardial infarction.

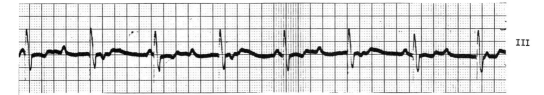

III

Figure 16-25. Anterograde A-V block with normal retrograde (V-A) conduction. The basic rhythm is sinus with AV dissociation and ventricular electronic pacing. The second, fourth, and sixth QRS complexes are followed by retrograde P waves with a coupling interval to the pacemaker stimulus of 160 ms. An atrial fusion between retrograde and sinus P wave follows the sixth QRS complex. V-A conduction is possible because the atria are no longer refractory, the preceding P wave having been inscribed 640 ms earlier. QRS complexes 1, 3, and 5 fail to reach the atria because the latter is still refractory, the result of the immediately preceding sinus impulse. It is also possible that failure of retrograde conduction is due to concealed conduction of sinus P waves into the junction, which blocks the retrograde conduction.

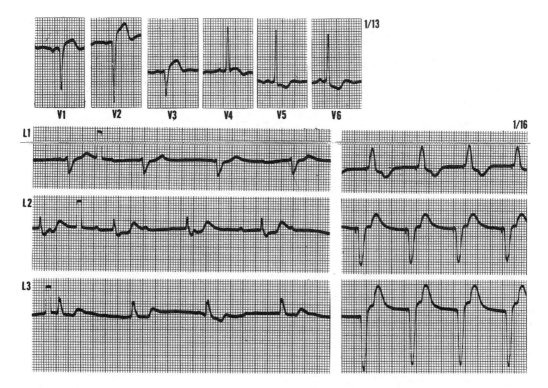

Figure 16-26. Complete anterograde A-V block with normal V-A conduction. An anterior myocardial infarction with sinus rhythm was recorded on 1/13. The left and right panels of the lower tracing were recorded on 1/16, immediately before (left) and after (right) insertion of a transvenous pacemaker. Complete A-V block with a P-P interval of 800 ms and an R-R interval of 1200 ms is noted in the left panel. In the right panel, the ventricle is paced at a cycle length of 780 ms with a 1:1 V-A conduction with a pacemaker to retrograde P wave interval of 220 ms. This figure indicates that the electrophysiological basis for anterograde and retrograde conduction may differ.

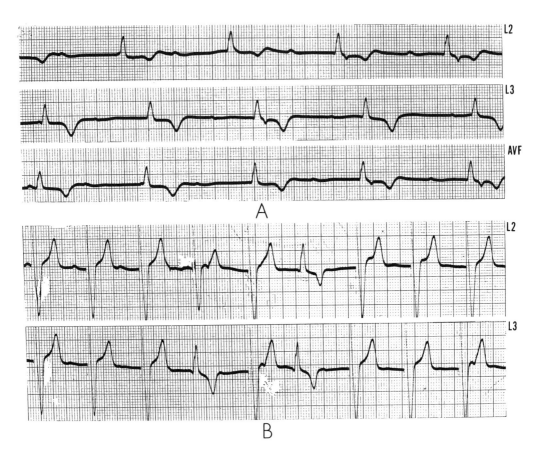

Figure 16-27. Complete anterograde A-V block with normal V-A conduction. The basic rhythm in panel A is complete third degree A-V block. QRS complexes 3 and 4 in L2, QRS 3 in L3, and QRS 4 and 5 in AVF conduct retrogradely, inscribing a negative P wave. The R to the retrograde P is approximately 200 ms. In panel B, the heart, paced electronically, is interrupted by three spontaneous QRS complexes. The fourth QRS complex in L2 and fifth and ninth QRS complex in L3 are conducted retrogradely with a stimulus to retrograde P of approximately 260 ms. Failure of retrograde conduction in panel B may be due to anterograde concealed conduction of the preceding sinus P wave.

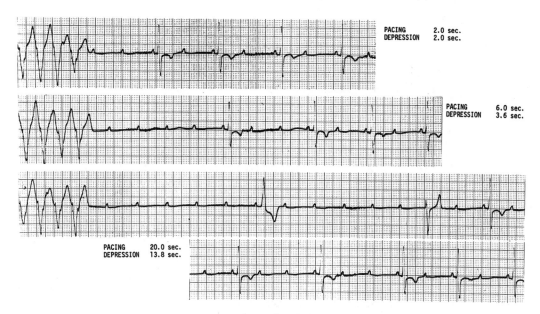

Figure 16-28. Overdrive suppression of A-V conduction. The basic rhythm is sinus with a 2:1 A-V block. The P-P and P-R intervals measure 680 ms and 120 ms, respectively. In the top, middle, and bottom tracings, pacing at cycles of 0.40 seconds for 2, 6, and 20 seconds is followed by A-V block of 2, 3.6, and 13.8 seconds, respectively. The duration of the depression of A-V conduction exhibits an almost linear relationship with the duration of the pacing as illustrated in Figure 16-29.

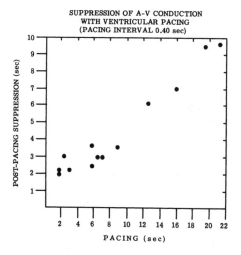

Figure 16-29. Duration of pacing and A-V suppression. The data shown in this figure were obtained from Figure 16-28 and compare the duration of pacing on the abscissa with duration of postpacing suppression of A-V conduction on the ordinate. The duration of postpacing A-V block maintains a linear relationship with the duration of the pacing.

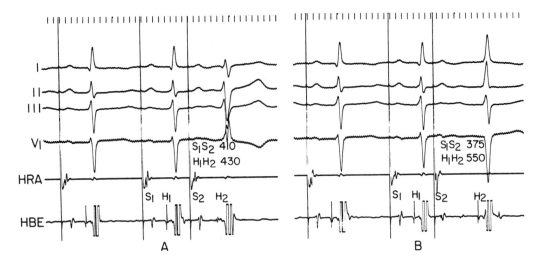

Figure 16-30. AV nodal GAP. The figure includes leads I, II, III, V₁, high right atrial (HRA), and His bundle electrogram (HBE). The basic pacing cycle length in panels A and B is 700 ms. In panel A, at an S1–S2 interval of 410 ms, the H1–H2 is prolonged to 430 ms, due to a 20-ms prolongation of the A-H interval. At this point, the impulse conducts with RBBB. In panel B, further shortening of the S1–S2 interval to 375 ms prolongs the H1–H2 interval to 550 ms, and causes an A-H prolongation of 175 ms. At this point the QRS complex is normal. The increasing prematurity of S2 with prolongation of conduction in the AV (A-H) node allows for recovery of the RBB conduction and the paradoxical normalization of the QRS complex.

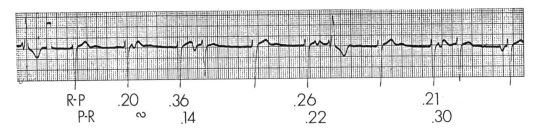

Figure 16-31. AV junctional GAP. The basic rhythm is sinus with a P-P interval of 1200 ms, AV dissociation, and a regular junctional rhythm with an R-R interval of approximately 1040 ms. The respective R-P, P-R, and R-R intervals are indicated in seconds. At an R-P interval of 0.20 s, the P wave is blocked. At an R-P interval of 0.36 s, the P-R interval is 0.14 s, the R-R interval is 0.50 s, and the QRS complex is normal. RBBB is recorded at an R-P interval of 0.26 s, a P-R interval 0.22 s, and an R-R interval of 0.48 s. At a shorter R-P of 0.21 s, the P-R interval is 0.30 s, the R-R interval is 0.51 s, and the QRS complex is normal. The fact that an R-P interval of 0.26 s is followed by an RBBB while an R-P interval of 0.21 s is followed by a normal QRS complex is unexpected. This paradox is due to that fact that at an R-P interval of 0.26 s, A-V conduction is more rapid, as indicated by a P-R interval of 0.22 s. As a result, the impulse arrives at the RBB after an R-R interval of only 0.48 s, and finds the RBB refractory. Conversely, at an R-P interval of 0.21 s, the P-R interval is prolonged to 0.30 s. Because of this, the impulse arrives at the RBB after a longer R-R interval of 0.51 s, the RBB has a chance to recover, and a normal QRS complex is inscribed. This delay in A-V conduction that allows for recovery of distal tissue and results in normal bundle branch conduction is referred to as the "GAP" phenomenon. The determinant of bundle branch conduction is not the R-P interval but the R-R interval, more correctly the H-H interval. The R-P interval of 0.26 s is accompanied by an R-R interval of 0.48 s, while the R-P interval of 0.21 s is accompanied by an R-R interval of 0.51 s. Consequently, the R-R interval of 0.48 s conducts with an RBBB, while the shorter R-P of 0.21 s with an R-R of 0.51 conducts normally.

References

1. Lewis T, Master AM. Observations upon conduction in the mammalian heart. A-V conduction. *Heart* 1925;12:209.
2. Wenckebach KF. Zur Analyse Des Unrezelmasigen Pulses. II. Uber Den regelmasig Intermitterenden Pulse. *Zscher Klin Med* 1899;37:475.
3. Wenckebach KF. Beitrage Zur Kenntnis der Menschlichen Herztatigkeit. *Arch Anat Physiol (Physiol Abtheilung)* 1906;297.
4. Hay J. Bradycardia and cardiac arrhythmia produced by depression of certain functions of the heart. *Lancet* 1906;1:139.
5. Mobitz W. Ober die unvollstandige Storung der Erregungsuberleitung zwischen Vorhof und Kammer des Menschlichen herzens. *Z Ges Exp Med* 1924;41:180.
6. Narula OS, Scherlag BJ, Samet P, Javier RP. Atrioventricular block. Localization and classification by His bundle recordings. *Am J Med* 1971;50:146.
7. Rosen KM, Lieb HS, Gunnar RM, Rahimtoola SH. Mobitz Type II block without bundle branch block. *Circulation* 1971;41:1111.
8. Wenckebach KF, Winterberg H. *Die Unregelmassige Herztatigkeit.* Leipzig: W Engelmann; 1927:313.
9. Narula OS, Samet P. Wenckebach and Mobitz Type II A-V block due to block within the His bundle and bundle branches. *Circulation* 1970;41:947.
10. Rosenbaum MB, Nau GJ, Levi RJ, Halpern SM, Elizari MV, Lazzari JO. Wenckebach periods in the bundle branches. *Circulation* 1969;40:79.
11. Schamroth L, Dove E. The Wenckebach phenomenon in sinoatrial block. *Br Heart J* 1966;28:350.
12. Omori Y. Repetitive multifocal paroxysmal atrial tachycardia: With cyclic Wenckebach phenomenon under observation for thirteen years. *Am Heart J* 1971;83:527.
13. Fisch C, Knoebel SB. Recognition and therapy of digitalis toxicity. *Prog Cardiovasc Dis* 1970;13:71.
14. Greenspan K, Anderson GJ, Fisch C. Electrophysiologic correlate of exit block. *Am J Cardiol* 1971;28:197.
15. Denes P, Levy L, Pick A, Rosen KM. The incidence of typical and atypical A-V Wenckebach periodicity. *Am Heart J* 1975;89:26.
16. Halpern MS, Nau GJ, Levi RJ, Elizari MV, Rosenbaum MB. Wenckebach periods of alternate beats—clinical and experimental observations. *Circulation* 1973;48:41.
17. Amat-Y-Leon R, Chuquimia R, Wu D, et al. Alternating Wenckebach periodicity: A common electrophysiologic response. *Am J Cardiol* 1975;36:757.
18. Langendorf R, Pick A. Concealed conduction. Further evaluation of a fundamental aspect of propagation of the cardiac impulse. *Circulation* 1956;13:381.
19. Kosowsky BD, Latif P, Radoff AM. Multilevel atrioventricular block. *Circulation* 1976;54:914.
20. Gallagher JJ, Damato AN, Varghese PJ, Lau SH. Manifest and concealed reentry. A mechanism of A-V nodal Wenckebach in man. *Circulation* 1973;47:752.
21. Langendorf R, Cohen H, Gozo EG. Observations on second degree atrioventricular block, including new criteria for the differential diagnosis between Type I and Type II block. *Am J Cardiol* 1972;29:111.
22. Strasberg B, Lam W, Swiry S, et al. Symptomatic spontaneous paroxysmal AV nodal block due to localized hyperresponsiveness of the AV node to vagotonic reflexes. *Am Heart J* 1982;103:795.
23. Lewis T. Single and successive extrasystoles. *Lancet* 1909;1:382.
24. Lewis T. The experimental production of paroxysmal tachycardia and the effect of ligation of the coronary arteries. *Heart* 1909;1:98.
25. Goldreyer BN, Bigger JT Jr. Ventriculo-atrial conduction in man. *Circulation* 1970;41:935.
26. Akhtar M, Gilbert CJ, Wolf FG, Schmidt D. Retrograde conduction in the His-Purkinje system. *Circulation* 1979;59:1252.
27. Cohn AE, Fraser FR. Occurrence of auricular contractions in a case of incomplete and complete heart block due to stimuli received from the contracting ventricles. *Heart* 1914;5:141.

28. Winternitz M, Langendorf R. Auriculo-ventricular block with ventriculo-auricular response. *Am Heart J* 1944;27:301.
29. Castellanos A, Castillo C, Agha AS. Mechanisms of retrograde activation of the His bundle, atria, ventricular echoes and reciprocating tachycardia. In Krikler DM, Goodwin JF (eds): *Advances in Electrocardiography*. New York: Grune and Stratton; 1972:221.
30. Khalilullah M, Singhal N, Gupta U, Padmavati S. Unidirectional complete heart block. *Am Heart J* 1979;97:608.
31. Langendorf R, Pick A. Artificial pacing of the human heart. Its contribution to the understanding of the arrhythmias. *Am J Cardiol* 1971;28:516.
32. Wald RW, Waxman MB. Depression of distal AV conduction following ventricular pacing. *PACE* 1981;4:84.
33. Moe GK, Mendez D, Han J. Aberrant A-V impulse propagation in the dog heart: A study of functional bundle branch block. *Circ Res* 1965;16:261.
34. Durrer D. Electrical aspects of human cardiac activity: A clinical-physiological approach to excitation and stimulation. *Cardiovasc Res* 1968;2:1.
35. Wit AL, Damato AN, Weiss MB, Steiner C. Phenomenon of the gap in atrioventricular conduction in the human heart. *Circ Res* 1970;27:679.
36. Gallagher JJ, Damato AN, Caracta AR, Varghese PJ, Josephson ME, Lau SH. Gap in the A-V conduction in man: Type I and Type II. *Am Heart J* 1973;85:78.
37. Agha AS, Castellanos A Jr, Wells D, Ross MD, Befeler B, Myerburg RJ. Type I, Type II, and Type III gaps in bundle branch conduction. *Circulation* 1973;47:321.
38. Akhtar M, Damato AN, Caracta AR, Batsford WP, Lau SH. The gap phenomena during retrograde conduction in man. *Circulation* 1974;49:811.

17

Dual Atrioventricular Conduction

Dual A-V conduction, a prerequisite for reentry, is most likely a variant of normal A-V conduction with one pathway having a shorter refractory period and one a longer conduction time.

The earliest ECG recording of reentry was published by White[1] in 1915; he later proposed dual A-V conduction as the mechanism of the reentry.[2] Subsequently, isolated clinical ECG tracings consistent with anterograde dual A-V conduction recorded during sinus rhythm have been reported.

With the advent of intracardiac stimulation techniques—discontinuous curves with discrete "jumps" in A-V conduction time—occasional reentry and reentrant tachycardia have been recorded in humans. These observations further support the concept of functional longitudinal dissociation of AV node conduction.[3–7]

Recent observations made during catheter ablation of reentrant arrhythmias and, more specifically, identification of an anatomically discrete slow conduction pathway, thought to be located in the posteroinferior aspect of the right atrium in the area adjacent to the coronary sinus, provide strong and direct evidence for dual A-V conduction.[8–11]

Electrocardiographic Manifestations of Dual Atrioventricular Conduction

The following are the ECG manifestations of dual AV nodal conduction during normal sinus rhythm: 1) spontaneous prolongation of the P-R interval (Figure 17-1); 2) abrupt prolongation and normalization of the P-R interval due to an APC and atrial tachycardia (Figure 17-2); 3) prolongation of the P-R interval with resumption of normal conduction due to an interpolated VPC (Figure 17-3); 4) slow pathway conduction initiated by an interpolated VPC (Figure 17-4); 5) interpolated VPC-induced P-R interval prolongation terminated by reentry (Figure 17-5); 6) P-R prolongation induced by VPCs and terminated by an APC (Figure 17-6); 7) sinus rhythm with alternans of the P-R interval and a paradoxical R-P to P-R relationship (Figure 17-7); 8) sinus rhythm with P-R alternans, Type I block in the slow pathway, and 2:1 block in the fast pathway (Figure 17-8); and 9) simultaneous conduction along the fast and slow pathway (Figure 17-9).

Mechanisms

To initiate conduction along the slow nodal pathway, an atrial impulse must arrive during the refractory period of the fast pathway. Abrupt P-R interval prolongation can be induced by an APC (Figure 17-2) and by atrial tachycardia, interpolated JPCs, VPCs (Figure 17-4), ventricular pacing, and, rarely, during normal sinus rhythm without ectopic beats (Figure 17-1). VPCs conduct retrogradely into the fast pathway, thus blocking fast pathway anterograde conduction and forcing conduction along the slow pathway. Although it is possible that the prolonged A-V conduction is due to the short R-P interval that follows the interpolated VPC, the evidence against a short R-P interval as the mechanism of slow A-V conduction with prolongation of the P-R interval is threefold: 1) electrophysiological studies in humans designed to elicit persistent prolongation of the P-R interval with interpolated VPCs have met with failure; 2) if the prolonged P-R interval was caused by a short R-P interval, one would expect this phenomenon to be observed more often because of the relative frequency of interpolated VPCs; and 3) a prolonged R-P interval is followed by a prolonged P-R—the opposite of that which is expected.

To sustain conduction along a slow pathway, it is necessary to invoke repetitive concealed reentry from the slow to the fast pathway and, thus, a continued refractoriness of the fast pathway. This mechanism is supported by the relatively common occurrence of manifest atrial reentry; therefore, it is reasonable to assume that concealed reentry may be responsible for continued fast pathway refractoriness and, consequently, sustained slow pathway conduction. Concealed conduction of ectopic impulses into the slow pathway will terminate the slow pathway conduction and shift conduction to the fast pathway. Similarly, absence of retrograde concealment from the fast to the slow pathway is prerequisite for slow pathway conduction.

P-R interval alternans, once ascribed to supernormal nodal conduction or to concealed intranodal reentry, is more likely due to dual AV node conduction (Figure 17-7).

The Type I conduction delay in the slow pathway observed in Figure 17-8 supports the postulate that the pathway contains specialized AV node-like tissue. Similarly, changing of slow pathway conduction in parallel with that of the sinus rate suggests a vagal effect and, thus, the presence of specialized tissue in the slow pathway.

That the two pathways are probably anatomical structures is suggested by termination of reentrant tachycardia with ablation of the slow pathway located in the atrium. Furthermore, persistent simultaneous conduction along both pathways (Figures 17-9 and 17-10) may result in a nonreentrant tachycardia with a manifest ventricular rate twice that of the atrial rate. Reentrant tachycardia, if present, would be relatively slow because of the participation of the slow pathway in the reentrant circuit.

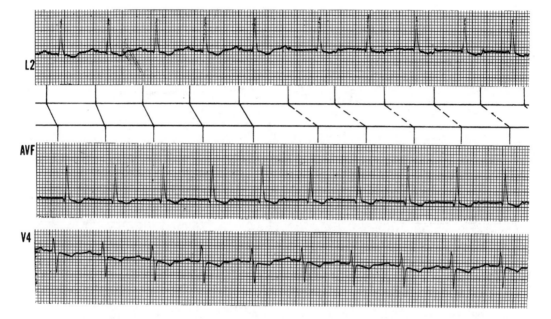

Figure 17-1. Dual AV nodal conduction. Spontaneous, abrupt prolongation of the sixth P-R interval from 200 to 400 ms is recorded in lead L2 but without any recognizable change in the R-P or the P-P interval. It is possible that there is a minimal shortening of the P-P interval that is sufficient to cause a "jump" of conduction to the slowly conducting pathway of the dual pathway system but that is not recognizable in the ECG. It is also possible that changes in autonomic tone altered the refractoriness or conduction or both of the fast pathway, shifting conduction to the slow pathway. Perpetuation of the slow pathway conduction is more likely due to repetitive concealment of conduction from the slow pathway to the fast pathway, causing block of conduction in the fast pathway. From Fisch C, Mandrola JM, Rardon DP. Electrocardiographic manifestations of dual AV nodal conduction during sinus rhythm. *J Am Coll Cardiol* 1997;29:1015.

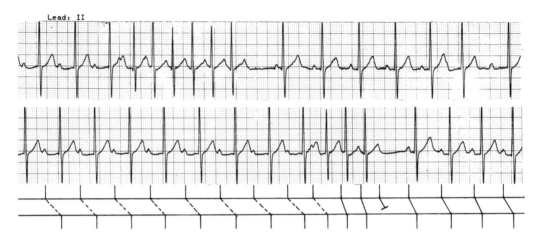

Figure 17-2. Dual AV nodal conduction. Shortening of the P-R interval caused by an APC and an atrial tachycardia is illustrated in this tracing. Sinus rhythm with a P-R interval of 320 ms is interrupted by an APC and atrial tachycardia, with shortening of the P-R interval to 160 ms. The last APC recorded in the top tracing is followed by a sinus impulse with R-P and P-R intervals of 560 and 340 ms, respectively. These simultaneously long R-P and P-R intervals prove that a shorter R-P interval is not the cause of the long P-R interval; rather, the long P-R interval reflects dual AV nodal conduction with a "jump" of conduction to the slow pathway. A repetitive concealment from the slow pathway to the fast pathway blocks fast pathway conduction, thus perpetuating slow pathway conduction. In the bottom tracing, the short P-R interval follows three consecutive APCs. From Fisch C, Mandrola JM, Rardon DP. Electrocardiographic manifestations of dual AV nodal conduction during sinus rhythm. *J Am Coll Cardiol* 1997;29:1015.

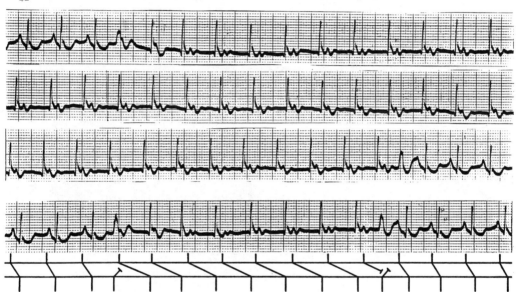

Figure 17-3. Dual AV nodal conduction. The first interpolated VPC in the bottom row blocks fast pathway conduction, shifting to conduction along the slow pathway. The second interpolated VPC either blocks slow pathway conduction or prevents concealed conduction from the slow pathway to the fast pathway, thus shifting conduction to the fast pathway. The top three rows illustrate an interpolated VPC causing a shift of conduction from fast to slow pathway, persistence of slow pathway conduction, and an interpolated PVC shifting conduction to the fast pathway. From Mamlin JJ, Fisch C. Sustained A-V conduction delay due to interpolated ventricular premature systole. *Am J Cardiol* 1965;16:765–766.

L2

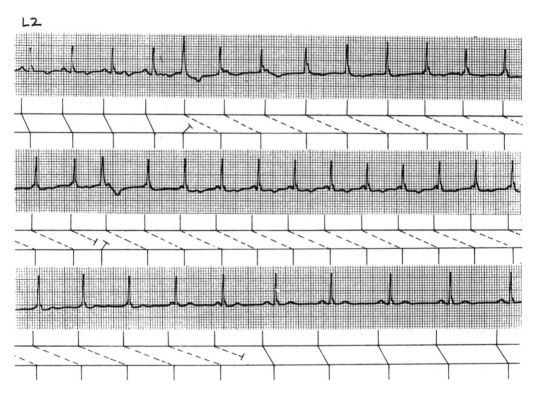

Figure 17-4. Dual AV nodal conduction. The basic rhythm, recorded at the beginning of the top tracing and at the right half of the bottom tracing, is sinus with a P-R interval of 160 ms. Beginning with the interpolated VPC in the top row, the P-R interval lengthens gradually from approximately 600 ms to 840 ms, with P wave conduction blocked in the bottom row. Beginning with the fourth from the last P wave in the top row, the P-R interval is longer than the P-P interval and, thus, the P waves are "skipped." The last skipped P wave in the bottom row fails to conceal from the slow pathway to the fast pathway with conduction along the fast pathway. Parallel with slowing of the sinus rate, the slow pathway conduction slows, with a gradual prolongation of the P-R interval from 640 ms in the second row to 840 ms in the bottom row. The delay in slow pathway conduction concomitant with sinus slowing suggests that the slow pathway is under the influential parasympathetic innervation and most likely contains AV node-like tissue. From Fisch C, Mandrola JM, Rardon DP. Electrocardiographic manifestations of dual AV nodal conduction during sinus rhythm. *J Am Coll Cardiol* 1997;29:1015.

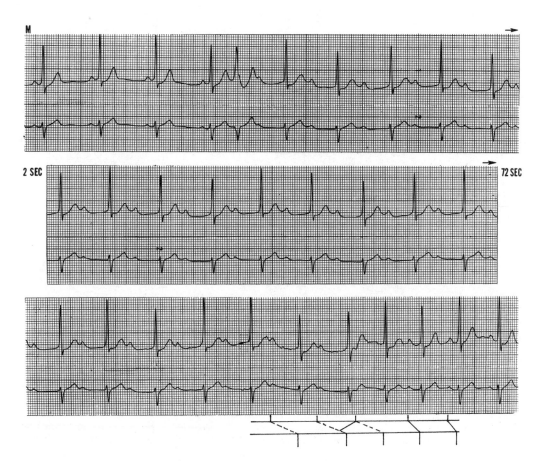

Figure 17-5. Dual AV nodal conduction. In the top row, an interpolated VPC initiates conduction along the slow pathway. In the bottom row, the slow conduction is terminated by retrograde conduction, and atrial reentry manifest by an inverted P wave. This in turn is followed by a ventricular reentry conducting along the slow conducting pathway (interrupted line). Failure of the latter to conceal into the fast pathway shifts conduction to the fast pathway; hence, the short P-R interval. From Fisch C. *Electrocardiography of Arrhythmias.* Philadelphia: Lea and Febiger; 1990:388.

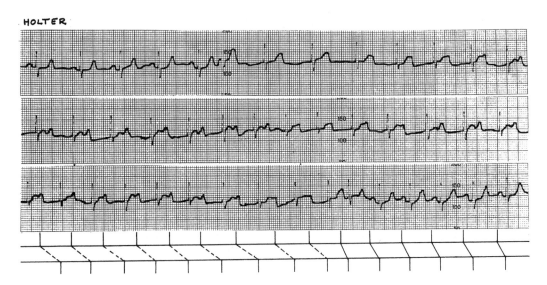

Figure 17-6. Dual AV nodal conduction. In the top tracing, following the interpolated VPC, the P-R interval prolongs from 160 to 600 ms. In the bottom tracing, the P-R interval normalizes. The prolonged P-R interval shortens gradually from 600 to 400 in parallel with shortening of the P-P interval from 800 to 680 ms, suggesting that the slow pathway conduction is under the influence of the autonomic nervous system. From Fisch C, Mandrola JM, Rardon DP. Electrocardiographic manifestations of dual AV nodal conduction during sinus rhythm. *J Am Coll Cardiol* 1997;29:1015.

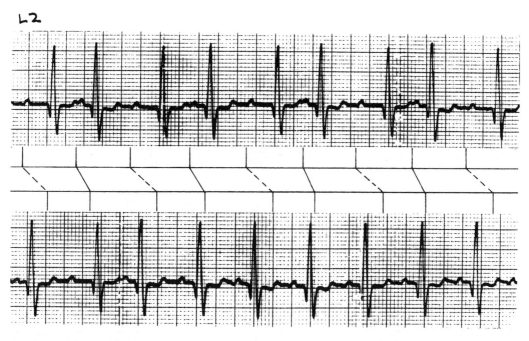

Figure 17-7. Dual AV nodal conduction. This tracing illustrates AV alternans. The paradoxical R-R to P-R interval relation (a long P-R interval following a long R-P interval) rules out shortening of the R-P interval as the cause of the longer P-R interval. Similarly, concealed intranodal reentry is unlikely, as indicated by the consecutive P-R intervals of 160 ms in the bottom row. The latter represents fast pathway conduction time that is identical to the short P-R intervals during alternans. These observations indicate that the short P-R interval, with or without alternans, reflects A-V conduction along the same pathway—namely, the fast pathway. From Fisch C, Mandrola JM, Rardon DP. Electrocardiographic manifestation of dual AV node conduction during sinus rhythm. *J Am Coll Cardiol* 1997;29:1015.

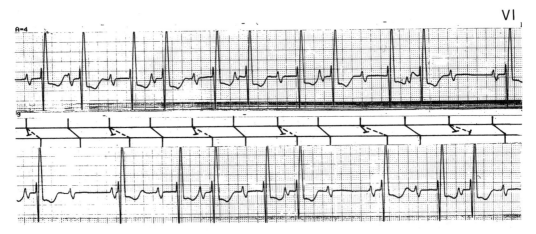

Figure 17-8. Dual AV nodal conduction with Type I A-V block. The analysis is that of the top tracing. There is a regular sinus rhythm with a P-P interval of 840 ms with alternans of the P-R intervals. The shorter of the two P-R intervals measures approximately 240 ms and remains constant
(solid line). The longer P-R interval (broken line), on the other hand, prolongs gradually from 320
to 560 ms, with the last P wave of the sequence blocked. While an escape cannot be ruled out, it
is unlikely because the next P wave conducts at an R-R interval that is longer than the established
escape interval. The escape interval is illustrated by the second QRS complex in the bottom tracing. From Fisch C. An unusual pattern of AV conduction. *J Cardiovasc Electrophysiol* 1996;7:277.

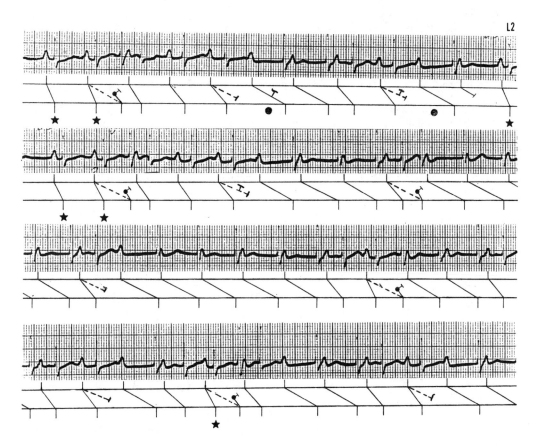

Figure 17-9. Dual AV nodal conduction. Simultaneous conduction of a single atrial impulse along both fast and slow pathways inscribing two QRS complexes is the least common ECG manifestation of dual AV node conduction. A probable example of this phenomenon is shown in this tracing. The long and short P-R intervals with paradoxical R-P to P-R relationship, namely, a short R-P interval followed by a short P-R interval and a long R-P interval followed by a long P-R interval, are best explained by dual A-V conduction. The normal P-R intervals are labeled with stars. In the top row, the first P wave conducts normally. The second P wave is assumed to conduct simultaneously along the fast pathway (solid line) and the slow pathway (broken line). There is a progressive prolongation of the P-R interval (Type I A-V block) in the fast pathway, with shift to the slow pathway (solid circle). The third row illustrates shift of conduction from slow pathway to fast pathway (eighth P wave). The ninth P wave conducts simultaneously along the slow and the fast pathways. The bottom tracing illustrates anterograde block in the fast pathway, with shifts of conduction of the third P wave to the slow pathway. Failure to conceal from slow pathway to fast pathway allows the fourth P wave to conduct along the fast pathway. The fifth P wave conducts along both pathways. From Fisch C, Zipes DP, McHenry PL. Electrocardiographic manifestations of concealed junctional ectopic impulses. *Circulation* 1976;53:217. By permission of the American Heart Association, Inc.

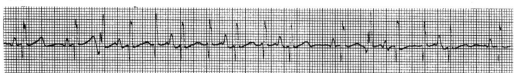

Figure 17-10. Dual AV nodal conduction. The rhythm appears to be sinus with a P-P of 800 ms interrupted by what appear to be interpolated junctional complexes. There are three P-P cycles without the junctional ectopic impulses. The P-P interval encompassing the JPC is equal to the P-P without the JPC, the sinus interval. A mechanism of this arrhythmia is similar to one suggested in Figure 17-9, namely the simultaneous conduction of the sinus P wave along the fast pathway with a P-R interval of approximately 200 ms and along the slow pathway with a P-R interval of approximately 600 ms. This is obviously an assumption that cannot be proven from the surface ECG. Evidence supporting simultaneous dual A-V conduction rather than JPCs is the fact that the JPCs do not alter the P-R interval of the sinus impulse. If these were JPCs, one would expect some P-R and P-P interval prolongation, with the P-P interval longer than the sinus interval.

References

1. White PD. A study of AV rhythm following auricular flutter. *Arch Intern Med* 1915;16:516.
2. White PD. The bigeminal pulse in AV rhythm. *Arch Intern Med* 1921;28:213.
3. Schuilenburg RM, Durrer D. Atrial echo beats in the human heart elicited by induced atrial premature beats. *Circulation* 1968;37:680.
4. Goldreyer BN, Bigger JT Jr. Site of reentry in paroxysmal supraventricular tachycardia in man. *Circulation* 1971;43:15.
5. Denes P, Wu D, Dhingra RC, Chuquimia R, Rosen KM. Demonstration of dual AV node pathways in patients with paroxysmal supraventricular tachycardia. *Circulation* 1973;48:549.
6. Witt AL, Weiss MB, Berkowitz WD, Rosen KM, Steiner L, Damato AN. Patterns of AV conduction in the human heart. *Circ Res* 1970;27:345.
7. Rosen KM, Menta A, Miller RA. Demonstration of dual AV nodal pathways in man. *Am J Cardiol* 1974;33:291.
8. Lee MA, Morady F, Kadish A, et al. Catheter modification of the atrioventricular junction with radiofrequency energy for control of atrioventricular nodal reentrant tachycardia. *Circulation* 1991;83:827.
9. Scheinmann MM. Catheter ablation: Present role and projected impact on health care for patients with cardiac arrhythmias. *Circulation* 1991;83:2146.
10. Jackman WM, Beckman KJ, McClelland JH, et al. Treatment of supraventricular tachycardia due to atrioventricular nodal reentry, by radiofrequency catheter ablation of slow-pathway conduction. *N Engl J Med* 1992;822:313.
11. Fisch C, Mandrola JM, Rardon DP. Electrocardiographic manifestations of dual nodal conduction during sinus rhythm. *J Am Coll Cardiol* 1997;29:1015.

18

Alternating and Bilateral Bundle Branch Block

A-V delay or block caused by BBB was demonstrated experimentally by Scherf and Shookhoff[1] in 1925. By sectioning one bundle branch and compressing the contralateral bundle, they were able to elicit a spectrum of A-V block ranging from prolongation of A-V conduction to complete A-V block. The concept of first, second, and third degree BBB was subsequently applied to ECG interpretation (Figure 18-1).[2–5]

Alternating BBB can manifest as: 1) bilateral BBB with abnormal A-V conduction (Figures 18-2 to 18-8); 2) RBBB with normal QRS (Figure 18-9); 3) RBBB with incomplete RBBB (IRBBB) (Figures 18-10, 18-11, and 18-12); 4) RBBB with LAFB or LPFB or both (Figures 18-13 to 18-16); 5) LBBB with a normal QRS complex (Figures 18-17, 18-17A, and 18-18; 6) LBBB with Wenckebach block (Figure 18-1); 7) LBBB with incomplete LBBB (Figure 18-19); 8) RBBB with LBBB (Figures 18-2, 18-3, 18-4, 18-5, 18-7, 18-8, 18-20); and 9) intraventricular conduction block (Figure 18-21) (see Table 18-1).

As a rule, A-V conduction delay or block can be assumed to be caused by BBB only in the presence of an alternating or intermittent RBBB and LBBB with a changing P-R interval (Figures 18-2 to 18-7). Not infrequently, the bilateral BBB is due to acceleration-dependent aberration (Figures 18-3, 18-5, 18-6, 18-8, and 18-18).

The ECG diagnosis of A-V block caused by bilateral BBB is based primarily on analysis of the conduction in the two bundles. The exact basic electrophysiological mechanism responsible for the conduction abnormalities in any one case is not clear because of the many variables that may affect conduction. Some of these include changing heart rate, refractoriness, influence of cycle length on refractoriness, "cross-over" of bundle branch refractoriness, concealed bundle branch penetration, geometry of the bundle, the GAP phenomenon, supernormality, autonomic influence, hemodynamic alterations, and electrolyte changes. Rarely, when a prolonged P-R interval with a normal QRS complex gives way to a shorter P-R interval with BBB, a diagnosis of first degree BBB block is tenable. In this situation, the equal delay in the bundles with a normal QRS complex gives way to more rapid conduction in one bundle and, thus, block in the opposite bundle. However, when the P-R interval is prolonged and constant, a diagnosis of a contralateral first degree BBB cannot be made because the prolongation of the P-R interval may be due to AV nodal delay.[6,7]

Table 18-1

Intraventricular Conduction Abnormalities

Bundle Branch Block	Figure
Bilateral BBB with block	18-2 through 18-8
RBBB with normal QRS	18-9
RBBB with IRBBB	18-10 through 18-12
RBBB with LAFB, LPFB	18-13 through 18-16
LBBB with normal QRS	18-17 and 18-18
LBBB with Wenckebach	18-1
RBBB with LBBB	18-2 through 18-5, 18-7 and 18-8, and 18-20
IVCD	18-21

ID: 001381103   10-AUG-1997

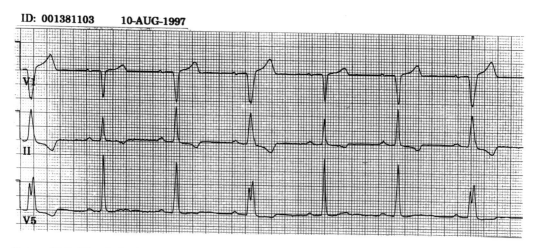

Figure 18-1. Wenckebach block in the LBBB. The basic rhythm is sinus with a P-P interval of 1100 ms and a normal P-R interval. The QRS prolongs gradually from 80 ms to 120 ms, from normal QRS to LBBB. Secondary ST-T changes parallel the changing QRS complex.

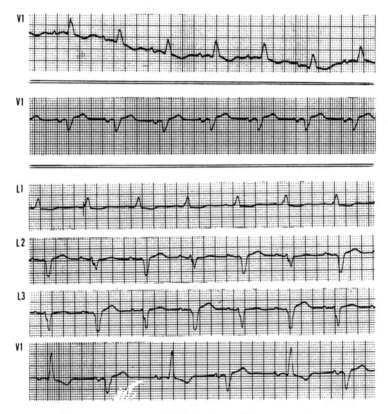

Figure 18-2. Alternating P-R interval and BBB. The basic rhythm is sinus. The three sections were recorded on different days. In the upper two sections, the P-R interval preceding the RBBB and LBBB measure 280 ms and 180 ms, respectively. In the lower section, the respective P-R intervals are 220 ms with RBBB and 180 ms with LBBB. There is an obligatory alternation of the R-R interval. In lead V_1, the R-R interval of 1000 ms terminates with LBBB and the R-R interval of 1120 ms terminates with RBBB. The assumption is that the changes in the P-R interval reflect differences in bundle branch conduction, with normal conduction in the LBB and delayed conduction in RBB. The mechanism responsible for the alternation of the A-V conduction is unclear. From Fisch C. *Electrocardiography of Arrhythmias.* Philadelphia: Lea and Febiger; 1990;433.

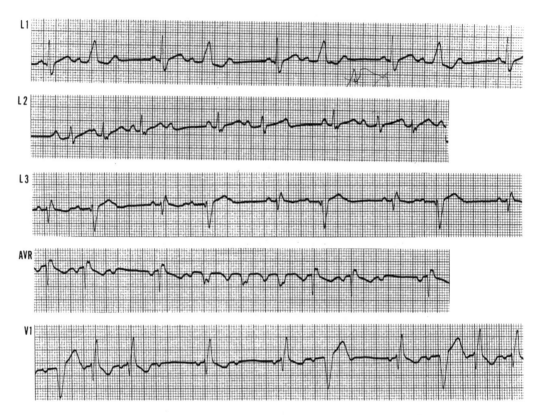

Figure 18-3. Type II A-V block due to bilateral BBB. The A-V conduction is predominantly 3:2 with occasional 1:1, 2:1, and 4:3 ratios. The most likely explanation for the events recorded in this figure is an intermittent acceleration-dependent LBBB in the presence of a fixed RBBB. Consequently, in the presence of LBBB, the prolonged P-R interval reflects the depressed RBB conduction. The depression of RBB conduction is less pronounced than that of the LBB. Following the longer pauses, LBB conduction recovers and the normal P-R interval is followed by the RBBB. In 3:2 Type II A-V block, the block of the P wave is due to bilateral BBB.

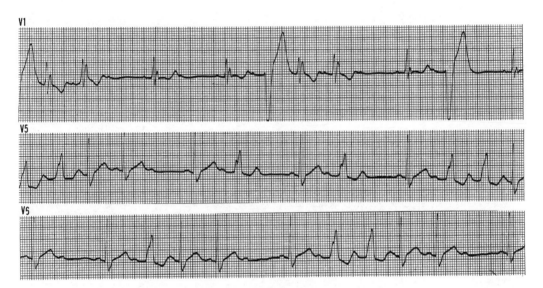

Figure 18-4. Type II A-V block caused by bilateral BBB. The basic rhythm is sinus with a P-P interval of approximately 600 ms. The P waves are blocked without prolongation of the P-R interval, indicating Type II A-V block. All pauses are terminated with RBBB and a P-R interval of approximately 160 ms. These are then followed by LBBB with a P-R interval of 240 ms. The P-R intervals of 160 ms with RBBB and 240 ms with LBBB indicate a longer conduction of the RBBB as compared with that of the LBB. Importantly, the criteria for bilateral BBB, namely alternating BBB with changing P-R interval, are satisfied.

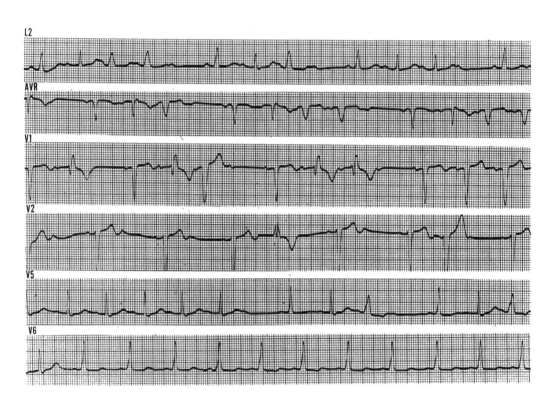

Figure 18-5. Type II A-V block caused by acceleration-dependent bilateral BBB. In lead V_6, the control QRS pattern is that of an incomplete LBBB with a P-P interval of approximately 800 ms. In lead V_5, when the P-P shortens to approximately 700 ms, RBBB appears. In lead V_2 at a P-P interval of 680 ms, 2:1 A-V block, RBBB, and LBBB are recorded. In general, at a P-P interval of 760 ms or longer, at 660 to 760 ms and at 560 to 640 ms, the QRS configuration is that of LBBB, RBBB, and LBBB, respectively. At a P-P interval of approximately 620 ms, there is bilateral BBB with block of A-V conduction. The P-R interval with LBBB is longer than the P-R interval with RBBB, indicating a greater delay of conduction in the RBBB. The mechanism of the longer P-P interval with RBBB and the shorter P-P interval with LBBB is unclear. It may reflect the "cross-over" of refractoriness, where the RBBB refractoriness is longer at slower rates and LBBB refractoriness is longer at faster rates.

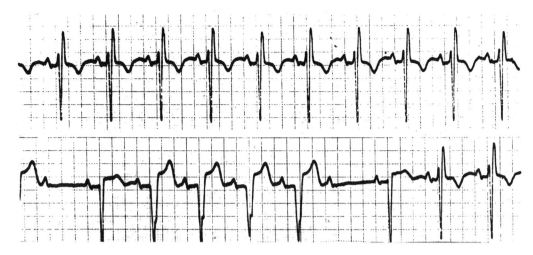

Figure 18-6. Type II A-V block caused by acceleration-dependent bilateral BBB. The P-P interval in the top and bottom tracings is regular at 800 ms. RBBB is present in the top tracing. In the lower tracing, the two long cycles are terminated by normal QRS complexes followed by LBBB with a P-R interval of 240 ms and RBBB with a P-R interval of 170 ms, respectively. The criteria for bilateral BBB, namely alternating BBB with a changing P-R interval, are present. The exact mechanism responsible for the changing P-R and bundle branch conduction is unclear. The normalization of the QRS complex following the longer cycle due to 2:1 Mobitz II A-V block indicates that the BBBs are acceleration-dependent.

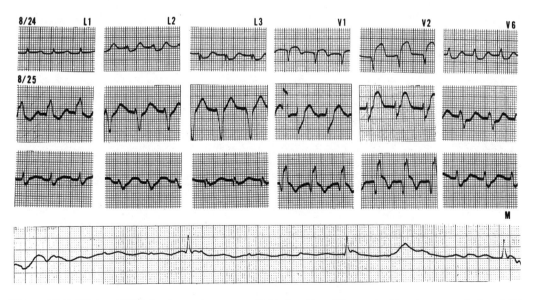

Figure 18-7. Bilateral BBB due to acute myocardial infarction. The control tracing recorded on 8/24 shows an acute anterior myocardial infarction. The top tracing, recorded on 8/25, shows LBBB with LAFB masking the myocardial infarction. The third tracing demonstrates RBBB and an acute anterior infarction. Bilateral BBB manifest by complete A-V block and an idioventricular rhythm is recorded in the bottom tracing.

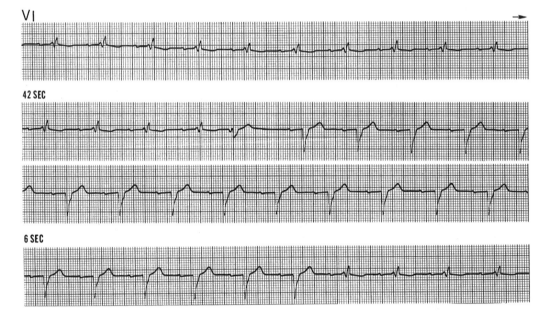

Figure 18-8. Bilateral BBB. The tracing is continuous with 42- and 6-second sections deleted for purposes of mounting. RBBB with a P-R interval of approximately 240 ms and an R-R interval of approximately 880 ms are recorded at more rapid rates. When the rate slows and is interrupted by a VPC, the conduction changes to LBBB with a P-R interval of 280 ms. The latter persists until, in the bottom row, the R-R interval shortens to 880 ms, at which time RBBB reappears. Although the conduction is probably delayed in both bundles, at slower heart rates the conduction in the LBB is slower than that of the RBB, and LBBB is recorded. At faster rates, the conduction in the RBB is delayed more than in the LBB, and RBBB is recorded. The change in the P-R that reflects the differences in duration of the bundle branch conduction is small, but sufficient to alter the BBBs.

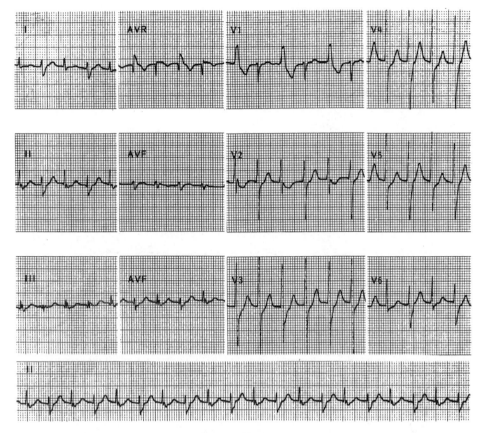

Figure 18-9. Alternating normal QRS complex and RBB conduction. The basic rhythm is an SVT with a rate of approximately 150 ms. The QRS complexes alternate between RBBB and normal.

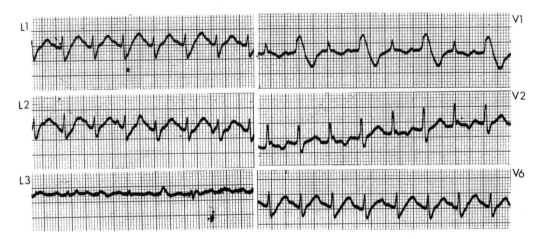

Figure 18-10. Alternation of IRBBB with complete RBBB. The basic rhythm is a sinus tachycardia with a P-P interval of 480 ms and a P-R interval of approximately 140 ms. The QRS complex alternates between IRBBB and complete RBBB.

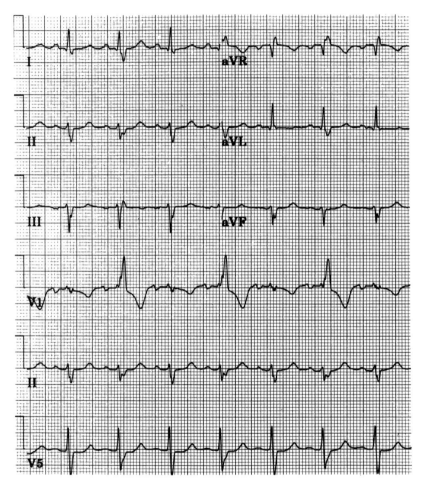

Figure 18-11. Alternation of RBBB and normal QRS complexes. The basic rhythm is sinus with a rate of approximately 100 per minute with LAFB. The QRS with the fixed LAFB alternates with RBBB. The P-R interval is constant at 160 ms.

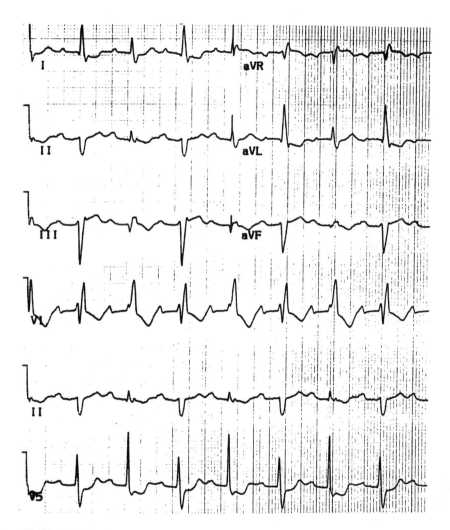

Figure 18-12. RBBB with alternating LAFB. The basic rhythm is sinus with a P-P interval of approximately 640 ms. Fixed RBBB with a normal axis alternates with LAFB. The P-R interval is 240 ms.

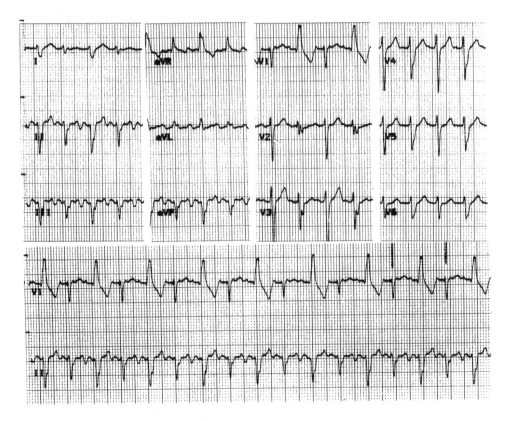

Figure 18-13. QRS complexes with LAFB alternating with RBBB. The basic rhythm is an atrial flutter with a 2:1 A-V conduction with a ventricular rate of approximately 150 per minute. There is a fixed LAFB with an alternating RBBB.

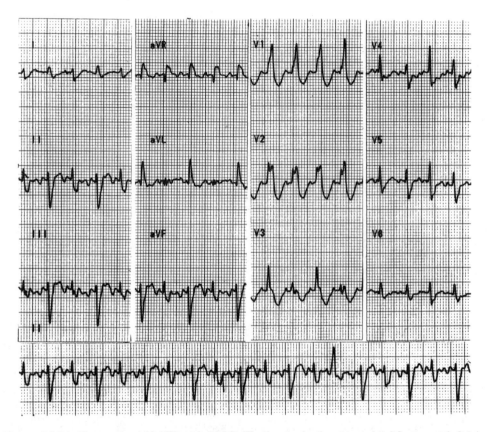

Figure 18-14. Alternation of LAFB with RBBB. The basic rhythm is an atrial flutter with 2:1 A-V conduction and a ventricular rate of approximately 160 per minute. There is a fixed RBBB, while LAFB alternates with a normal QRS complex.

ID: 001375920   01–JUL–1997

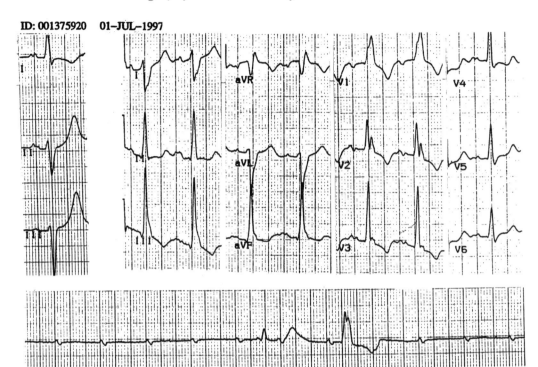

Figure 18-15. Trifascicular block. The basic rhythm is sinus with a rate of approximately 100 per minute. An RBBB with LAFB is recorded in the left panel and RBBB with LPFB in the right panel. The P-R is 200 ms. The bottom tracing shows complete A-V block with ventricular standstill. The mechanism of the A-V block is trifascicular block, namely RBBB, LAFB, and LPFB.

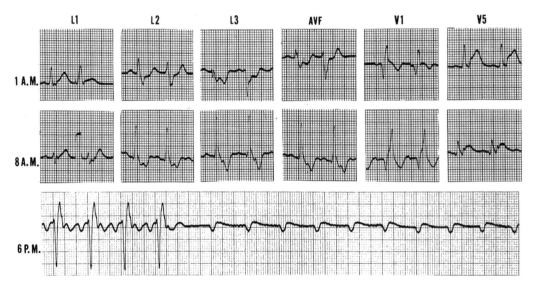

Figure 18-16. Trifascicular block complicating an acute anterior myocardial infarction. RBBB with a P-R of 160 ms and VPCs are recorded at 1:00 A.M. At 8:00 A.M., the pattern is that of RBBB with LPFB without change in the P-R interval. An abrupt complete A-V block with ventricular asystole is recorded in the bottom tracing. The mechanism of the block is trifascicular block.

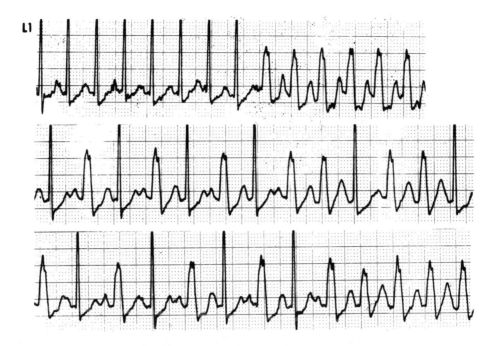

Figure 18-17. Alternation of LBBB and normal QRS complexes. Sinus tachycardia with a normal QRS complex at a rate of approximately 160 per minute is recorded in the top tracing. In the middle tracing, LBBB and normal QRS complexes alternate with two consecutive LBBB patterns recorded in the middle section. In the bottom tracing, alternation of LBBB with a normal QRS complex changes to LBBB.

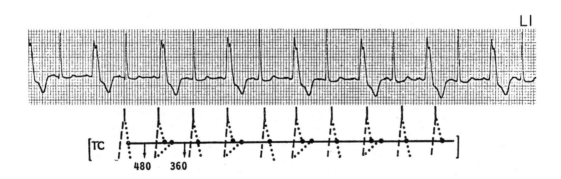

Figure 18-17A. Alternating LBBB due to concealed transseptal and supernormal conduction. In the presence of LBBB and delayed concealed transseptal activation of the LBB, the recovery curve shifts to the right, allowing the sinus impulse to reach the LBB during the supernormal period of LBB recovery. This results in a normal QRS complex. With the normal QRS complex, the recovery curve of the LBB shifts to the left, the impulse falls during the refractory period of the LBB, and LBBB results. As long as the sinus rate, transseptal conduction, and "position" of recovery remain constant, the alternation of LBBB may persist. From Fisch C. The electrocardiogram and arrhythmias: Limitation of a technique. *Circulation* 1987;75:48. By permission of the American Heart Association, Inc.

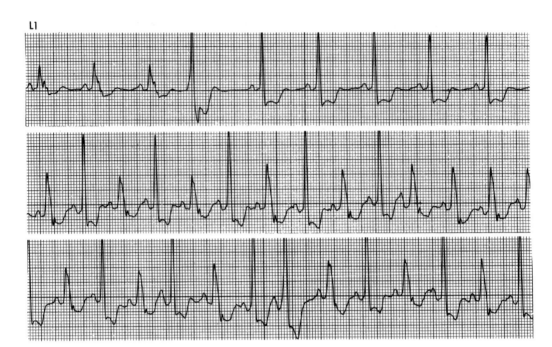

Figure 18-18. Acceleration-dependent LBBB and alternation of LBBB with normal QRS complexes. LBBB at a rate of 75 per minute is present in the top tracing. As the rate slows, the LBBB gives way to a slightly prolonged QRS complex. In the middle and the bottom tracings, the LBBB alternates with a minimally prolonged QRS. For possible mechanisms, see Figure 18-17A.

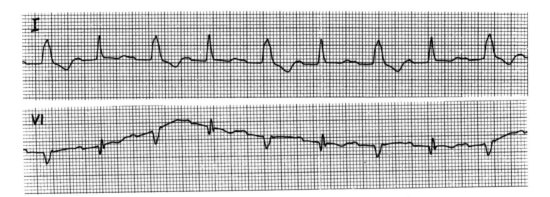

Figure 18-19. Alternation of LBBB and normal QRS complexes. The basic rhythm is sinus with a P-R interval of 280 ms and a rate of 88 per minute. LBBB alternates with normal QRS complexes (see Figure 18-17).

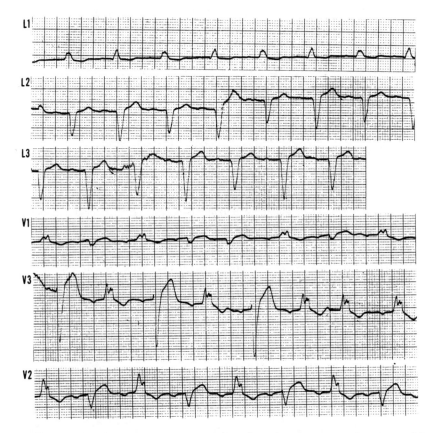

Figure 18-20. Alternation of RBBB and LBBB. The basic rhythm is regular sinus with a rate of approximately 75 per minute. The P-R interval is 240 ms. There is a fixed LAFB with alternation of RBBB and LBBB. The persistent LBBB-like pattern in the limb leads and alternating RBBB and LBBB in the precordial leads is characteristic of so-called masquerading bilateral BBB.

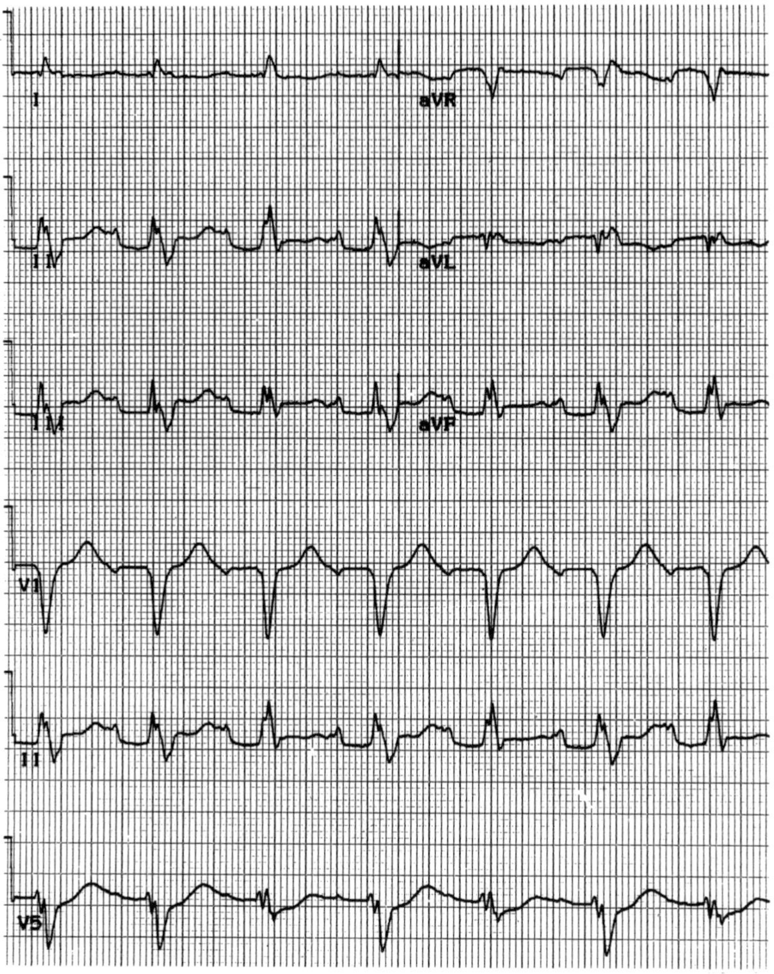

Figure 18-21. Alternation of duration of intraventricular conduction delay. The basic rhythm is sinus with a P-P interval of 740 ms. The nonspecific intraventricular conduction delay alternates between 140 and 200 ms.

References

1. Scherf D, Shookhoff C. Reitzleitungs-strorungen in Bundel. II. Mitteilung, Wein. *Arch Intern Med* 1925;11:425.
2. Lenegre J. Bilateral bundle branch block. *Cardiologia* 1966;48:134.
3. Rosenbaum MB, Lepeschkin E. Bilateral bundle branch block. *Am Heart J* 1955;50:38.
4. Vesell H, Leveine J. 2:1 bundle branch block. Classification with special reference to the critical heart rate. *Am J Cardiol* 1960;6:963.
5. Berkowitz WD, Lau SH, Patton RD, Rosen KM, Damato AN. The use of His bundle recordings in the analysis of unilateral and bilateral bundle branch block. *Am Heart J* 1971;81:340.
6. Lepeschkin E. Electrocardiographic diagnosis of bilateral bundle branch block in relation to heart block. *Prog Cardiovasc Dis* 1964;6:445.
7. Delon WU, Denes P, Dhingra RC, et al. Electrophysiological and clinical observations in patients with alternating bundle branch block. *Circulation* 1976;53:464.

Additional Electrocardiograms

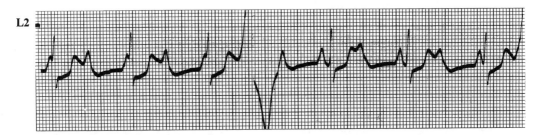

AE-1. Triple ectopic rhythm. Atrial tachycardia at a rate of 120 per minute, junctional rhythm at a rate of 60 per minute, and a VPC.

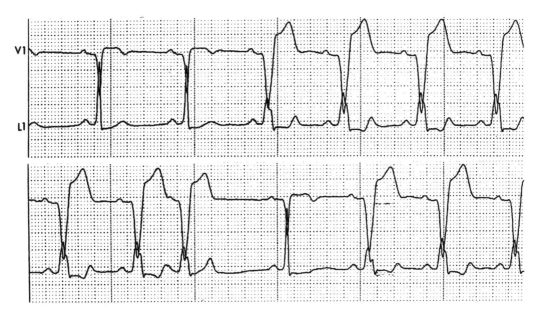

AE-2. Acceleration-dependent aberration. In the top row, with acceleration of the rate from 58 to 65 per minute, LBBB appears. In the bottom row, following the APC and a compensatory pause, the QRS complex normalizes. The LBBB recurs as the rate accelerates. Note the extremely slow rates at which LBBB appears.

L2

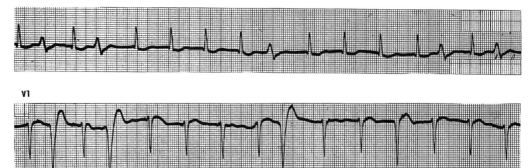

V1

AE-3. NPJT at a rate of 88 per minute and a ventricular parasystole at a rate of 56 per minute. The basic rhythm is atrial fibrillation.

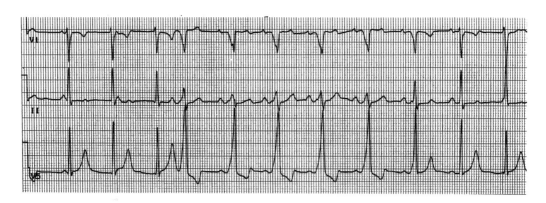

AE-4. Junctional tachycardia (first three QRS complexes) at a rate of 79 per minute with AV dissociation followed by WPW and normalization of the QRS complex at the end of the record. The third complex from the end is a fusion between a junctional impulse and an impulse conducting along the bypass, as indicated by a delta wave. The fusion is further supported by the altered T wave.

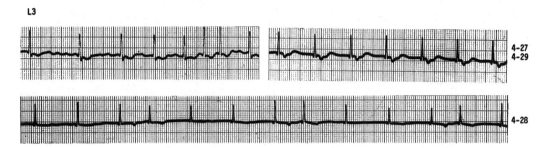

AE-5. Atrial fibrillation is shown in the top left panel, NPJT with retrograde P waves are recorded in the top right panel. The bottom tracing illustrates NPJT, with what are most likely retrograde P waves with ventricular reentry.

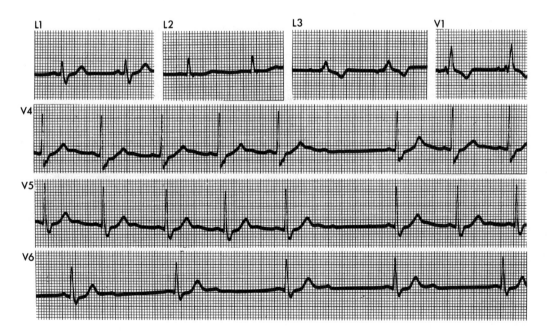

AE-6. Mobitz II Type II A-V block with RBBB.

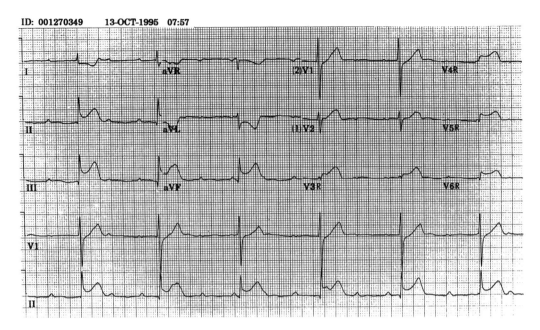

AE-7. Acute inferior and right ventricular myocardial infarction with a complete A-V block.

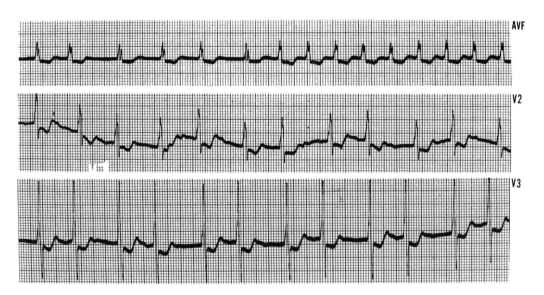

AE-8. The basic rhythm is junctional tachycardia at a rate of approximately 150 per minute illustrated in the right part of lead AVF. A bigeminal junctional rhythm is recorded in leads V_2 and V_3. The sum of a short–long cycle equals three basic cycles recorded in lead AVF. The short–long cycle reflects a 3:2 Wenckebach exit from the junctional focus. The Wenckebach structure is suggested by the short R-R being longer than the basic R-R recorded in AVF and the long R-R being shorter than the two preceding cycles.

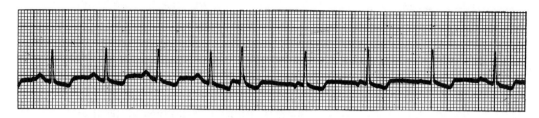

AE-9. Sinus rhythm with an APC followed by a shift of the site of origin of the atrial pacemaker. The second P wave from the end is fusion between the ectopic and the upright (sinus?) P wave.

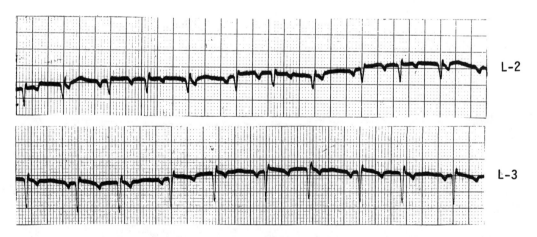

AE-10. Atrial or junctional tachycardia at a rate of 150 per minute with a 3:2 Wenckebach Type I A-V conduction. For additional comments see Figure AE-8.

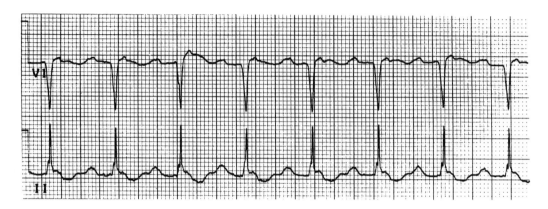

AE-11. Atrial tachycardia at a rate of 167 per minute with a 2:1 A-V conduction.

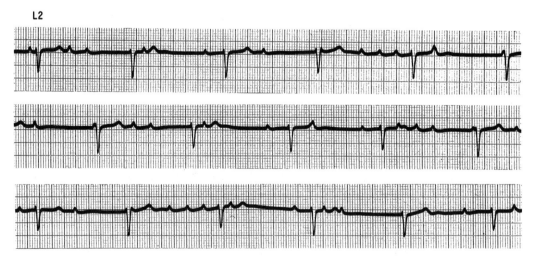

AE-12. Complete A-V block with a regular ventricular rate of 41 per minute with ectopic atrial complexes, some in runs (atrial flutter).

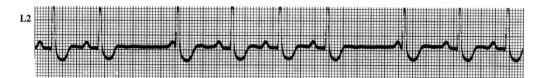

AE-13. Sinus rhythm at a rate of 88 per minute with pauses, an exact multiple of the basic sinus cycle indicative of a 2:1 Type II exit block from the sinus node. The pauses are terminated by junctional escape.

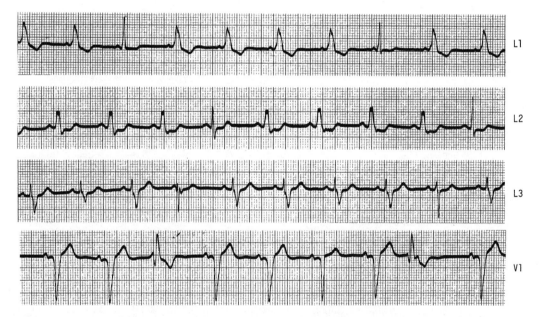

AE-14. Sinus rhythm with LBBB and VPC with RBBB configuration. The narrow QRS complexes, some nearly normal, present in each of the leads represent a fusion between the RBBB-like VPC and the LBBB. The left ventricular VPC discharges at the same time as the sinus impulse reaches and activates the right ventricle, resulting in a normal or near normal appearing QRS complex.

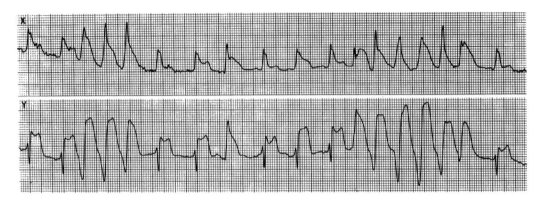

AE-15. Prinzmetal's angina manifest by short runs of VT, a current of injury with alternans of the ST segment and the T wave.

ID: 001131995   14-FEB-92 08:45

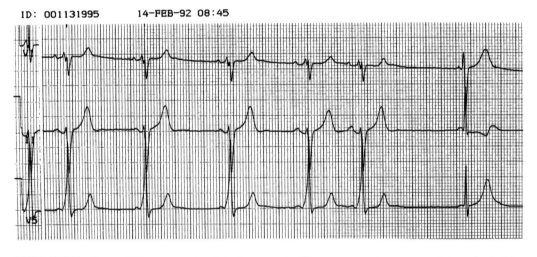

AE-16. WPW with an APC suppressing the sinus node. The compensatory pause is terminated by a junctional escape.

L-2

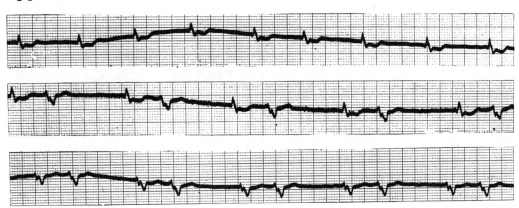

AE-17. The basic rhythm, illustrated in the top row, is atrial fibrillation with an occasional junctional escape at an R-R interval of 940 ms. Ventricular bigeminy is noted in the middle row. In the bottom row, the bigeminal rhythm consists of VPC couplets. The long pause is a multiple of the short pause, indicating a 3:2 Mobitz II Type II exit block from the ventricular focus.

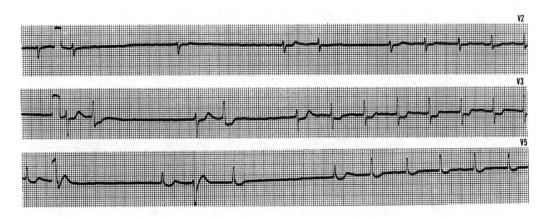

AE-18. The basic rhythm is an atrial fibrillation with NPJT, the latter indicated by the short, regular R-R intervals. The long R-R intervals are an exact multiple of the short R-R intervals, indicating Mobitz II Type II exit block.

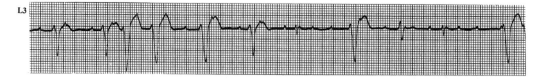

AE-19. The basic rhythm is an atrial tachycardia interrupted by a ventricular parasystole. The parasystolic interval is 880 ms. The long pauses are an exact multiple of this basic interval. The third ventricular impulse does not disturb the rhythmicity. The third QRS complex from the right is a fusion between the parasystolic QRS complex and the supraventricular, low amplitude QRS complex.

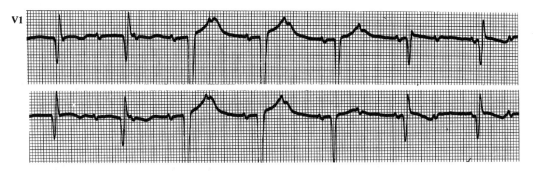

AE-20. Complete A-V block with two idioventricular foci with RBBB and LBBB configuration. In the top row, the fifth and the sixth QRS complexes are fusions between the two idioventricular complexes. In the bottom row, the fifth QRS complex is similarly a fusion. It is unlikely that the fifth QRS complex is a sinus capture.

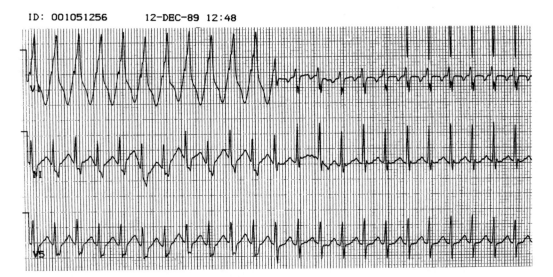

AE-21. SVT, most likely a sinus tachycardia, with RBBB aberration giving way to normal intraventricular conduction. The normalization of the QRS complex may be due to shortening of the refractory period secondary to the tachycardia or it may be due to failure of concealed transseptal conduction from the left bundle to the right bundle to maintain the aberration.

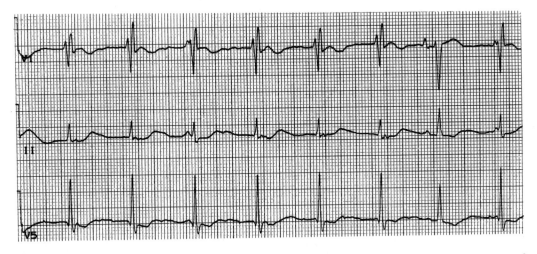

AE-22. Idioventricular rhythm at an R-R interval of 800 ms with rare sinus P waves. The second from the right is a sinus-initiated QRS complex (capture).

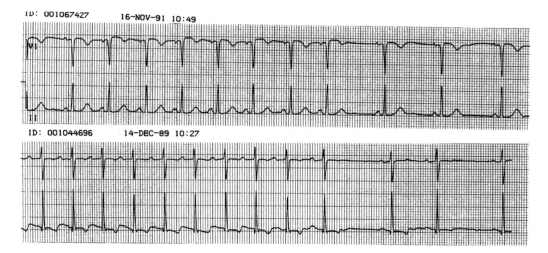

AE-23. SA nodal reentrant tachycardia. This arrhythmia is characterized by P waves similar to the sinus P wave and most often a sudden onset and sudden termination.

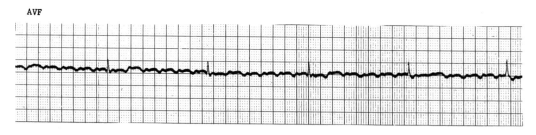

AE-24. Atrial flutter or a rapid atrial tachycardia with a complete A-V block. The junctional R-Rs measure 1700 ms and are regular.

LI

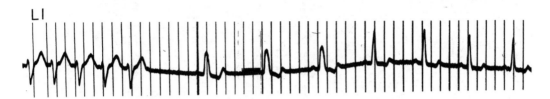

AE-25. Overdrive suppression of the left bundle by VT. The VT suppresses LBB conduction with gradual normalization of QRS conduction as the sinus rate accelerates.

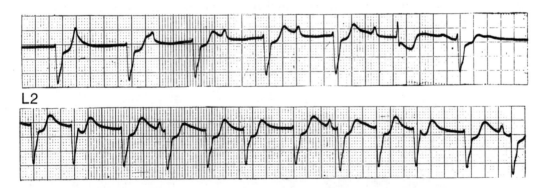

AE-26. A high degree of A-V block with one conducted P wave is recorded in the top strip. In the bottom tracing, the VT is manifest in the form of "group beating," gradual shortening of the R-R interval with the longer R-R less than the sum of the two R-R cycles, indicative of Type I Wenckebach exit from the ventricular focus. The recognition of the Wenckebach exit block depends on recognition of the repetitive pattern, "group beating," described above.

LI

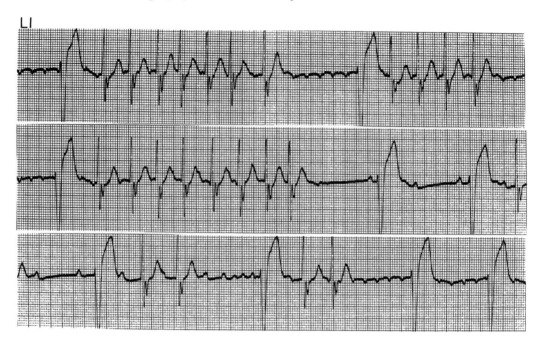

AE-27. The basic rhythm is atrial flutter with atrial flutter converting to sinus with high degree of A-V block and, in the bottom row, the sinus rhythm converting again to flutter. The narrow, rapid QRS complexes are supraventricular. Each run of SVT follows an idioventricular complex. The relation of the supraventricular complex to the idioventricular complex is in keeping with conduction during the supernormal period induced by the idioventricular impulse. Each subsequent impulse falls during the supernormal period of the previous QRS complex and, thus, supraventricular QRS conduction is perpetuated.

ID: 001235215   26-JUN-94

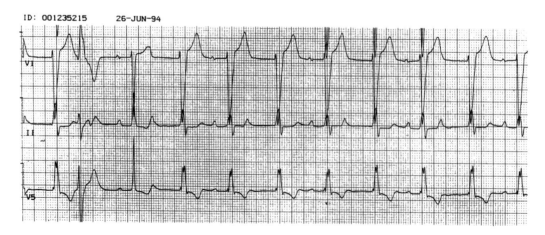

AE-28. Sinus with what appears to be a 3:2 Type I Wenckebach A-V block. Each third P wave of the Wenckebach sequence is buried within the QRS complex. The configuration of the QRS complex is that of the LBBB. Following the VPC and the compensatory pause, the QRS complex normalizes, indicating that the LBBB is acceleration-dependent.

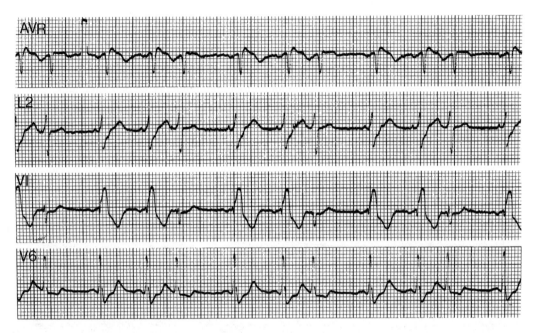

AE-29. Sinus rhythm with RBBB and atrial trigeminy. The APC is conducted with a normal QRS complex. The paradox of normalization after a short R-R interval is due to conduction during the supernormal phase of RBB recovery.

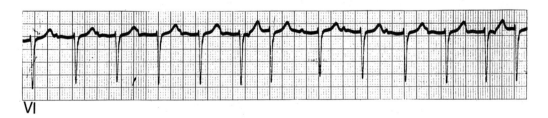

AE-30. Sinus rhythm with Type I Wenckebach A-V block, retrograde conduction, and ventricular reentry. The retrograde P waves are followed by ventricular reentry.

IUMC 452530

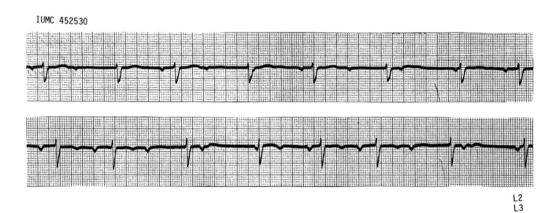

L2
L3

AE-31. Double junctional rhythm with high degree of A-V block. This is best illustrated in the bottom row, where the first two P waves conduct with an increasing P-R interval. The next two QRS complexes are junctional escapes and are followed by two conducted P waves and junctional escape. The negative P wave in L2w and L3 originate in the junction. The normal duration QRS complex similarly originates in the junction; thus, a double junctional rhythm.

Appendix

Abbreviations Used in this Book

APC = atrial premature complex
AV = atrioventricular (node)
A-V = atrioventricular (conduction)
AVNRT = AV nodal reentrant tachycardia
AVRT = AV reentrant tachycardia
BBB = bundle branch block
ECG = electrocardiogram
HBE = His bundle electrocardiography
IRBBB = incomplete right bundle branch block
JPC = junctional premature complex
LAF = left anterior fascicle
LAFB = left anterior fascicular block
LBB = left bundle branch
LBBB = left bundle branch block
LPF = left posterior fascicle
LPFB = left posterior fascicular block
NPJT = nonparoxysmal junctional tachycardia
PSVT = paroxysmal supraventricular tachycardia
RBB = right bundle branch
RBBB = right bundle branch block
SA = sinoatrial
SAN = sinoatrial node
SVT = supraventricular tachycardia
TAP = transmembrane action potential
TP = threshold potential
TRP = transmembrane resting potential
V-A = ventriculoatrial
VPC = ventricular premature complex
VT = ventricular tachycardia
WPW = Wolff-Parkinson-White syndrome

Index

Numbers in italics indicate figures. Numbers followed by *t* indicate tables.